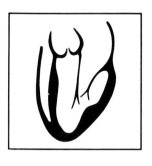

ECHOCARDIOLOGY
SELECTED PAPERS

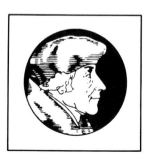

PRESENTED DURING THE FOURTH
SYMPOSIUM AT ERASMUS UNIVERSITY,
ROTTERDAM, JUNE 24-26, 1981

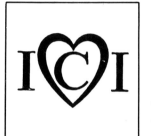

INTERUNIVERSITY INSTITUTE OF
CARDIOLOGY, AMSTERDAM

DEVELOPMENTS IN
CARDIOVASCULAR MEDICINE

VOLUME 13

Other volumes in this series:

series ISBN 90-247-2336-1

ECHOCARDIOLOGY

edited by

HANS RIJSTERBORGH

Thoraxcenter, Erasmus University, Rotterdam
Interuniversity Institute of Cardiology, Amsterdam

1981

MARTINUS NIJHOFF PUBLISHERS

THE HAGUE / BOSTON / LONDON

Distributors:

for the United States and Canada

Kluwer Boston, Inc.
190 Old Derby Street
Hingham, MA 02043
USA

for all other countries

Kluwer Academic Publishers Group
Distribution Center
P.O. Box 322
3300 AH Dordrecht
The Netherlands

Library of Congress Cataloging in Publication Data   CIP

Main entry under title:

Echocardiology.

    (Developments in cardiovascular medicine; v. 13)
    Proceedings of the 4th Symposium on Echocardiology.
    Includes indexes.
    1. Ultrasonic cardiography-Congresses.
I. Rijsterborgh, Hans. II. Symposium on Echocardiology (4th: 1981: Erasmus University,
Rotterdam) III. Series.
RC683.5.U5E25   1981   616.1'207543   81-38415

ISBN 90-247-2491-0 (this volume)
ISBN 90-247-2336-1 (series)

PRINTED IN THE NETHERLANDS

FOREWORD

This symposium is the fourth of a series of scientific meetings in the field of echocardiology, held at the Erasmus University, Rotterdam.* The series was initiated by Klaas Bom, who organized the first two meetings, and was continued by Charles Lancée. These previous symposia met with great success.

These proceedings comprise most of the invited lectures and free communications which had their 'live performance' during the 4th Symposium on Echocardiology.

We decided, again, to maintain one of the most striking features of the last meetings: having the proceedings available at the time of the meeting. As a consequence, the authors-to-be were confronted with a very tight schedule. The editing time was also limited and therefore neither terminology nor units have been completely standardized. However, as a result, these proceedings do reflect the 'state of the art' in echocardiology.

This is not a textbook on echocardiology, but cardiologists and technicians, with experience in the field of echocardiology, will certainly appreciate the educational features of this book.

This symposium was organized in association with
— Interuniversity Institute of Cardiology, Amsterdam, the Netherlands.
— Dutch Society of Ultrasound in Medicine and Biology
— Dutch Heart Foundation, The Hague, the Netherlands
— European Society of Cardiology

Financial support was given by
— Interuniversity Institute of Cardiology, Amsterdam, the Netherlands
— University-fund Rotterdam Foundation, Rotterdam, the Netherlands
— Dutch Heart Foundation, The Hague, the Netherlands.

Rotterdam, June 1981   HANS RIJSTERBORGH

---

* The second symposium has been published as: Bom N, ed: Echocardiology. Martinus Nijhoff Publishers, The Hague/Boston/London: 1977. The third symposium has been published as: Lancée CT, ed: Echocardiology. Martinus Nijhoff Publishers, The Hague/Boston/London: 1979.

ACKNOWLEDGEMENTS

A book of this size is naturally the work of a large team. First of all, I wish to express my gratitude to, and my admiration of, all the lecturers who provided me with their carefully prepared manuscripts, in some cases at very short notice. Without their excellent cooperation this book would not exist.

I am especially indebted to Mary Rose Hoare, who contributed heavily to the editing and correcting of the material. Without her critical support, this book would have looked quite different.

My colleagues of the organizing committee, Klaas Bom, Jos Roelandt, Charles Lancée and Paul Hugenholtz were always available for assistance and advice, for which I am very grateful.

Furthermore, I have to thank our secretaries Corrie de Bruijn, Ineke van Lieshout and Ria Willemstein who cheerfully invested many hours in the preparation of this book.

Thanks are also due to Hans Eggink who spent hours on the preparation of the very long list of contributors and to Egbert Bos and Paul Voogd who helped in reading manuscripts and in explaining the finer points of pediatric cardiology to me.

Finally, I would like to pay a special tribute to Martinus Nijhoff Publishers, whose achievement, the publication of a book of this type within a period of six months, should be in the Guinness Book of Records.

HANS RIJSTERBORGH

CONTENTS

B. Applications in left ventricular function analysis

II. PEDIATRIC ECHOCARDIOLOGY

III. TECHNOLOGICAL ASPECTS OF ECHOCARDIOLOGY

CONTRIBUTORS

Abbate, A. L'., CNR Clinical Physiology Institute and University of Pisa, Pisa, Italy.

Abitbol, G., Dept, of Cardiology, Fondation A. de Rothschild, Paris, France.

Allen, H.D., University of Arizona, Tucson, Arizona, USA.

Anderson, R.H., Cardiothoracic Institute, Brompton Hospital, London, England.

Anliker, M., Institute for Biomedical Engineering, University and ETH, Zürich, Switzerland.

Azzolina, G., Tuscan Heart and Chest Center, Florence, Italy.

Bardos, P., Dept. of Cardiovas. Surgery, Rheinisch-Westfälische Technische Hochschule, Aachen, FRG.

Bastiaans, O.L., University of Technology, Delft, The Netherlands.

Becker, A.E., Dept. of Pathology, University of Amsterdam, Wilhelmina Gasthuis, Amsterdam, The Netherlands.

Behrenbeck, D.W., Med. Clinic and Policlinic, Dept. of Cardiology, University of Cologne, Cologne, FRG.

Beller, G., University of Virginia, Charlottesville, Virginia, USA.

Blair, S., Stanford University, Stanford, California, USA.

Bloch, A., Cardiac Center, University Hospital, Geneva, Switzerland.

Blom, J.A., Dept. of Obstetrics, Erasmus University, Rotterdam, The Netherlands.

Bogunovic, N., Gollwitzer Meier Institut, Bad Oeynhausen, FRG.

Bommer, W., Sect. of Cardiovascular Medicine, School of Medicine, Davis, California, USA

Bonzel, T., Abt. Kardiologie, Medizinische Universitätsklinik, Freiburg, FRG.

Brandestini, M.A., University of Washington, Seattle, Washington, USA.

Breda Vriesman, P.C.J. van, Dept. of Pathology, University of Leiden, Leiden, The Netherlands.

Busch, H.J., Dept. of Pediatric Cardiology, University of Nijmegen, Nijmegen, The Netherlands.

Carabello, B., University of Virginia, Charlottesville, Virginia, USA.

Carnahan, Y., University of Arizona, Tucson, Arizona, USA.

Cosyns, J., Cliniques Universitaires Saint-Luc, Brussels, Belgium.
Daly, K., Cardiac Dept. King's College Hospital, London, England.
Daniëls, O., Dept. of Pediatric Cardiology, University of Nijmegen, Nijmegen, The Netherlands.
Davidson, D.M., Stanford University, Stanford, California, USA.
Davies, M.J., Cardiac Dept. St. George's Hospital, London, England.
Dawson, J.R., Hillingdon Hospital, Uxbridge, Middlesex, England.
Delatte, D., Cliniques Universitaires Saint-Luc, Brussels, Belgium.
DeMaria, A.N., Section of Cardiovascular Medicine, School of Medicine, Davis, California, USA.
Distante, A., CNR Clinical Physiology Institute and University of Pisa, Pisa, Italy.
Durrer, D., Dept. of Cardiology, Wilhelmina Gasthuis, Amsterdam, The Netherlands.
Effert, S., Dept. of Internal Medicine I, Rheinisch-Westfälische Technische Hochschule, Aachen, FRG.
Erbel, R., Dept. of Internal Medicine I, Rheinisch-Westfälische Technische Hochschule, Aachen, FRG.
Eyll, Ch. van, Cliniques Universitaires Saint-Luc, Brussels, Belgium.
Ezekowitz, M.D., University of Oklahoma, Health Sciences Center, Oklahoma City, Oklahoma, USA.
Farjon, M., Dept of Cardiology, Fondation A. de Rothschild, Paris, France.
Fassbender, D., Gollwitzer Meier Institut, Bad Oeynhausen, FRG.
Fehr, R., Central Research Units, F. Hoffmann-La Roche & Co, Basel, Switzerland.
Feigenbaum, H., Dept. of Medicine, University of Indiana, Indianapolis, Indiana, USA.
Fox, W.W., Div. of Neonatology, Children's Hospital of Philadelphia, School of Medicine, Philadelphia, Pennsylvania, USA.
Gewitz, M.H., Div. of Cardiology, Children's Hospital of Philadelphia, School of Medicine, Philadelphia, Pennsylvania, USA.
Gibson, D.G., Cardiac Dept. Brompton Hospital, London, England.
Gleichmann, U., Gollwitzer Meier Institut, Bad Oeynhausen, FRG.
Godman, M.J., Royal Hospital for Sick Children, Edinburgh, Scotland.
Goldberg, S.J., University of Arizona, Tucson, Arizona, USA.
Greene, H.L., Harborview Medical Center, University of Washington, Seattle, Washington, USA.
Gross, B.W., Harborview Medical Center, University of Washington, Seattle, Washington, USA.
Guerin, F., Hôpital Cochin, Paris, France.
Guichard, J.P., Dept. of Cardiology, Fondation A. de Rothschild, Paris, France.

Guiney, T.E., Dept. of Cardiology, St. George's Hospital, London, England.

Gussenhoven, W.J., Interuniversity Cardiology Institute and Thoraxcenter, Erasmus University, Rotterdam, The Netherlands.

Hatle, L., Regional Hospital, Trondheim, Norway.

Hanrath, P., Dept. of Cardiology, University Hospital Hamburg, Hamburg, FRG.

Hansmann, M., Univ. Kinderklinik und Poliklinik Bonn, Bonn, FRG.

Haskell, W.L., Stanford University, Stanford, California, USA.

Hilger, H.H., Medical Clinic and Policlinic, Dept. of Cardiology, University of Cologne, Cologne, FRG.

Ho, P., Stanford University, Stanford, California, USA.

Hoeks, A., Dept. of Biophysics, Biomedical Centre, University of Limburg, Maastricht, The Netherlands.

Hoenecke, H., University of Arizona, Tucson, Arizona, USA.

Hombach, V., Medical Clinic and Policlinic, Dept. of Cardiology, University of Cologne, Cologne, FRG.

Hopman, J.C.W., Dept. of Pediatric Cardiology, University of Nijmegen, Nijmegen, The Netherlands.

Hunter, S., Regional Cardiothoracic Centre, Freeman Hospital, Newcastle upon Tyne, England.

Jackson, G., Cardiac Dept., King's College Hospital, London, England.

Janko, C.L., Harborview Medical Center, University of Washington, Seattle, Washington, USA.

Jansen, W.C., Medical Clinic and Policlinic, Dept. of Cardiology, University of Cologne, Cologne, FRG.

Jenni, R., Medical Policlinic, Dept. of Cardiology, University Hospital, Zürich, Switzerland.

Jewitt, D.E., Cardiac Dept. King's College Hospital, London, England.

Kalmanson, D., Fondation A. de Rothschild, Paris, France.

Kan, G., Dept. of Cardiology, Wilhelmina Gasthuis, Amsterdam, The Netherlands.

Kanaly, P.J., University of Oklahoma Health Sciences Center, Oklahoma City, Oklahoma, USA.

Kawabori, I., University of Washington, Seattle, Washington, USA.

Krayenbuehl, H.P., Medical Policlinic, University Hospital Zürich, University and ETH, Zürich, Switzerland.

Kremer, P., Dept. of Cardiology, University Hospital Hamburg, Hamburg, FRG.

Lambertz, H., Dept. of Internal Medicine I, Rheinisch-Westfälische Technische Hochschule, Aachen, FRG.

Lancée, C.T., Thoraxcenter, Erasmus University, Rotterdam, The Netherlands.

Langenstein, B.A., Dept. of Cardiology, University Hospital Hamburg, Hamburg, FRG.
Leech, G.J., Cardiac Dept. of St. George's Hospital, London, England.
Lutfalla, G., Hôpital Cochin, Paris, France.
Macartney, F.J., Dept. of Paediatric Cardiology, Hospital for Sick Children, London, England.
Magherini, A., Tuscan Heart and Chest Center, Florence, Italy.
Martin, R.P., University of Virginia, Charlottesville, Virginia, USA.
Maseri, A., CNR Clinical Physiology Institute and University of Pisa, Pisa, Italy.
Mason, D.T., Section of Cardiovascular Medicine, School of Medicine, Davis, California, USA.
Matsumoto, M., Dept. of Cardiology, University Hospital Hamburg, Hamburg, FRG.
Mayor, Ch., Cardiac Center, University Hospital, Geneva, Switzerland.
McCabe, D., University of Washington, Seattle, Washington, USA.
McGhie, J., Thoraxcenter, Erasmus University, Rotterdam, The Netherlands.
Minale, S., Dept. of Internal Medicine I, Rheinisch-Westfälische Technische Hochschule, Aachen, FRG.
Meijboom, E.J., Div. of Cardiology and Neonatology, Children's Hospital of Philadelphia, School of Medicine, Philadelphia, Pennsylvania, USA.
Meyer, J., Dept. of Internal Medicine I, Rheinisch-Westfälische Technische Hochschule, Aachen, FRG.
Medema, D.K., University of Washington, Seattle, Washington, USA.
Meltzer, R.S., Thoraxcenter, Erasmus University, Rotterdam, The Netherlands.
Merier, G., Cardiac Center, University Hospital Geneva, Switzerland.
Messmer, B.J., Dept. of Cardiovascular surgery, Rheinisch-Westfälische Technische Hochschule, Aachen, FRG.
Monaghan, M.J., Cardiac Dept. King's College Hospital, London, England.
Moritz, W.E., University of Washington, Seattle, Washington, USA.
Monsjou, L.K., Dept. of Cardiology, University of Leiden, Leiden, The Netherlands.
Niehues, B., Medical Clinic and Policlinic, Dept. of Cardiology, University of Cologne, Cologne, FRG.
Palombo, C., CNR Clinical Physiology Institute and University of Pisa, Pisa, Italy.
Parker, D.E., University of Oklahoma Health Sciences Center, Oklahoma City, Oklahoma, USA.
Parker, D.J., Cardiac Dept. St. George's Hospital, London, England.
Pearlman, A.S., University of Washington, Seattle, Washington, USA.
Peer, P.G.M., Dept. of Statistical Consultation, University of Nijmegen,

Nijmegen, The Netherlands.

Popp, R.L., Stanford University, Stanford, California, USA.

Ports, T.A., Cardiovascular Research Institute, University of California, San Francisco, California, USA.

Raphael, D., Cliniques Universitaires Saint-Luc, Brussels, Belgium.

Razor, J., Section of Cardiovascular Medicine, School of Medicine, Davis, California, USA.

Redel, D.A., Universitäts Kinderklinik und Poliklinik Bonn, Bonn, FRG.

Reneman, R.S., Dept. of Physiology, Biomedical Centre, University of Limburg, Maastricht, The Netherlands.

Roelandt, J.R.T.C., Thoraxcenter, Erasmus University, Rotterdam, The Netherlands.

Rovai, D., CNR Clinical Physiology Institute and University of Pisa, Pisa, Italy.

Ruissen, C., Dept. of Biophysics, Biomedical Centre, University of Limburg, Maastricht, The Netherlands.

Sahn, D.J., University of Arizona, Tucson, Arizona, USA.

Sainte-Beuve, D., Dept. of Cardiology, Fondation A. de Rothschild, Paris, France.

Schicht, I., Dept. of Nephrology, University of Leiden, Leiden, The Netherlands.

Schiller, N.B., Cardiovascular Research Institute, University of California, San Francisco, California, USA.

Scherer, E., Medical Clinic and Policlinic, Dept. of Cardiology, University of Cologne, Cologne, FRG.

Schweizer, P., Dept. of Internal Medicine I, Rheinisch-Westfälische Technische Hochschule, Aachen, FRG.

Serruys, P.W., Thoraxcenter, Erasmus University, Rotterdam, The Netherlands.

Silverman, N.H., Cardiovascular Research Institute, University of California, San Francisco, California, USA.

Skjærpe, T., Regional Hospital, Trondheim, Norway.

Smallhorn, J.F., Dept. of Paediatric Cardiology, Hospital for Sick Children, London, England.

Smeets, F., Dept. of Biophysics, Biomedical Centre, University of Limburg, Maastricht, The Netherlands.

Smith, E.O., University of Oklahoma Health Sciences Center, Oklahoma City, Oklahoma, USA.

Snider, A.R., Cardiovascular Research Institute, University of California, San Francisco, California, USA.

Stamm, R.B., University of Virginia, Charlottesville, Virginia, USA.

Stevenson, J.G., University of Washington, Seattle, Washington, USA.

Stoelinga, G.B.A., Dept. of Pediatric Cardiology, University of Nijmegen,

Nijmegen, The Netherlands.

Speck, S.M., Harborview Medical Center, University of Washington, Seattle Washington, USA.

Sutherland, G.R., Regional Cardiothoracic Centre, Freeman Hospital, Newcastle upon Tyne, England.

Sutton, G.C., Hillingdon Hospital, Uxbridge, Middlesex, England.

Taylor, G., University of Virginia, Charlottesville, Virginia, USA.

Tickner, E.G., Ultra Med. Inc. (formerly Rasor Associates Inc.), Sunnyvale, California, USA.

Trieb, G., Gollwitzer Meier Institut, Bad Oeynhausen, FRG.

Tommasini, G., Dept. of Paediatric Cardiology, Hospital for Sick Children, London, England.

Toussaint, M., Hôpital Cochin, Paris, France.

Tucker, C.R., Stanford University, Stanford, California, USA.

Turina, J., Medical Policlinic, University Hospital Zürich, University and ETH, Zürich, Switzerland.

Valdes-Cruz, L.M., University of Arizona, Tucson, Arizona, USA.

Verbeek, P.W., University of Technology Delft, Delft, The Netherlands.

Vernejoul, Fl. de, Hôpital Cochin, Paris, France.

Veyrat, C., Dept. of Cardiology, Fondation A. de Rothschild, Paris, France.

Vieli, A., Institute for Biomedical Engineering, University and ETH, Zürich, Switzerland.

Visser, C.A., Dept. of Cardiology, Wilhelmina Gasthuis, Amsterdam, The Netherlands.

Voogd, P.J., Dept. of Cardiology, University of Leiden, Leiden, The Netherlands.

Vosters, R., Dept. of Obstetrics and Gynaecology, Erasmus University, Rotterdam, The Netherlands.

Watson, D., University of Virginia, Charlottesville, Virginia, USA.

Weiss, J.L., Heart Station, The Johns Hopkins Hospital, Baltimore, Maryland, USA.

Wells, P.N.T., Bristol General Hospital, Bristol, England.

Werner, J.A., Harborview Medical Center, University of Washington, Seattle, Washington, USA.

Wieken, L.R. van der, Dept. of Cardiology, Wilhelmina Gasthuis, Amsterdam, The Netherlands.

Wilson, D.A., University of Oklahoma Health Sciences Center, Oklahoma City, Oklahoma, USA.

Wladimiroff, J.W., Dept. of Obstetrics and Gynaecology, Erasmus University, Rotterdam, The Netherlands.

Wood, D.C., Div. of Cardiology, The Children's Hospital of Philadelphia, School of Medicine, Philadelphia, Pennsylvania, USA.

Wood, P.D., Stanford University, Stanford, California, USA.

I. ECHOCARDIOLOGY IN ADULTS

A. GENERAL APPLICATIONS

1. ECHOCARDIOGRAPHY AS THE DIAGNOSTIC INVESTIGATION BEFORE CARDIAC SURGERY

D.G. GIBSON

Cardiac surgery has made remarkable strides since the introduction of cardiopulmonary bypass in the late 1950's. This would not have been possible without the accurate preoperative diagnostic information from cardiac catheterization and angiography. Since then, it has been widely held that cardiac catheterization is a necessary preliminary to operation. However, correlation of this same information with symptoms and physical signs led to a very significant improvement in the efficacy of the clinical method, a development particularly associated with the work of Paul Wood [1]. It thus became possible to make an accurate clinical diagnosis not only of the presence of valve or simple congenital heart disease, but also of the extent of the disturbances to flow, pressure and pulmonary arterial resistance. Unfortunately, in some institutions, the clinical tradition has not been acquired, or has been lost, so that these simple methods are not used as widely as they deserve, and reliance is placed on more elaborate and less cost-effective investigations. Another major contribution of invasive methods has been to form the basis of comparison against which other, more recently introduced techniques are introduced. These new methods and, in particular, echocardiography have developed to the extent that they are now able to give much anatomical and physiological information which has hitherto been inaccessible to simple clinical examination, or even, more recently, to cardiac catheterization itself. An unfortunate side effect has been that invasive methods have become invested with an aura of infallibility, which has led to results being accepted uncritically in individual cases and has, at the same time, actively discouraged studies of their specificity, sensitivity or reproducibility. With the new knowledge available from alternative techniques, the role of cardiac catheterization as an invariable precursor to cardiac surgery can now be questioned in relation to congenital, valvular, and coronary artery disease.

CONGENITAL HEART DISEASE

Preoperative cardiac catheterization can be dispensed with in two separate sets of circumstances in patients with congenital heart disease. The first is in

Rijsterborgh H, ed: Echocardiology, p 3-8. All rights reserved.
Copyright © 1981 Martinus Nijhoff Publishers, The Hague/Boston/London.

complex congenital heart disease, particularly in neonates and infants, when a palliative shunt procedure is planned to increase pulmonary blood flow and accurate intracardiac diagnosis is not required. All that may be necessary here is to confirm the presence of anatomical abnormalities compatible with the clinical picture. Definitive diagnosis is better deferred until corrective surgery is planned. The second is in certain forms of simple congenital heart disease. This group includes patients, particularly older children or adults, with ostium secundum atrial septal defects, bicuspid aortic valve causing significant aortic stenosis, coarctation of the aorta and persistent ductus arteriosus. Indeed, in the last two of these conditions, the diagnosis can readily be established on simple clinical criteria, and even echocardiography adds little additional information. In atrial septal defect, again, the clinical picture is usually clear-cut, but reversed septal motion can be demonstrated by M-mode, and a right to left shunt or a negative jet is present in the right atrium after a peripheral venous contrast injection. Although pulmonary valve motion gives some information about pulmonary artery pressure, this can more reliably and simply be obtained from straightforward clinical examination.

In contrast to the above conditions, two-dimensional echocardiography has shown itself to be an essential prelude to surgery, in association with invasive methods, in all forms of complex congenital heart disease. This reflects its ability to define the presence and position of an interventricular or trabecular septum, and its relation to one or two atrioventricular valves. It is probably the only method that can define the attachments of subvalve apparatus, information that is inaccessible to angiography, even using non-standard projections. Indeed, it is probably now true to say that corrective surgery should not be performed on such patients without high quality preoperative two-dimensional echocardiography in addition to invasive studies. While it would be inappropriate to review the field in detail, the value of the method can be illustrated by the results of a study of 80 cases of univentricular heart [2]. It was possible to categorize them into right ventricular, left ventricular, or indeterminate from the position of the rudimentary chamber. In addition, the mode of atrioventricular connexion was established, either via two valves, a common valve or a straddling valve. Absent connexion could be distinguished from an imperforate valve, which occurred in 5 patients. In addition, echocardiography can be used to study ventricular function in such patients, a field which has hitherto been almost completely neglected. Developments in image processing also suggest that echocardiography can detect abnormalities in ventricular structure which may be major determinants of the quality of postoperative results.

Although the incidence of rheumatic fever is declining in the West, degenerative mitral valve disease, calcific aortic stenosis and infective endocarditis persist. In the Third World, the incidence of chronic rheumatic heart disease remains high [3]. In valvular heart disease, simple clinical methods allow an accurate diagnosis to be made in the majority of patients. It has been our experience that cardiac catheterization in valvular heart disease, although confirming the original diagnosis, rarely alters management. M-mode and two-dimensional echocardiography have increasingly taken on the role of confirming the initial diagnosis made on clinical grounds. Not only do these methods give anatomical information about valve pathology, but digitized M-mode echocardiography can be used to give a comprehensive analysis of systolic and diastolic function. For this reason, at Brompton Hospital, we have felt justified, for the last eight years, in dispensing with routine cardiac catheterization in any adult patients with valvular heart disease in whom clinical and echocardiographic assessments are in agreement.

In order to examine the working of this system of management, we have examined the operative results of all patients undergoing valve replacement at the Brompton Hospital in 1978. These numbered 306. Of these, 61 were catheterized routinely by the referring source, and form a control group. Of the remainder, 61 were catheterized electively, for the assessment of possible coronary artery disease or because clinical and echocardiographic assessments were discordant, and the remainder, 184, had no catheterization. Patient age, sex, and aetiology of the valve disease were similar in the three groups, although emergency operation was undertaken significantly more frequently without preoperative catheterization. Hospital mortality was low for first operations on mitral (2.5% of 113 cases), aortic (4.4% of 79 cases) and double (10% of 53 cases) valve disease. These figures include emergency operations for infective endocarditis. For second operations, mortality was higher (18% of 63 cases), although this group includes 13 emergencies. In elective operations the mortality was not significantly different between the non-catheterized and either of the catheterized groups of patients. In patients requiring emergency operation, however, mortality was significantly higher in catheterized patients. This reflects the haemodynamic effects of angiographic dye on left ventricular function in seriously ill patients and the delay to essential surgery caused by invasive investigation. In all patients, the preoperative diagnosis was confirmed at operation. Information obtained at routine cardiac catheterization did not (1) add to clinical and noninvasive findings or (2) influence diagnosis, patient management or operative mortality. We conclude, therefore, that preoperative cardiac catheterization need not be performed routinely before operation in patients with valvular heart disease, but can be reserved for specific indications in a minority of patients.

A problem in this group of patients is the possible existence of additional coronary artery disease, requiring correction at the time of operation. Although it is widely assumed that this should be sought, and dealt with if present, objective evidence to support this contention is lacking. Thus, in the only series reported in the literature in which comparable groups of patients with both valvular heart disease and coronary artery disease, there was no effect on either early or late mortality of the additional procedure [4, 5, 6]. Our own experience is that preoperative angina is always relieved when significant aortic stenosis is corrected, and this has been confirmed by standard exercise testing in 40 such patients at variable periods after operation [11]. The study of possible effects of additional bypass grafting is thus a suitable subject for investigation in selected centres, but there is no reason for taking hitherto unproved benefits as a reason for performing it routinely, in view of the additional resources required for its detection.

The question of the place of routine cardiac catheterization in the investigation of valvular heart disease assumes particular importance as cardiological facilities are set up in the Third World. Here rheumatic heart disease is common, and occurs in young patients, in whom the incidence of coronary artery disease is low. It seems undesirable to impose on these new centres an expensive pattern of practice based on that required for a much older patient population in a society prepared to devote considerable effort to avoiding a very small risk of mis-diagnosis. Rather, these scarce resources, both technical and human, should be devoted to areas where their effects on the well-being of the community are more commensurate with their cost.

CORONARY ARTERY DISEASE

Echocardiography has little place to play in the routine surgical management of patients with ischaemic heart disease. Arteriography appears a remarkably satisfactory method of delineating the interior of a coronary artery, the information required for successful saphenous bypass grafting. There are, however, several areas where the echocardiography can give useful information. When the main symptom is breathlessness, and there is clinical or radiological evidence of left ventricular disease, then the differential diagnosis is likely to lie between a ventricular aneurysm and diffuse disease or ischaemic cardiomyopathy. Two-dimensional echocardiography has been reported as being remarkably successful in this field, with findings of between 95% and 100% agreement with angiography [7, 8]. Our own experience has been rather less favourable than this. In some patients (approximately 10%) it is not possible to obtain adequate delineation of the apical region of the ventricle due to obesity or chest disease. A second problem is the lack of a rigorous definition of ventricular aneurysm, particularly in angiographic terms. Although such regions are frequently said to show paradoxical outward motion, this is frequently a subjective phenomenon, and when objective digitization of angiograms is undertaken [9], no such movement is found. Although reversal of curvature at the boundary of an aneurysm may be prominent, especially at the apex, this does not necessarily apply in other regions of the ventricle. There appears to be a group of patients in whom both two-dimensional echocardiography and angiography are unhelpful, and the correct diagnosis is only made by the demonstration of full thickness fibrosis of the ventricular wall at operation.

A second field where echocardiography may be of value here is in the patient, who develops a pansystolic murmur in the period following a myocardial infarction, when the differential diagnosis of acquired VSD or mitral regurgitation arises. In some cases of septal rupture, the defect itself can be visualized, using two-dimensional echocardiography in either the apical or subcostal view, associated with a negative jet in the right ventricle [10]. Again, it may not always be possible to obtain pictures of diagnostic standard, but if an increased amplitude of left ventricular wall motion can be demonstrated, this is a very good reason for performing left ventriculography, even in a seriously ill patient.

CONCLUSION

It is now possible to perform cardiac surgery safely without preoperative cardiac catheterization in a significant number of patients. These include the majority of those with valvular heart disease, single or multiple, of any aetiology. In seriosly ill patients with acute valvular regurgitation or infective endocarditis, avoidance of angiography appears to have significant advantages in terms of increased postoperative survival. In complex congenital heart disease, the indication for routine two-dimensional echocardiography is that it can provide information about the relation between the atrioventricular valves and the interatrial and interventricular septa much more reliably than by angiography. Here the two techniques should be regarded as complementary. It is suggested that noninvasive techniques, and in particular M-mode and two-dimensional echocardiography have displaced invasive techniques from their dominant role in this field. Future studies might look more closely at the exact contribution of cardiac catheterization and angiography to the clinical decision-making process in order that expensive facilities can be used in a more cost effective way.

8

ACKNOWLEDGEMENT

I am grateful to my medical, paediatric, and surgical colleagues for permission to quote results obtained at Brompton Hospital.

REFERENCES

1. Wood P: Diseases of the Heart and Circulation. 2nd Edition, Eyre and Spottiswoode, London, 1955.
2. Rigby ML, RH Anderson, ODH Jones, EA Shinebourne, DG Gibson, MC Joseph: Two-dimensional echocardiographic categorization of univentricular heart: ventricular morphology, type and mode of atrioventricular connection. Br Heart J 43:722–723, 1980.
3. Editorial: Community control of rheumatic heart disease in developing countries: 1. A major public health problem. WHO Chron 34:336–345, 1980.
4. Riner RN, A Tajik, RB Wallace, RL Frye: Aortic valve disease and myocardial revascularization. Am J Cardiol 41:412, 1978.
5. Jang GC, EW Hancock: Aortic stenosis and coronary artery disease: long term survival after aortic valve replacement. Am J Cardiol 43:368, 1979.
6. Bonow RO, KM Kent, DR Rosing, LC Lipson, CL McIntosh, AG Morrow, SE Epstein: Aortic valve replacement in patients with combined aortic valvular and coronary artery disease: the case against routine myocardial revascularization. Circulation 59:II-222, 1979.
7. Grison D, G Lassabe, P Dumeny, B Descoings, A Sacrez: L'echocardiographie bidimensionnelle de l'aneurysme ventriculaire. Arch Mal Cœur 72:1337–1345, 1979.
8. Weyman AE, SM Peskoe, ES Williams, JC Dillon, H Feigenbaum: Detection of left ventricular aneurysms by cross-sectional echocardiography. Circulation 54:936–944, 1976.
9. Gibson DG, TA Prewitt, DJ Brown: Analysis of left ventricular wall movement during isovolumic relaxation and its relation to coronary artery disease. Br Heart J 38:1010–1019, 1976.
10. Farcot C et al.: Two-dimensional echocardiographic visualization of ventricular septal rupture after acute anterior myocardial infarction. Am J Cardiol 45:370–377, 1980.
11. Dawkins KD, DG Gibson: Digitized M-mode echocardiography in the assessment of patient following aortic valve replacement; a comparison with exercise testing. 4th Symposium on Echocardiology, Rotterdam, 1981 (abstract).

2. INTRAOPERATIVE APPLICATIONS OF TWO-DIMENSIONAL AND CONTRAST TWO-DIMENSIONAL ECHOCARDIOGRAPHY FOR EVALUATION OF CONGENITAL, ACQUIRED AND CORONARY HEART DISEASE IN OPEN-CHESTED HUMANS DURING CARDIAC SURGERY

DAVID J. SAHN

1. INTRODUCTION

Echocardiography has traditionally been most widely applied and praised as a noninvasive way for deriving cardiac structural and functional information. With increasing resolution and increasing utility, however, M-mode and two-dimensional echocardiography have, in recent years, been applied as measurement techniques in animal models and in basic science experimentation. The anatomic detail of externally performed two-dimensional echocardiographic cardiac imaging is of major assistance in confirming a patient diagnosis and describing fine points of anatomy, often complementarily to angiography. However, certain anatomical details and certain portions of the cardiac silhouette (for instance, the coronary arteries) have not been adequately imaged externally in many patients. Several recent studies of echocardiographic evaluation of the human heart during open-heart surgery for assessment of cardiac function or evaluation of the effects and adequacy of the surgical procedure itself, such as coronary artery bypass surgery, have been described [1, 2, 3, 4, 5]. Syracuse and coworkers first applied a sterilized M-mode transducer directly to the ventricular septum after myotomy-myectomy for idiopathic hypertrophic subaortic stenosis, to measure the width of the remaining septum and aid in the decision making process as to the adequacy of repair [1]. Waggoner et al. applied intracardiac M-mode echocardiography for evaluation of septal motion and thickening at surgery [2]. Related efforts to evaluate cardiac function at surgery have been published by Wong and Spotnitz, who used two-dimensional ultrasound to study pressure/volume relationships in open-chested humans to assess the deleterious effect of cardiac surgery on cardiac muscle function [3, 4]. Kisslo described an application of operative scanning to identify the location of a bullet embedded in the myocardium in which echocardiography was of direct benefit to the patient in guiding the surgical procedure [5]. Other than these preliminary reports, a comprehensive or ongoing evaluation of the utility of two-dimensional scanning during cardiac surgery has not been undertaken.

Rijsterborgh H, ed: Echocardiology, p 9-23. All rights reserved.
Copyright © 1981 Martinus Nijhoff Publishers, The Hague/Boston/London.

2. METHODOLOGY

Over the past twelve months, in conjunction with Sir Brian Barratt-Boyes and the Cardiothoracic Surgical Unit at Green Lane Hospital, Auckland, New Zealand, we explored applications of echocardiographic scanning at cardiac surgery in several settings. We have performed two-dimensional sector-scanning echocardiography intraoperatively to evaluate cardiac anatomy, providing details of diagnostic importance and allowing time for the surgeon to explore additional areas of the heart by substituting an echocardiographic scan in place of more time consuming dissection. Intraoperative anatomic information was obtained which had not been imaged with traditional external echocardiography or angiography, such as chordal fusion in mitral stenosis, presence of membranous subaortic stenosis or prolapsed aortic leaflets, or location of muscular ventricular septal defects.

A second class of echocardiographic investigation, also using sector-scan instrumentation during surgery, has allowed imaging of valvular contours before or after aortic or mitral valvulotomy and for assessment of the adequacy of positioning of prosthetic valves implanted in the heart. Imaging combined with contrast injections in the aorta, left ventricle, or left or right atrium has been used to assess valvular insufficiency after valvulotomy, adequacy of ventricular septal defect closure, and contour configuration and adequacy of Mustard baffles after surgical correction of transposition of the great arteries.

The third intrasurgical application we have explored has involved the use of a 9 MHz electronically-focused water path near-field scanner, placed directly over the surface of the heart. This device has allowed significantly detailed imaging of the coronary vascular tree, aiding surgical decision making about placement of saphenous vein bypass grafts, defining additional coronary lesions, localizing angiographically visualized lesions, and clarifying the status of coronary arteries when the angiogram has been ambiguous. It will be the purpose of this paper to present examples of these utilities derived from these ongoing studies.

It has been our experience that most array transducers withstand gas sterilization without damage and that they are insulated well enough to prevent electrical discharge to the surface of the heart. Over 50 open-chested imaging studies in humans have been obtained at the time of writing, with no significant complications. There have been no infections and no arrhythmias. The surgeons who are most adept at handling the heart and manipulating it during surgery have quickly learned the techniques of open-chested two-dimensional scanning, planning which patients can best benefit by these applications at presurgical conferences.

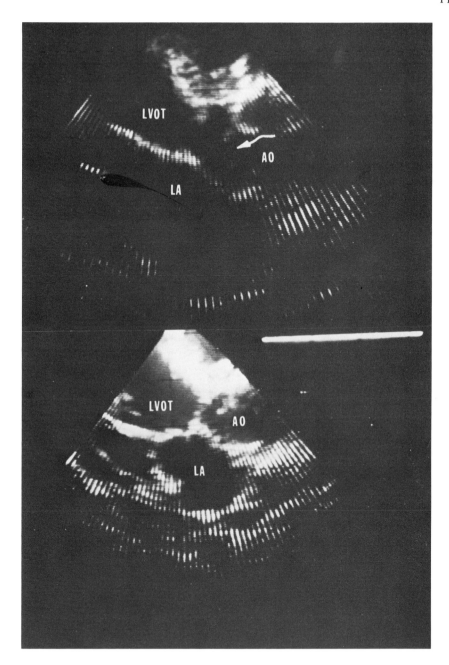

Figure 1. The upper panel shows the prolapsing aortic leaflet (arrow) inferiorly in the left ventricular outflow tract just above a partially imaged subaortic membrane arising from the septum. Alteration of scanning technique (lower panel) at surgery allowed complete imaging of discrete subaortic stenosis, a diagnosis that had been missed in the preoperative evaluation due to apposition of the prolapsing aortic cusp to the membrane on angiography.

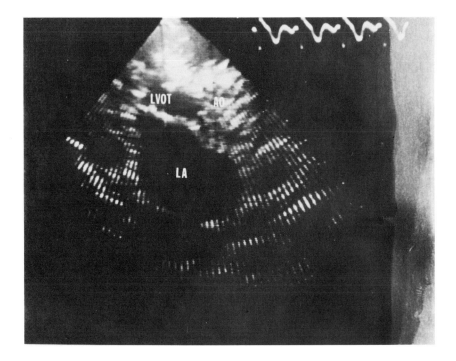

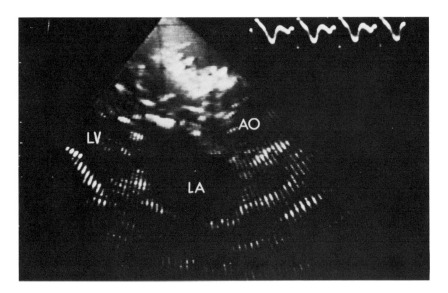

Figure 2. The upper panel shows the beginnings of a contrast injection in the aortic root in the patient whose echo is shown in Figure 1. The lower panel shows that significant aortic insufficiency still exists, as shown by generous filling of the left ventricle with contrast material.

3. AORTIC INSUFFICIENCY WITH VALVE REPLACEMENT

The first utility may be illustrated by the following case. A nine-year-old youngster was followed for evaluation of an initially suspected diagnosis of ventricular septal defect with aortic insufficiency. At cardiac catheterization, the ventricular septal defect had apparently closed and aortic insufficiency was present. The patient was referred for cardiac surgery, with precatheterization and preoperative two-dimensional echocardiography showing only nonspecific findings. In the operating room, before placing the patient on cardiopulmonary bypass, a gas-sterilized transducer from a phased-array instrument was placed directly on the heart and long-axis images were obtained. Initial observation suggested that the non coronary leaflet of the aortic valve prolapsed inferiorly toward the left ventricular outflow tract and a specific suggestion about the type of aortic insufficiency was therefore made (top panel, Figure 1). A septal abnormality beneath the aortic valve was suggested which, with change of transducer angulation, was imaged as a subaortic diaphragm beneath the aortic valve (bottom panel, Figure 1). When the aorta was surgically opened, the posterior coronary cusp was fenestrated and prolapsed into the left ventricle. Exploration of the subaortic area revealed a moderately tight discrete membrane lying against the prolapsed aortic leaflet, accounting for the fact that, while the leaflet prolapse was visualized angiographically, the diagnosis of subaortic stenosis was missed. The valve cusp was supported and repaired and cardiopulmonary bypass was discontinued. Assessment of the adequacy of the valve repair was made at surgery using two-dimensional echocardiography combined with aortic injection of indocyanine green dye for echo contrast. The degree of aortic insufficiency was still judged moderate on the basis of this study (Figure 2) and the decision was therefore made to replace the aortic valve.

4. AORTIC VALVULOTOMY

Another example of the utility of operative scanning is suggested in Figure 3 by the pre and postoperative appearances of the aortic valve orifice imaged in short-axis at the level of the aorta in a patient with aortic stenosis. The surgeon was concerned about producing significant aortic insufficiency during the valvulotomy and performed it quite conservatively. On contrast injection after surgery, aortic insufficiency appeared minimal and the aortic orifice had been enlarged from $70 \, mm^2$ to $120 \, mm^2$, as measured by planimetry of the short-axis view of the aortic orifice. The change in commissural configuration and orifice size are shown in Figure 3. In this case, a decision that the surgical endeavor had been adequately performed was aided by the two-dimensional echocardiogram.

14

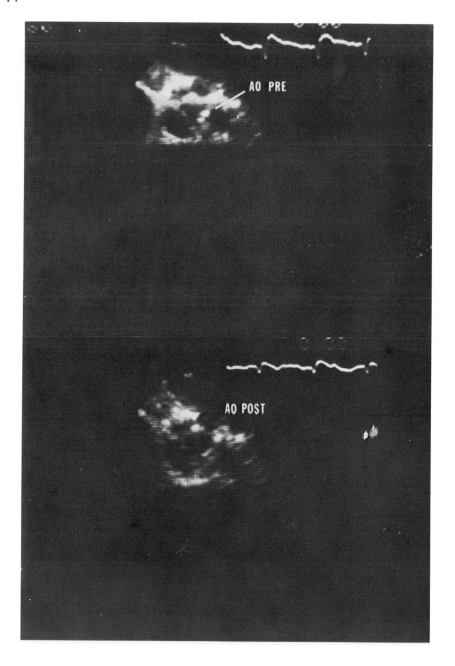

Figure 3. The upper panel shows the aortic valve orifice imaged in short axis in an open-chested human before aortic valvulotomy. The lower panel shows enlargement of the aortic cross-sectional orifice area after the valvulotomy had been performed.

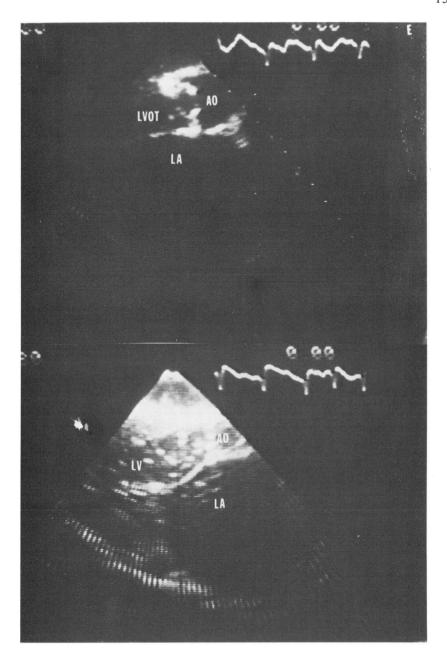

Figure 4. A patient with aortic stenosis, mitral stenosis and insufficiency is shown. The aortic dome is seen in the upper panel. Aortic echo contrast injection shows aortic insufficiency with filling of the left ventricle and significant regurgitation of contrast material across the mitral valve into the left atrium.

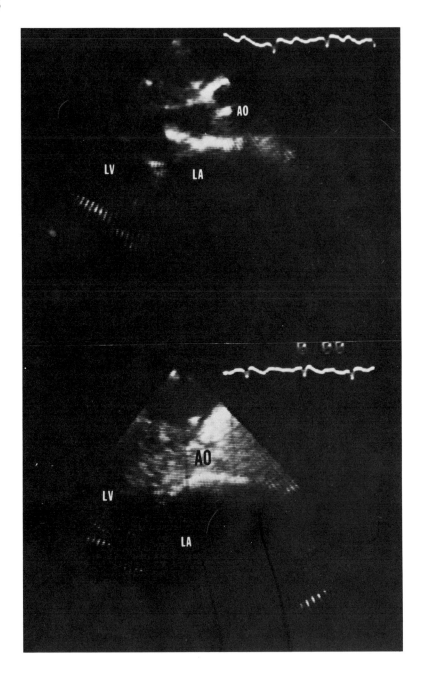

Figure 5. The postoperative evaluation of the patient whose echo is shown in Figure 4 shows adequate positioning of the porcine heterograft valve which is not angled too close to the septum (upper panel). In the lower panel, there is mild aortic insufficiency with contrast only filling the upper portion of the left ventricle after aortic contrast injection.

5. AORTIC AND MITRAL INSUFFICIENCY

An additional example of evaluation of valvular disease is the case of a young adult referred with mitral and aortic valvular disease. At catheterization, he had moderately severe mitral insufficiency and a suspicion of mild mitral stenosis as well. His aortic stenosis appeared moderate by hemodynamic and angiographic evaluation. At cardiac surgery, the two-dimensional echocardiographic image of the aortic valve suggested that it was moderately severely affected and doming, but that the cusps were indeed thin and pliable (Figure 4). Intraoperative contrast injections suggested aortic insufficiency and mitral insufficiency as left ventricle and left atrium filled generously with contrast material after aortic contrast injection (bottom panel, Figure 4). Aortic valvulotomy and mitral valve replacement were performed. A postoperative two-dimensional echocardiogram, performed in the operating room shortly after cardiopulmonary bypass was discontinued showed the position of the mitral valve porcine xenograft to be adequate. Contrast injection performed at this time showed mild aortic insufficiency with no mitral insufficiency; the patient's operative result was deemed adequate (Figure 5).

These individual case vignettes show how the surgeon can use two-dimensional echocardiography to aid in diagnosis and help in decision making regarding the adequacy and results of open-heart surgery. While surgeons use pressure measurements, calculations of cardiac output or green dye curves for evaluation of residual shunts or valvular insufficiency in the operating room, two-dimensional echocardiography, combined with contrast techniques, provides direct anatomical imaging information about the contour of surgically repaired or replaced valves, as well as information about the site and severity of valvular insufficiency. This information can be obtained safely and without significant difficulty by the surgeon at a time when it can be of assistance in the decision-making process.

6. CORONARY ARTERY IMAGING

Echocardiography has also been applied for imaging the left main coronary artery. It is unclear how effectively noninvasive two-dimensional echocardiography images the coronary tree when studies are evaluated. It appears that the noninvasive application of echocardiography for evaluation of the coronary bed itself is limited, and this application of two-dimensional echocardiography remains controversial. The coronary vascular tree is a complicated vascular bed in space, making it difficult to evaluate by planar imaging techniques because the vessels are small; the left main coronary artery is only approximately 4 to 5 mm in size. Coronary angiography remains the "gold standard" for evaluation of coronary disease, yet not

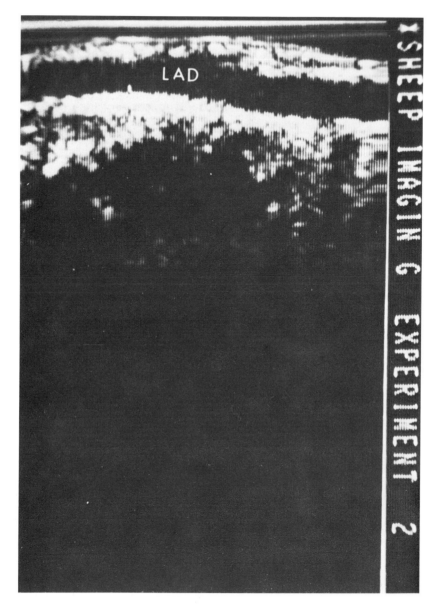

Figure 6. Imaging of the left anterior descending coronary artery in the interventricular sulcus of a sheep performed as an open-chested imaging experiment is shown. The left anterior descending vessel in this animal is approximately 2 mm.

infrequently portions of the coronary bed are not well defined even on selective coronary injections, either because they are obscured by other coronary structures or because they fill poorly, being downstream from other obstructive lesions. As such, the usual patient is referred to cardiac surgery

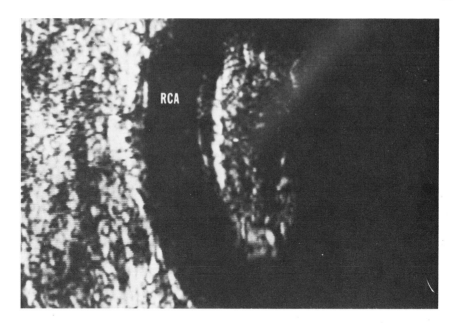

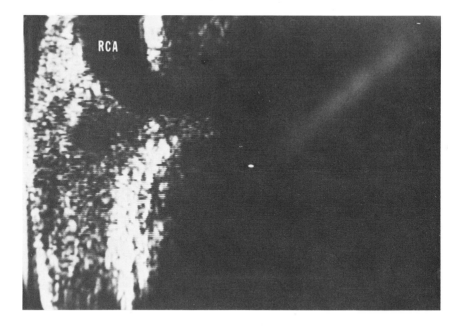

Figure 7. Imaging of the right coronary artery orifice is shown (lower panel) in an image derived from an open-chested human. The upper panel shows the more distal course of the right coronary artery. In all these and subsequent coronary studies, the image orientation is inverted. The superior direction is at the bottom of the scan and the inferior direction at the top of the scan. This image inversion is necessitated by the geometry of the transducer. The normal right coronary artery is $4\frac{1}{2}$ to 5 mm in size and good endothelial definition is obtained.

for 3, 4, or 5 bypasses, with the surgeon usually always performing the higher number of saphenous vein bypass grafts. Localizing the angiographically shown lesions and determining their location on the surface of the heart is difficult because the surgeon cannot evaluate the lumen size or patency of the coronary arteries at surgery. We have, therefore, explored ultrasound techniques for evaluating coronary vascular anatomy at the time of cardiac surgery. Initial studies were performed with a 9 MHz water path scanner in open-chested sheep with placement of the transducer over the interventricular sulcus (the external marker for the position of the left anterior descending coronary), resulting in high quality imaging data (Figure 6). After contrast echocardiographic validation of imaging of coronary veins and arteries in the animal model, human patients were selected for intraoperative scanning with the goal of imaging normal coronary arteries in humans and applying the technique to evaluate coronary disease. Comparative studies were obtained of appearance of known coronary vascular lesions with angiographic/open-chested echo correlations resulting in a learning curve for this technique. The appearance of the normal right coronary artery by this technique is shown in Figure 7; the lower panel shows the orifice of the right coronary artery and the upper panel its distal course. The coronary artery imaged here is 4 mm in size and there is good endothelial detail in a patient with an angiographically normal right coronary artery. In contrast, Figure 8 shows the echocardiographic appearance of a 75% obstructive lesion of the right coronary artery. The lesion not only narrows the lumen but casts an ultrasonic shadow. Open-chested imaging of the left main coronary artery and the proximal left anterior descending and left circumflex arteries have been more difficult since they lie between the aorta and pulmonary artery in an area difficult to access with the near-field scanner. This problem has been alleviated by using the pulmonary artery as a window for imaging the proximal left coronary circulation. The transducer is placed obliquely and transversely across the pulmonary artery and angled down onto the superior surface of the heart where the left main coronary artery leaves the aorta and bifurcates. Representative images of a normal left main coronary artery are shown in Figure 9. In one of our recent patients, there was clear angiographic indication that coronary artery bypass grafting involving the left circumflex and right coronary artery circulation was indicated; a very proximal left anterior descending lesion was also demonstrated. The rest of the left anterior descending coronary artery tree, however, was poorly visualized on biplane angiography because it was poorly filled and there was concern as to the presence of additional left anterior descending lesions. As shown in Figure 10, when the left anterior descending coronary artery was followed down the interventricular sulcus, an additional obstructive lesion was visualized distal to the septal perforators and the first diagonal. At surgery, the saphenous vein bypass graft was applied in such a way as to bypass both the proximal

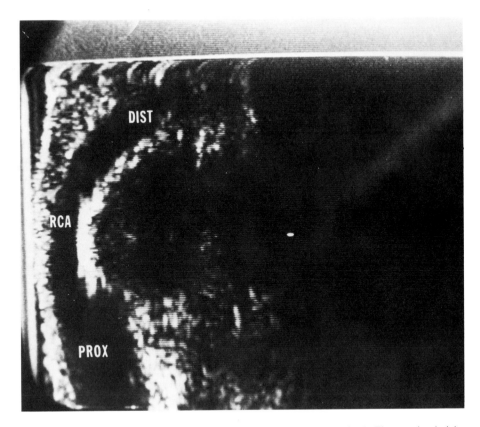

Figure 8. An obstructive coronary lesion of the right artery is visualized. The proximal right coronary is at the bottom, the distal segment at the very top of the image. The lesion arises primarily from the posterior wall of the coronary artery and casts an echocardiographic shadow.

and distal left anterior descending lesions. In summary, it appears that open-chested imaging of the coronary vascular system can be achieved and that it may help clarify coronary vascular anatomy and assist the planning of saphenous vein coronary bypass grafts.

7. SUMMARY

The application of these new intraoperative techniques in open-chested humans at Green Lane Hospital has suggested to us that two-dimensional echocardiography with echo contrast for the evaluation of cardiac chamber and valvular anatomy, as well as for the clarification of coronary vascular anatomy, can be of significant use in planning heart surgery. Also, this

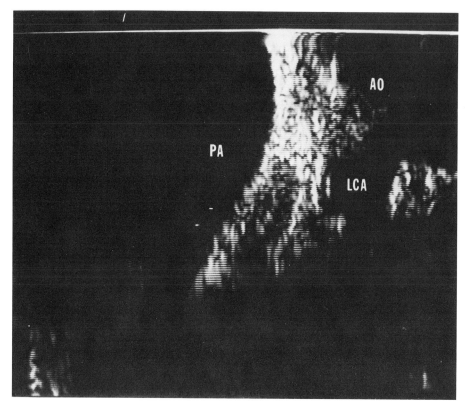

Figure 9. A transverse plane image shows the plane of the pulmonary artery with the origin of the left coronary from the aorta behind the pulmonary artery in an open-chested human.

combination of contrast and two-dimensional echocardiography is of significant importance for immediate postoperative verification that surgical endeavors have been adequately and successfully performed.

The results of our studies at Green Lane have suggested that cardiac surgeons, who have excellent understanding of the spatial anatomy of the heart, learn two-dimensional echocardiography very quickly and that its intraoperative application is without significant mortality or morbidity. Specific engineering and technical changes will, however, be necessary to design ultrasound probes for intraoperative application which will be less bulky and easier to apply; we expect that these new applications will serve as an impetus for development of surgically appropriate ultrasound scanning devices.

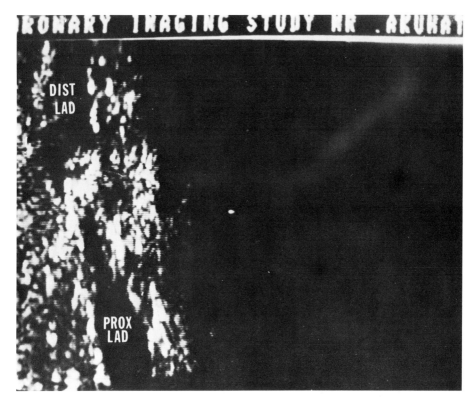

Figure 10. Again, an inverted image shows the proximal left anterior descending artery at the bottom of the image and the distal left anterior descending artery at the top with 100% obstruction. This diagnosis had not been made angiographically because of inadequate filling of the left anterior descending coronary artery due to a more proximal lesion.

REFERENCES

1. Syracuse DS, VA Audiani, DG Kastl, WL Henry, AG Morrow: Intraoperative, intracardiac echocardiography during left ventriculomyotomy and myectomy for IHSS. (abst) Circulation 56:27, 1977.
2. Waggoner AD, AA Shah, JS Schuessler, ES Crawford, RR Miller, MA Quinones: Effect of cardiac surgery on echocardiographic septal motion: Assessment by intraoperative and postoperative echocardiography. (abstr) Circulation 62:20, 1980.
3. Wong CYH, HM Spotnitz: Effect of nitroprusside on end-diastolic pressure-diameter relations of the human left ventricle after pericardiotomy. Am J Cardiol 45:393, 1980.
4. Spotnitz HM, CYH Wong, AJ Spotnitz, RH Collins: Intraoperative left ventricular performance evaluated by two-dimensional ultrasound. (abstr) Circulation 62:329, 1980.
5. Kisslo JA: personal communication, 1980.

3. LONG-TERM CONTROL OF LEFT VENTRICULAR FUNCTION AFTER AORTOCORONARY BYPASS SURGERY BY TWO-DIMENSIONAL ECHOCARDIOGRAPHY

R. Erbel, P. Schweizer, P. Bardos, J. Meyer, S. Minale, B.J. Messmer, and S. Effert

1. INTRODUCTION

Noninvasive methods are needed for serial measurements of left ventricular function, particularly in follow-up studies.

Because of regional myocardial dysfunction, M-mode echocardiography cannot be used for evaluation of left ventricular function in patients with coronary artery disease [4, 5]. After open-heart surgery, paradoxical septal motion develops, thus further limiting the possibilities of using M-mode echocardiography for studying the left ventricular funcion after aortocoronary bypass surgery.

These methodological problems were overcome by two-dimensional echocardiography. Even in patients with coronary artery disease, high correlations between left ventricular volumes and ejection fraction determined by two-dimensional echocardiography and by cineangiography were found [1, 3, 8].

Two-dimensional echocardiography was therefore used for a follow-up study in patients with coronary artery disease. Left ventricular function was analysed before and after aortocoronary bypass surgery.

2. METHODS

2.1. Patients

The study was performed in 31 patients (27 men, 4 women) with a mean age of 51.9 years (range 40 to 63 years). A mean of 2.3 bypass grafts were inserted, 28 to the anterior descending branch and 14 to the circumflex branch of the left coronary artery, 5 to the diagonal branch of the anterior ascending artery, 13 to the right coronary artery and 11 to the marginal branch of the right coronary artery.

In 29/31 patients two-dimensional echocardiograms of acceptable quality could be recorded 10 to 14 days postoperatively; 6 months postoperatively 22/31, and 18 months postoperatively 23/31 patients could be reexamined.

26

2.2. Echocardiography

Two-dimensional echocardiography was performed using a phased-array wide-angle sector-scanner, Varian V-3000 A. A 2.25 MHz transducer was used. Real-time two-dimensional echocardiograms were recorded at 30 frames/sec on video tape.

Recordings were made by placing the transducer on the apex impulse location and aiming the beam towards the left atrium (Figure 1). In the four-chamber view, left atrium, left ventricle, right atrium and right ventricle were scanned. The interventricular septum was clearly visualized.

After recording on video tape, left ventricular endocardial contour was traced with a lightpen system. Computer-assisted left ventricular volumes

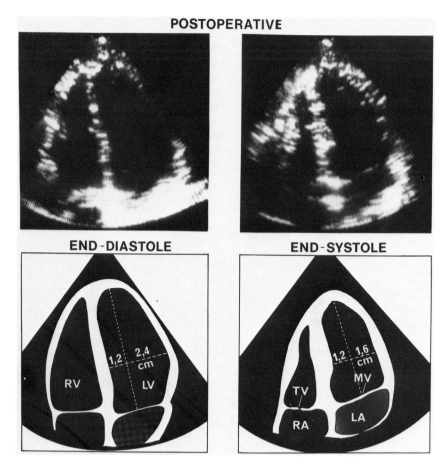

Figure 1. End-diastolic and end-systolic four-chamber view, early postoperatively, demonstrating akinetic septal motion despite systolic thickening. Left ventricular diameter is divided by the long-axis in a septal and posterolateral half-axis for evaluation of wall motion.

were calculated using Simpson's rule. End-diastolic (peak of R wave) and end-systolic (end of T wave and smallest left ventricular silhouette) frames were defined in stop frame mode with reference to the ECG.

2.3. Calculations

Recent studies revealed a systematic underestimation of two-dimensional echocardiographically determined volumes, when compared to cineangiography, despite high correlation coefficients [3, 8]. Therefore, calculated end-diastolic and end-systolic volumes were corrected using regression equations, whose coefficients were obtained from volumes determined preoperatively using cineangiography (V_{angio}) and two-dimensional echocardiography (V_{echo}). The regression equation was given by $V_{echo} = 0.747 V_{angio} + 12.1$ ml.

2.4. Statistics

Statistical analysis was done using Student's t-test for unpaired data. A p-value of less than 0.05 was considered to be significant. All values are given with the standard error of the mean (s.e.m.).

3. RESULTS

Early postoperatively, 4/31 patients showed a pericardial effusion, which was drained in 2/4 patients. Six months postoperatively only 1/4 patients had a small pericardial effusion.

Blood pressure was preoperatively $17.5 \pm 0.5/11.1 \pm 0.3$ kPa, early postoperatively $17.4 \pm 0.5/11.4 \pm 0.4$ kPa, 6 months later $18.7 \pm 0.6/12.0 \pm 0.2$ kPa, and 18 months postoperatively $17.6 \pm 0.7/11.0 \pm 0.4$ kPa. Systolic and diastolic blood pressures were not significantly different over the study.

Changes in heart rate (HR), end-diastolic volume (EDV), end-systolic volume (ESV), stroke volume (SV), and ejection fraction (EF) are listed in Table 1.

Table 1. Values for HR, EDV, ESV, SV, and EF preoperatively (1.), 10–14 days (2.), 6 months (3.), and 18 months postoperatively (4.).

	HR(Hz)	EDV(ml)	ESV(ml)	SV(ml)	EF(%)
1.	1.2 ± 0.04	172.3 ± 9.1	70.1 ± 8.2	102.2 ± 3.7	59.4 ± 2.7
2.	1.6 ± 0.04	155.8 ± 9.2	77.8 ± 7.8	78.0 ± 3.5	50.1 ± 2.6
3.	1.3 ± 0.05	155.5 ± 12.5	59.9 ± 8.5	95.7 ± 4.6	61.5 ± 2.3
4.	1.2 ± 0.03	171.7 ± 12.8	75.6 ± 8.2	96.1 ± 5.4	56.0 ± 1.6

28

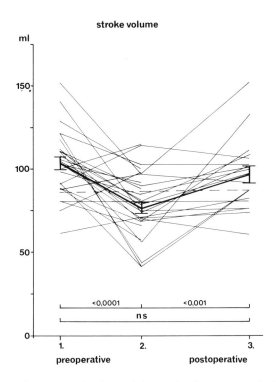

stroke volume

ml

150

100

50

0

<0,0001   <0,001

ns

1.   2.   3.
preoperative   postoperative

Figure 2. Stroke volume before (1.), early (2.), and 6 months (3.) postoperatively. The mean values ± s.e.m. are shown together with all individual values. Stroke volume decreased after aortocoronary bypass surgery early postoperatively and reached the starting point 6 months later.

End-diastolic and end-systolic volume changes were not significant. As shown in Figure 2, a highly significant decrease in stroke volume was found, except in 6 patients early postoperatively. 6 months later, stroke volume had nearly reached the initial level and was not significantly different from the preoperative values. Calculated cardiac output remained constant pre and postoperatively 7.44 ± 0.01 l/min versus 7.39 ± 0.01, 7.43 ± 0.13 and 6.90 ± 0.01 l/min. Changes in EF were similar to changes in stroke volume.

Early postoperatively, wall motion abnormalities, particularly of the septum, were observed. For quantitative analysis, fractional shortening of septal and postero-lateral half-axis were calculated (Figure 3) as illustrated in Figure 1. Early postoperatively, septal wall motion decreased significantly from $34.8 \pm 3.4\%$ to $14.2 \pm 3.2\%$ ($p < 0.01$), whereas postero-lateral wall motion increased from 24.7 ± 3.2 to $28.9 \pm 2.8\%$ (not significant). Six months later, septal half-axis shortening was $17.5 \pm 3.5\%$ and postero-lateral half-axis shortening $28.6 \pm 1.4\%$. 18 months postoperatively septal shortening

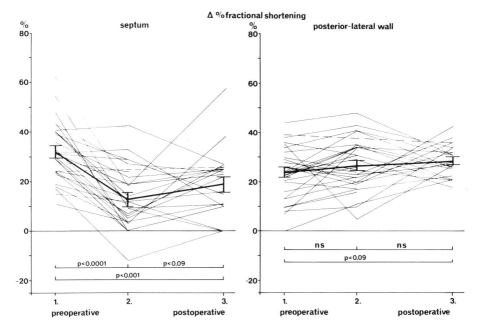

Figure 3. Fractional shortening of septum and postero-lateral wall preoperatively (1.), early postoperatively (2.), and 6 months postoperatively (3.). Individual and mean values are illustrated.

improved to $30.7 \pm 2.2\%$, while postero-lateral wall motion remained nearly constant at $26.7 \pm 1.6\%$.

4. DISCUSSION

Whereas M-mode echocardiography cannot be used for evaluation of left ventricular function after open-heart surgery because of paradoxical septal motion, apical two-dimensional echocardiography has overcome these methodological limitations.

In 29/31 patients two-dimensional echocardiograms of acceptable quality could be obtained. In 4 patients a pericardial effusion was detected, which was not otherwise suspected in 2/4. Thus pericardial effusion may be expected in about 5% to 10% of the patients after aortocoronary bypass surgery. Similar results have been reported by other authors [10]. Based on the two-dimensional echocardiograms an estimation of the amount of fluid could be obtained.

Early postoperatively left ventricular stroke volume decreased significantly, because end-diastolic volume decreased and end-systolic volume increased. Thus ejection fraction decreased, too. Because of the decrease in stroke volume, heart rate increased significantly as a compensatory mechanism keeping cardiac output constant. During the follow-up, stroke volume increased and consequently heart rate decreased. Similar results were obtained using tantalum markers. Mintz et al. [6] reported a significant increase in heart rate early postoperatively. They also found an increase in stroke volume during the postoperative period.

The reason for the decrease of stroke volume is the disturbed septal wall motion, already observed by M-mode echocardiography [2, 7]. Because septal systolic thickening was diminished, it could be shown that not only septal motion but also septal myocardial function was depressed. Similar results were reported by Vignola et al. [10], using M-mode echocardiography and radionuclide methods. In our study these earlier results were confirmed by two-dimensional echocardiography. A significant reduction in septal inward movement was found early postoperatively, accompanied by a compensatory increase in posterior wall motion, which could not, however, prevent the decrease in stroke volume. Similar results were obtained with epicardial markers by Serruys et al. [9]. Following these authors we were also able to show, that in the follow-up period regional, and consequently left ventricular, function improved. Surgery related problems like ischemia, cardioplegia, and open pericardium are the reason for depressed regional myocardial function.

5. CONCLUSION

After aortocoronary bypass surgery, two-dimensional echocardiography revealed early postoperatively a depressed septal wall motion resulting in a decrease of stroke volume. As a compensatory mechanism heart rate increased. Thus, cardiac output remained constant. During the follow-up period septal wall motion improved, stroke volume increased and heart rate decreased.

REFERENCES

1. Carr K, R Engler, J Forsythe, A Johnson, B Gosink: Measurement of left ventricular ejection fraction by mechanical cross-sectional echocardiography. Circulation 59:1196, 1979.
2. Corallo S, A Pezzano, M Castognone, B Brusoni, L Ladelli, F Rovelli: Left ventricular behaviour before and after coronary artery bypass graft. Echocardiographic study. In: Europ. Congr. on Ultrasonic in Medicine, Bologna, Edizione centro, minerva medica, 287, 1978.

3. Erbel R, P Schweizer, J Meyer, H Grenner, W Krebs, S Effert: Bestimmung der Volumina und der Ejektionsfraktion des linken Ventrikels aus dem zweidimensionalen Echokardiogramm bei Patienten mit koronarer Herzerkrankung. Z Kardiol 69:52, 1980.

4. Erbel R, P Schweizer: Diagnostischer Stellenwert der Echokardiographie bei der koronaren Herzerkrankung – I. M-Mode Echokardiographie. Z Kardiol 69:391, 1980.

5. Linhart JW, GS Mintz, BL Segal, N Kawai, MN Kotler: Left ventricular volume measurements by echocardiography: Fact or fiction? Am J Cardiol 36:114, 1975.

6. Mintz LJ, NBJr Ingles, GT Daughters II, EB Stinson, EL Alderman: Sequential studies of left ventricular function and wall motion after coronary arterial bypass surgery. Am J Cardiol 45:210, 1980.

7. Righetti A, MH Crawford, RA O'Rourke, H Schelbert, PO Daily, J Ross Jr.: Interventricular septal motion and left ventricular function after coronary bypass surgery. Am J Cardiol 39: 372, 1977.

8. Schiller NB, H Acquatelle, TA Ports, D Drew, J Goerke, H Ringertz, NH Silverman, B Brundage, R Boswelle, E Carlsson, WW Parmley: Left ventricular volume from paired biplane two-dimensional two-dimensional echocardiography.Circulation 60:574, 1979.

9. Serruys PW, RW Brower, HJ ten Kate, M vd Brand, PG Hugenholtz: Early myocardial depression after coronary artery bypass surgery. In: Coronary heart surgery. Roskamm H., M. Schmutzler (ed.) Berlin-Heidelberg-New York: Springer 349, 1978.

10. Vignola PA, ChA Boucher, GD Curfman, HJ Wolter, WH Shea, RE Dinsmare, GM Pohost: Abnormal interventricular septal motion following cardiac surgery: Clinical, surgical, echocardiographic and radionuclide correlates. Am Heart J 97:27, 1979.

4. EVALUATION OF THE ST. JUDE MEDICAL VALVE PROSTHESIS IN THE MITRAL POSITION

W.C. Jansen, B. Niehues, V. Hombach, E. Scherer, D.W. Behrenbeck, and H.H. Hilger

Due to advances in cardiac surgery, the number of patients with artificial cardiac valves has increased and both quality and expectancy of life have been considerably improved. The main goal of postoperative control of these patients is to recognize dysfunction as early as possible and to differentiate it from cardiac failure. Of the noninvasive methods, echocardiography plays a major role in the function control of the cardiac valve prosthesis. Due to various constructional properties, evaluation of valve function by echocardiography is sometimes very difficult.

Since 1978 our cardiac surgery department has increasingly often implanted the St. Jude Medical valve prosthesis (SJM) in the aortic and mitral positions, because of its superior hemodynamic qualities [1] (Figure 1).

This type of prosthesis is quite different from the tilting-disc prosthesis, because it consists of two half discs moving like a folding door around the central hinges.

In the opening position, the valve provides three nearly equal areas for the blood to flow through. Since the SJM is made from pyrolytic carbon, a highly-polymerized inert hydrocarbon, it normally cannot be visualized fluoroscopically and therefore echocardiography plays a major role in the evaluation of valve function and recognition of dysfunction.

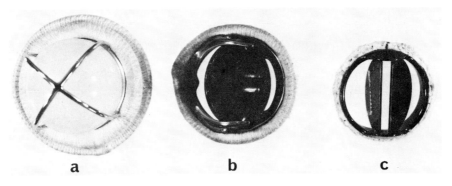

a   b   c

Figure 1. a Starr-Edwards caged-ball prosthesis, b Lillehei-Kaster prosthesis, c St. Jude Medical prosthesis.

Rijsterborgh H, ed: Echocardiology, p 33-38. All rights reserved.
Copyright © 1981 Martinus Nijhoff Publishers, The Hague/Boston/London.

34

In 40 patients, age from 23 to 65, with an SJM in the mitral position, valve function was routinely evaluated echocardiographically 3 to 6 weeks post-operatively, by means of the ECHOCARDIOVISOR 01 (Organon Teknika, Munich) (transducer 2.25 MHz, diameter 13 mm, focal distance 75 mm). The transducer was positioned for the echo beam to be directed in parallel to the suture ring and perpendicular to the leaflets in the opening position. In 30 patients, echocardiograms and phonocardiograms were recorded simultaneously.

The following parameters were measured:
1. Opening (MOV) and closing velocity (MCV) (mm/sec)
2. Excursion of the posterior leaflet (mm)
3. A_2 closing to mitral opening interval (A_2-MPO) (ms)
4. Time interval from Q-wave to mitral closing sound (Q-MPC) (ms)

RESULTS

In 32 patients (80%), the motion pattern of the leaflets could be well visualized. With an SJM in the mitral position, the echo beam in diastole is parallel to the suture ring and perpendicular to the opened leaflets. Thus the leaflets are visualized on the M-mode as two, almost congruent, triangles, when studied in an ideal position of the prosthesis. During systole, i.e. with the leaflets closed, the echo beam is incident in parallel to the suture ring and to the leaflets. Thus immediately after the onset of the ORS-complex, the

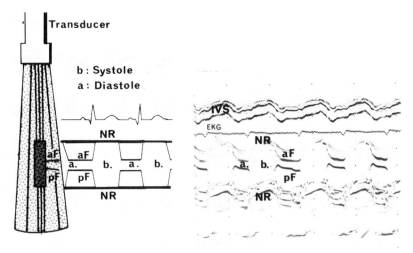

Figure 2. The echocardiographic motion pattern of the SJM prosthesis in mitral position. NR = suture ring, aF = anterior leaflet, pF = posterior leaflet, IVS = interventricular septum.

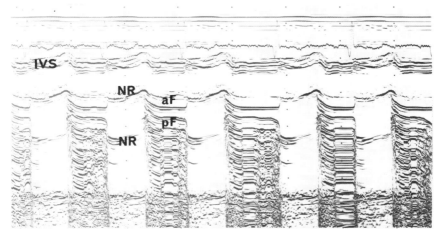

Figure 3. Echocardiogram (paperspeed 50 mm/sec) of an SJM prosthesis in mitral position
IVS = intraventrical septum, NR = suture ring, aF = anterior leaflet, pF = posterior leaflet.

echoes of the leaflets start to disappear (Figure 2). Figure 3 shows a
characteristic M-mode of an SJM in mitral position. The contours of the
suture ring (NR) are well visualized. In diastole, the opened anterior (aF) and
posterior (pF) leaflets are delineated as rectangles. An opening click is not
present in the SJM and a high frequency, high amplitude sound can be
recorded phonocardiographically, corresponding to the complete closure of
the prosthesis. Thus the echocardiographic motion pattern of the SJM is
quite different from that of the ball valve, tilting-disc and non tilting-disc
prostheses.

Due to recording characteristics, the MOV and MCV, as well as the
excursion amplitude of the anterior leaflet, were lower than those of the
posterior leaflet. The following motion characteristics of the posterior leaflet
were obtained:
Excursion amplitude: 8-14 mm (according to the specific model implanted),
MOV: 300-1400 mm/sec (mean 820 mm/sec), MCV: 480-2500 mm/sec
(mean 920 mm/sec). Though MOV and MCV varied widely the MCV was
always faster than the MOV, which was also found to be the case for the
Lillehei-Kaster [2] and Omniscience prostheses [3]. The interval between
aortic closing sound and complete opening of the posterior leaflet had a
mean of 65 ms and was thus shorter than in the ball or tilting-disc prostheses.
The closing sound of the mitral prosthesis was recorded at a mean of 70 ms
after the beginning of the QRS-complex. Figure 4 shows an echocardiographically interesting finding in a patient with second-degree, Wenkebach-type,
AV heart block. During the first 4 heart cycles the leaflets are closed by
80 ms prior to the onset of the QRS-complex. The 5th atrial excitation is
blocked, ventricular systole is lacking. Following the 6th atrial complex with

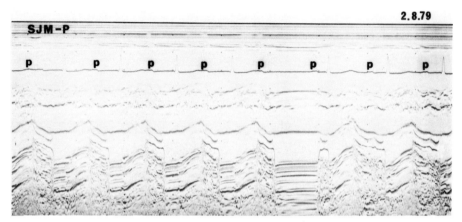

Figure 4. Echocardiogram of a patient with an SJM prosthesis in mitral position during phases of second degree AV heart block.

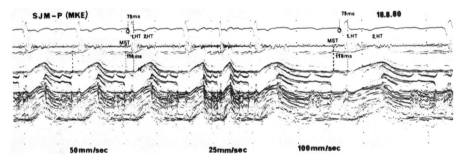

Figure 5. Echocardiogram of an SJM prosthesis in mitral position during a phase of atrial flutter and 4:1 AV-block.

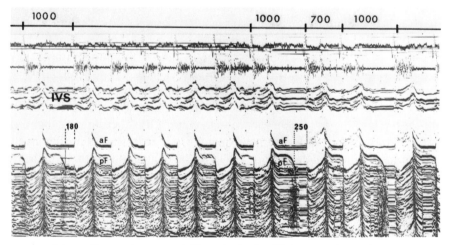

Figure 6. Echocardiogram (paperspeed 25 mm/sec) of a SJM prosthesis. During bradycardiac cycles in late diastole the posterior (pF) leaflet moves backwards prematurely.

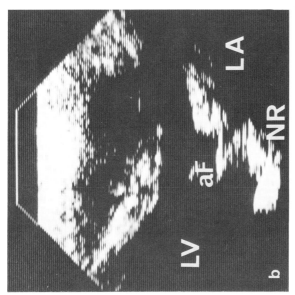

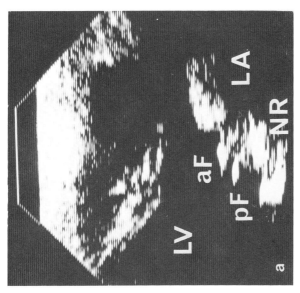

Figure 7. Two-dimensional echocardiograms of the SJM prosthesis. a) Both leaflets (aF, pF) are in the opening position in diastole. b) Only the anterior (aF) leaflet can be seen in the opening position in presystole.

atrial contraction the SJM opens briefly because of the rising atrial pressure. Figure 5 shows SJM valve function in a patient with atrial flutter and 4:1 AV-block. Valve closure appears prematurely, with the closing sound seen on the phonocardiogram (MST). Following the 4th P-wave the leaflets open briefly. The onset of mitral valve opening and closure, as well as the MOV and MCV, depend on the left atrial pressure, diastolic period, cardiac output and stroke volume. In patients with bradyarrhythmias, a late diastolic premature closure of the posterior leaflet can sometimes be seen (Figure 6).

In contrast, we have never seen a premature closure of the anterior leaflet. The following figures show the premature closure in a two-dimensional echocardiogram. In Figure 7a both leaflets are in the opening position in diastole however, in Figure 7b only the anterior leaflet can be seen in the opening position. The echo of the posterior leaflet disappears within the echo of the suture ring (NR).

CONCLUSIONS

Because of the superior hemodynamics of the SJM, this type of prosthesis has been used surgically more and more. In most patients, the motion pattern can be well visualized echocardiographically, provided the prosthesis has been implanted in a useful echocardiographic position, i.e. the rotation axis of the leaflets should be positioned in parallel to the ventricular septum. This cannot always be realized because of anatomical and surgical conditions. Thus, by means of simultaneous registration of phonocardiogram and echocardiogram, dysfunction of the SJM can be detected noninvasively.

REFERENCES

1. Niehues B, H Lübbing, W Jansen, DW Behrenbeck, M Tauchert, H Dalichau: Hämodynamische Frühergebnisse nach Implantation der St.-Jude-Medical-Klappenprothese. Therapiewoche 30:2045, 1980.
2. Gibson TC, PJK Starek, S Moos, E Craig: Echocardiographic and phonocardiographic characteristics of the Lillehei-Kaster mitral valve prosthesis. Circulation 49:434, 1974.
3. Jansen W, B Niehues, H Lübbing, M Tauchert, E Scherer, DW Behrenbeck, T Lie, H Dalichau: Echocardiographische und hämodynamische Befunde nach Implantation der Omniscience-Prothese. Z Kardiol 69:704, 1980.

5. ECHOCARDIOGRAPHY OF THE AORTIC VALVE

G.J. LEECH, T.E. GUINEY, M.J. DAVIES, and D.J. PARKER

INTRODUCTION

Although detection of echoes from the aortic cusps was described in the early days of echocardiography [1], its application in the diagnosis and management of aortic valve disease has remained limited. This partly is due to the difficulty in obtaining clear recordings of the valve cusps throughout the cardiac cycle; even in normal subjects, this is possible in only about 75 % of cases. It is also due to limitations of apparatus resolution, since the small size of the valve necessitates more accurate measurements if, for example, valve area is to be correlated with that found at surgery. Nevertheless, echocardiography can provide a good deal of useful information, which we shall attempt to review.

DETECTION OF LEFT VENTRICULAR OUTFLOW OBSTRUCTION

In the majority of cases of congenitally bicuspid aortic valve, some abnormality is evident from inspection of the valve echoes. As described by Nanda et al., the diastolic closure line is typically eccentric and comprises multiple echoes [2]. Use of simultaneous echo-phono recordings allows identification of the aortic ejection sound by demonstrating the coincidence between timing of the sound and maximal systolic cusp opening, a feature which we believe is invariably present in cases of mobile bicuspid valves [3] (Figure 1). Finally, two-dimensional echocardiography permits the "doming" of the valve during systole to be seen [4], a feature which can also be inferred from the abnormal presence of echoes from the cusps during systole when viewed by M-mode from the apex [3]. Taken together, these features give virtually 100 % sensitivity in detection of bicuspid valves. However, it must be stressed that routine M-mode recordings can give an entirely normal appearance in cases of bicuspid valves, even when there is severe stenosis.

With advancing age, a proportion of bicuspid valves become fibrotic and calcify, though the latter condition is rarely found under the age of 35 in the indigenous Northern European population. Stiffening and fibrosis restrict cusp separation. The thickened cusps generate more intense echoes, and

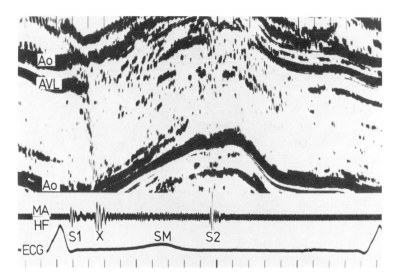

Figure 1. Magnified view of a bicuspid aortic valve recorded at 200 mm/sec paper speed. Note the coincidence of the onset of the ejection sound (X) with halting of the valve cusps as they reach their maximal opening.

calcium shows as multiple, parallel lines which usually obscure the cusp motion completely. Thickening and calcification, accompanied by commissural fusion, are also features of rheumatic aortic stenosis. Although the distribution of the calcium is different, being predominantly in the cusps in the case of a bicuspid valve and in the commissures in rheumatism, this distinction cannot usually be made by M-mode or two-dimensional echocardiography, and the echocardiographic appearances in later life are often identical, except that rheumatic disease virtually always manifests echocardiographic abnormality of the mitral valve.

Echocardiography is also a sensitive method for detecting both the discrete and hypertrophic types of subvalvar stenosis. In the former, the aortic cusps initially separate normally at the onset of ejection, but then almost immediately partly close and flutter rapidly for the remainder of systole. This finding is not specific, being associated also with aortic root aneurysm, low cardiac output and following correction of Fallot's Tetralogy, but when seen in the clinical context of left ventricular (LV) outflow obstruction, it is a sensitive method of differentiating subvalvar from valvar obstruction. Additional distinguishing features include absence of both ejection sound and systolic doming. In hypertrophic obstructive cardiomyopathy, the pattern of aortic cusp motion is usually somewhat different, with normal cusp separation being maintained until 1/3-1/2 way through systole, at which point the cusps begin to close with an irregular, coarse fluttering until they appose (contrary to many reports, reopening in late systole is very unusual in our experience). This pattern is also non-specific, since it simply represents premature cessation of ejection, and is seen in severe mitral regurgitation and in ventricular septal defect with large shunt. However, with the clinical signs of LV outflow obstruction and when associated with the other well-known echocardiographic features of hypertrophic cardiomyopathy, it is a reliable diagnostic sign [5].

Lastly, in the very rare condition of supra-valve stenosis, it has been reported [6] that narrowing of the proximal aorta can be detected on M-mode and, probably more reliably, by two-dimensional scanning in the parasternal long-axis plane [4].

SEVERITY OF AORTIC STENOSIS

Although echocardiography is useful for detecting LV outflow obstruction and for differentiating between its various causes, the primary need of the clinician is to know the severity, especially in view of the association with sudden death. Unfortunately echocardiography has so far been of little value in this respect. Several attempts to measure the aortic valve orifice area from two-dimensional echocardiograms [7] or to infer it from M-mode studies [8] have been reported. Such measurements are, however, fraught with technical problems: precise transducer angulation is necessary to transsect the orifice at its minimum diameter; transducer damping and amplifier gain must be optimised to prevent artefactual cusp thickening while maintaining adequate definition; reverberation echoes from calcium make it impossible to visualise the orifice clearly. Thus, while this method may be adequate to distinguish mild from severe stenosis in the paediatric clinic, it cannot be used to provide quantitative data in the majority of cases.

In older patients, the extent of calcification is a fairly good indicator of severity of stenosis. Work in progress in our laboratory suggests that there is a fairly good quantitative relationship between calcification, asssessed from cine-fluoroscopy, and pressure gradient. However, although echocardiography is equally sensitive for detection of calcium, our attempts to grade severity have not been so successful. Our studies have been based on M-mode recordings and better results might be expected from two-dimensional recordings. Another approach is to measure the degree of myocardial hypertrophy or stiffness as indications of wall stress and hence of peak LV pressure. One study [9] reported good correlation between measured valve gradient and the difference between peripheral arterial pressure and LV peak pressure estimated from wall stress. The results have not, however, been duplicated generally and in our hands the method has been unreliable. While there is no doubt that echocardiography can measure wall mass [10], and is probably superior to the ECG for assessing LV hypertrophy, the relationship

42

between wall mass and peak pressure seems more tenuous. Possibly this is because there is a time element in the development of hypertrophy, and possibly because of inter-individual differences in myocardial stress/strain relationships. The peak rate of increase of LV dimension in diastole gives some indication of myocardial stiffness, but his method suffers the same drawbacks as for the wall mass. Furthermore, both are complicated by co-existing aortic regurgitation or mitral valve disease, and by coronary disease or LV failure.

AORTIC REGURGITATION: DETECTION AND ASSESSMENT OF SEVERITY

Echocardiographic detection of aortic regurgitation rests primarily upon the finding of fluttering of the mitral valve apparatus or the septal endocardium, as a result of the turbulent regurgitant jet striking one or both during diastole. Good M-mode technique, using magnified recordings to show the flutter more clearly, is a sensitive detector of aortic regurgitation, and can be superior even to a skilled auscultator, particularly in the presence of other valve lesions. In the absence of other valve lesions or coronary disease, echocardiographically-derived left ventricular cavity dimensions can provide useful information both on the degree of regurgitation and on myocardial function. A large difference between end-diastolic and end-systolic dimensions, which can be expressed in terms of stroke volume if desired, indicates the degree of volume overload of the left ventricle. In the absence of mitral regurgitation or ventricular septal defect (which can be ruled out if there is no pansystolic murmur), the increased stroke volume can be attributed to the aortic regurgitation. Furthermore, LV inflow obstruction can be ruled out by a normal mitral valve echocardiogram and LV dysfunction due to coronary disease is unlikely if clinical examination and ECG studies are negative. Under these circumstances, echocardiographically-derived indices of myocardial function, such as shortening fraction, are valid. In the presence of volume overload, impairment of myocardial function manifests as an increase in end-systolic dimension and, as reported recently by Henry et al. [11], this measurement is both a good index of myocardial function and a valuable prognostic indicator of the risk of surgery.

ACCURACY OF ECHOCARDIOGRAPHY FOR DETERMINING THE PATHOGENESIS OF ISOLATED AORTIC REGURGITATION

It is helpful for the clinician to know the aetiology of aortic regurgitation. In cases of infective endocarditis, evidence of deteriorating LV function may indicate the need for surgery, even before infection can be controlled.

Marfan's disease and syphilis carry implications for medical and surgical management. Rheumatic disease may mask significant mitral stenosis, which can be missed both at cardiac catheterisation and at surgery. We have therefore reviewed all cases of aortic regurgitation requiring valve replacement at our hospital during the period 1976-79 inclusive, to see whether it would be possible to determine the pathogenesis by M-mode echocardiography.

Patients and methods

All the patients in this study had essentially "pure" aortic regurgitation; none had an aortic valve pressure gradient of more than 4.7 kPa (35 mmHg) (even in the presence of increased stroke volume) and none required mitral valvotomy or replacement. Some patients were eliminated due to lack of preoperative echo studies; none was eliminated solely on the grounds of technically inadequate studies, although in some cases these left a lot to be desired. Out of an original cohort of 92, analysis was possible in 72 cases, 57 males and 15 females, age range 19-72 years, median 52.

Routine preoperative echo and phonocardiograms had been recorded on a multichannel stripchart recorder at paper speeds of 50, 100 or 200 mm/sec. A 2.25 MHz focussed transducer and air-coupled crystal microphones were used. The recordings were reviewed in line with our current laboratory standards. Particular attention was paid to the following:

1. Aortic root diameter, measured at end-diastole using "top-to-top" criterion at the point where the cusp echoes were seen most clearly.
2. The appearance of the aortic wall and aortic valve cusp echoes.
3. The presence or absence of a high-frequency sound co-incident with maximal aortic cusp separation.
4. The appearance of the mitral valve, especially the motion of the posterior leaflet.

Excised valves and samples of aortic root tissue were examined histologically: cusp area was measured; root biopsies were stained to show elastic, smooth muscle, collagen and connective tissue mucins. Both the echocardiographic and pathological assessments were made independently, and without knowledge of the clinical or surgical findings. The echocardiographic findings were then reviewed in the light of the known pathology to determine which features correlated best with the pathology for each type of aetiology.

Results

Pathology

In almost all cases, examination of the excised cusps and root biopsies

44

allowed the pathogenesis to be established. A total of 19 patients (26%) had bicuspid valves. In one further case there were three equal-sized cusps, with the commissure between two of them completely fused. This has been described as an "acquired pseudo-congenital bicuspid valve" and is more likely to be of rheumatic origin.

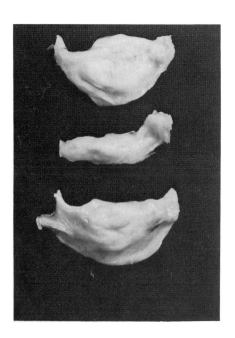 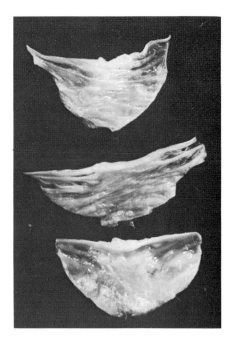

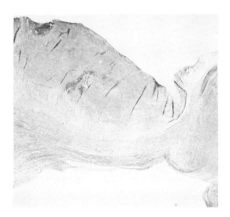 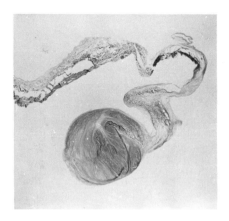

Figure 2. Gross appearance and cross-section of cusps in a case having rheumatic aetiology (left) and idiopathic aortopathy (right). In the rheumatic cusps, there is overall thickening. With idiopathic aortopathy, the cusps are translucent, with only the free margins thickened. This gives the cross-section a "tadpole" appearance.

Eight of the bicuspid valves were complicated by bacterial endocarditis and there were a further 7 patients who had infection on tricuspid aortic valves, giving a total of 15 (21%). In most instances one or more cusps were perforated; only one patient had florid vegetations; one case had a cusp completely destroyed and had developed a large mycotic aneurysm in the aortic wall, bulging posteriorly between the aorta and the left atrium.

There were 18 cases (25%) of rheumatic disease, producing thickening and retraction of the cusps. Sectioning (Figure 2) showed complete fibrous obliteration of the cusp architecture.

The aortic root biopsies revealed six cases (8%) of inflammatory disease: 3 syphilitic, 1 Reiter's disease, 1 giant cell arteritis and 1 non-specific. In two further cases there was some inflammation secondary to endocarditis. In 23 patients (32%), the biopsy showed varying degrees of destruction of the elastic laminae within the aortic media. The appearance was similar to that seen in Marfan's syndrome, but unlike that of post-stenotic dilatation, in which the media is stretched but the structural integrity of the elastic laminae is maintained. Loss of the elastic laminae allows systolic aortic pressure to dilate the region where the cusps are attached, with the result that the extent to which they overlap and rest against each other to maintain valve competence is reduced and one or more cusps prolapse during diastole. As a result, the cusps develop a characteristic "rolled" edge. The thick margin can be mistaken for rheumatic disease, but as shown in Figure 2, the body of the cusp remains thin, and there is no evidence of inflammation. We have named this type of non-inflammatory root disease "idiopathic aortopathy". Five of our cases had bicuspid valves in addition; in the other 18, the valves were tricuspid and quite normal, apart from rolling of the edges.

In the remaining 4 patients, although the valves were obviously abnormal, it was not possible to assign a definite pathogenesis. One had 3 cusps, with some calcium and normal root histology. There was no clinical or echo evidence of mitral valve abnormality. It may have been rheumatic, though there was no history of rheumatic fever and we believe that it is rare to find rheumatic disease confined to the aortic valve in patients from temperate climates. Another patient had one cusp with a thick edge, one with an aneurysmal bulge and one normal. It is possible that this was dual rheumatic and infective pathology. One patient had a normal tricuspid valve and normal root histology, but had ruptured one cusp; there was no history of chest trauma. Finally, one patient had a tricuspid valve with one rolled cusp and mild root disease, but a strong history of rheumatic fever and an abnormal mitral valve echo, again suggesting the possibility of dual pathology.

Echocardiography

Omitting the 4 patients in whom the pathology was uncertain, the

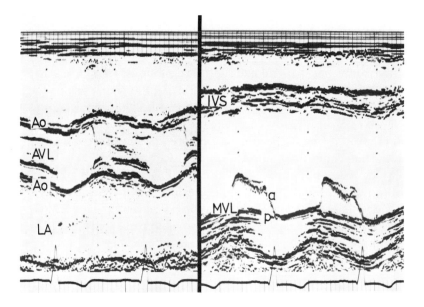

Figure 3. Aortic (left) and mitral valves from a case having rheumatic aetiology. Note the minimal mitral valve abnormality.

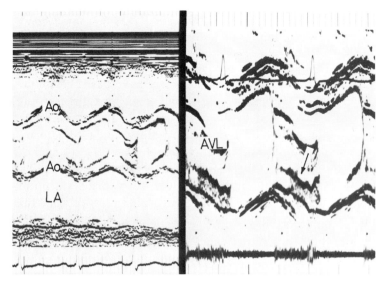

Figure 4. Aortic valve echoes from a patient with endocarditis on a tricuspid valve. Note the "shaggy" echoes during diastole on the magnified view.

independently generated echocardiographic data was compared with the pathological and surgical findings. The results for each sub-group are given below.

Rheumatic

The echocardiographic diagnosis of rheumatic pathology was based upon finding a combination of heavy or multiple echoes from the aortic valve with an abnormal mitral valve, though in many cases the mitral abnormality was slight and confined to restriction of posterior leaflet motion (Figure 3). Mean root diameter was 29 mm and, with one exception, was always less than 36 mm. In one case the root diameter was 46 mm and although the biopsy was reported as normal, review of the preoperative angiogram confirmed that the root was very large. Many of these patients had an aortic ejection sound on the phonocardiogram and it is interesting to note that the one with a "pseudo-congenital bicuspid valve" had an exceptionally loud click. The echocardiographic findings were completely correct in 16/18; in the other two it was not certain whether they were rheumatic or bicuspid (one of which was the pseudo-congenital bicuspid). Echo specificity was 100%.

Bacterial endocarditis

The echocardiographic features of bacterial endocarditis have been described elsewhere [12, 13]. In the present series, the most consistent finding was fluttering on the aortic valve cusps during diastole, suggestive of cusp perforation or tear. Only one of our patients had florid vegetations; although not well seen on the M-mode, these were excellently visualised by two-dimensional echocardiography. The seven cases having endocarditis on a tricuspid aortic valve were all identified, and the mycotic aneurysm was demonstrated (Figure 5). In one case having a normal root biopsy, the root diameter was 41 mm. The surgeon commented that the aorta was thin and suggested that the valve lesion was not the sole cause of the regurgitation. Of the eight cases of infection on bicuspid valves, only three were completely recognised. Two cases were thought to have a tricuspid valve, and in one case the infection was missed; two were thought to be calcified valves, in one of which the surgeon commented that old, calcified vegetations were present.

Bicuspid

The echocardiographic features of a bicuspid valve have been described earlier. Using these criteria, particularly the identification of an aortic ejection sound, the correct diagnosis was made in all the five cases having an uncomplicated bicuspid valve. In three of these, the root diameter was normal (under 36 mm), but two had marked root dilatation, which was confirmed by the angiogram in one (the film of the other has been mislaid).

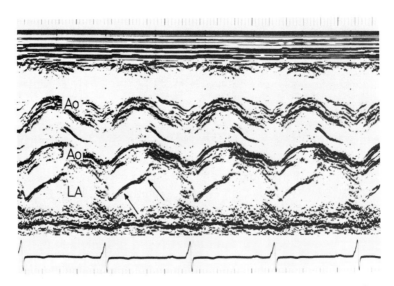

Figure 5. An infected tricuspid aortic valve which developed a large mycotic aneurysm (arrowed). This view does not show the cusp flutter, which was seen on other recordings.

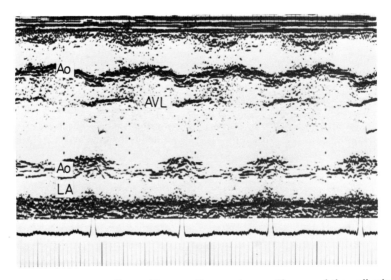

Figure 6. Inflammatory root disease. The root diameter is over 60 mm and the wall echoes are very thick.

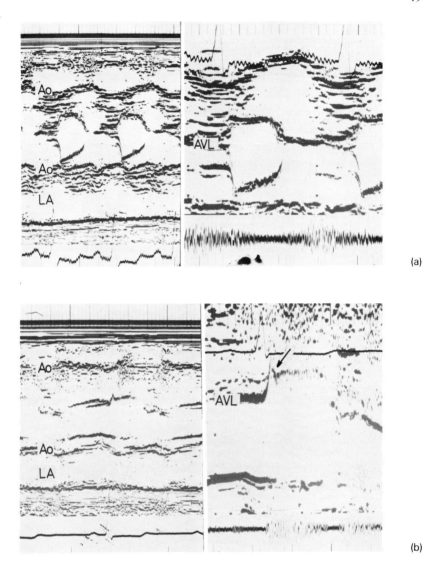

Figure 7. Idiopathic aortopathy. (a) The aortic root is dilated to 46 mm and there are multiple echoes from the rolled cusps. (b) Case with gross dilatation showing premature partial closure and flutter of the aortic cusps.

In the six patients with bicuspid valves and abnormal root biopsies, the echocardiogram demonstrated the abnormal valve and root dilatation in each, although in one the aortic wall was said to be inflamed. The eight cases of infected bicuspid valves have been discussed above; the proportion of completely correct echocardiographic diagnoses was lower with the dual pathology.

Inflammatory root disease

We attempted to detect this by the combination of root dilatation and abnormally thick echoes from the aortic walls. In all six cases, the root was enlarged (37-54, mean 43 mm). However, in only two were the aortic wall echoes thought to be abnormal. One patient was thought to have an ejection sound and was therefore labelled as bicuspid with root dilatation. Conversely, four patients with non-inflammatory root disease were thought to have thick aortic walls and were wrongly called inflammatory. It is obvious that the sensitivity and specificity of this sign are too low to be useful.

Idiopathic aortopathy

The characteristic echocardiographic features of this condition are an increased root diameter, often with multiple echoes arising from the rolled cusp edges, but with no ejection sound and a normal mitral valve (Figure 7). In all but one of the 18 cases, the root diameter on echo was greater than 37 mm, ranging from 38-60 (mean 44) mm. In the remaining case the echocardiographic diameter was only 33 mm; the pathology report stated that there was severe aortopathy, with evidence of a healed dissection tear. No reason for this discrepancy can be offered. Three of the cases appeared to have thick aortic wall echoes and were erroneously thought to have inflammatory disease. In two cases an aortic ejection sound was thought to have been recorded on the phonocardiogram and they were said to be bicuspid. One interesting case showed obvious diastolic flutter of the cusp echoes and it was suggested that there might be infection present. At surgery, a tear was found at the base of one cusp. In several cases, the aortic valve recordings showed that pattern of early partial cusp closure followed by fluttering once thought to be specific for subvalvar stenosis but now recognised in other situations, including root aneurysm (Figure 7).

Discussion

Echocardiography correctly determined the pathogenesis in 50/68 patients, was partially correct in 17 and was wrong in only one: the case of idiopathic aortopathy with an old dissection, in which the root diameter appeared normal. In many aspects, this study confirms other reports, but we believe that it makes two additional contributions. Thirty years ago, it was thought that isolated aortic valve disease was mainly of rheumatic aetiology. More recently, it has been realised that in the majority of cases it originates from a congenitally bicuspid aortic valve. We have shown that it is possible to distinguish these two with a high degree of accuracy on the basis that echocardiography is a very sensitive detector of rheumatic mitral valve disease. Rheumatic heart disease normally involves the mitral valve, partic-

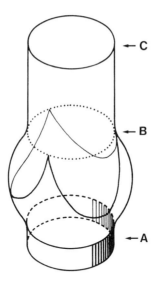

Figure 8. Diagram of the aortic root showing (A) lower annulus, (B) supra-aortic ridge, (C) proximal root.

ularly in the indigenous Northern European population. Therefore, if the mitral valve is echocardiographically normal, aortic regurgitation virtually never has rheumatic aetiology.

The second contribution of this study is to point out the significance of the echocardiographic measurement of aortic root diameter.

Figure 8 shows a diagram of the aortic valve. The leaflets are mounted within a sleeve of connective tissue, mainly collagen, which allows it to bulge outwards under pressure. Where the lower margin of this sleeve joins the ventricle, a distinct ring is felt when a finger is passed through the valve; this is used by the surgeon to attach a prosthesis. The radiologist assesses the size of the proximal aorta where it emerges from the cardiac shadow, above the valve. The echocardiographer, however, measures the aortic root where valve echoes are seen, that is at the level of the commissures, which in turn are level with the circular rim, known as the supra-aortic ridge, at the junction of the valve sleeve and the base of the aorta.

It is important to distinguish between these three regions and to understand the rôle of each [14]. Dilatation of the lower annulus is uncommon; dilatation of the proximal aorta is found in aortic stenosis and with widespread aortic wall disease, but does not necessarily indicate failure of the valve support ring. It is dilatation of the root at the level visualised by echocardiography which pulls the cusps apart, reducing their mutual support and permitting regurgitation (Figure 9).

The upper limit of normal aortic root diameter in our laboratory is 36 mm, and in younger subjects it is rarely more than 34 mm. To have a root

52

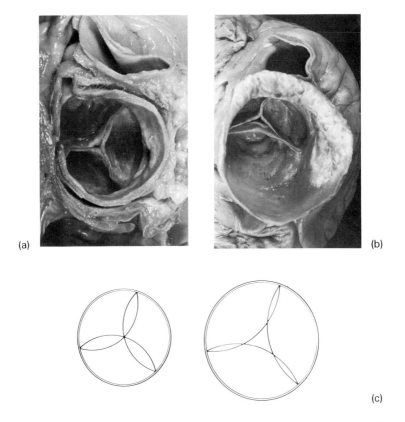

(a)

(b)

(c)

Figure 9. (a) Normal aortic valve, viewed from above. The supra-aortic ridge can clearly be seen. (b) A case of idiopathic aortopathy, showing dilatation of the aortic root and disappearance of the supravalve ridge. (c) Diagram showing how dilatation reduces the extent of cusp overlap.

diameter of 38 mm alone, can cause aortic regurgitation of sufficient severity to require valve replacement.

In this series, root dilatation was present in 32/68 cases. If patients from Southern Europe and the Middle East are excluded, 31/52 patients had root dilatation and idiopathic aortopathy was the most common aetiology (16 cases), followed by endocarditis (13) and rheumatic disease in only six cases.

Correct identification of the pathogenesis of valve disease is important in determining the prognosis and management. The ability of echocardiography to perform this function inexpensively and noninvasively is yet another application for this powerful diagnostic technique.

REFERENCES

1. Edler I, A Gustafson, T Karlefors, B Christensson: Ultrasound cardiography. Acta Med Scand (Suppl.) 370:68, 1961.
2. Nanda NC, R Gramiak, PM Shah, JA DeWeese: Echocardiographic recognition of the congenital bicuspid aortic valve. Circulation 49:870, 1974
3. Leech GJ, PG Mills, A Leatham: The diagnosis of a non-stenotic bicuspid aortic valve. Brit Heart J 40:941, 1978.
4. Weyman AE, H Feigenbaum, RA Hurwitz, DA Girod, JC Dillon, S Chang: Localization of left ventricular outflow obstruction by cross-sectional echocardiography. Amer J Med 60:33, 1976.
5. Shah PM, R Gramiak, AG Adelman, ED Wigle: Role of echocardiography in diagnostic and hemodynamic assessment of hypertrophic subaortic stenosis. Circulation 44:891, 1971.
6. Bolen JL, RL Popp, JW French: Echocardiographic features of supravalvular aortic stenosis. Circulation 52:817, 1975.
7. Leo LR, MJ Barrett, CL Leddy, NM Wolf, WS Frankel: Determination of aortic valve area by cross-sectional echocardiography. Circulation 59 & 60 Supp. II:203, 1979.
8. Yeh H-C, F Winsberg, EM Mercer: Echographic aortic valve orifice dimension: its use in evaluating aortic stenosis and cardiac output: J Clin Ultrasound 1:182, 1973.
9. Bennett DH, DW Evans, MVJ Raj: Echocardiographic left ventricular dimensions in pressure and volume overload. Their use in assessing aortic stenosis. Brit Heart J 37:971, 1975.
10. Devereux RB, N Reichek: Echocardiographic determination of left ventricular mass in man. Circulation 55:613, 1977.
11. Henry WL, RO Bonow, JS Borer, JH Ware, KM Kent, DR Redwood, CL McIntosh, AG Morrow, SE Epstein: Observations on the optimum time for operative intervention for aortic regurgitation. Circulation 61:471, 1980.
12. Roy P, AJ Tajik, ER Giuliani, TT Schattenberg, GT Gau, RL Frye: Spectrum of echocardiographic findings in bacterial endocarditis. Circulation 53:474, 1976.
13. Wray TM: The variable echocardiographic features in aortic valve endocarditis. Circulation 52:658, 1975.
14. Reeves WC, U Ettinger, K Thomson, N Nanda, R Gramiak, J DeWeese, S Stewart: Limitations in the echocardiographic assessment of aortic root dimensions in the presence of aortic valve disease. Radiology 132:411, 1979.

6. TWO-DIMENSIONAL SUPRASTERNAL ECHOCARDIOGRAPHY IN DISEASES OF THE THORACIC AORTA

P. Schweizer, R. Erbel, H. Lambertz, and S. Effert

1. INTRODUCTION

Although M-mode echocardiography may be useful for detecting aortic abnormalities, the method lacks spatial orientation. False positive or false negative findings may be artefacts of the direction of the single ultrasonic beam [1]. The better spatial orientation of cross-sectional echocardiography should enable more comprehensive examinations to be made.

The purpose of this study was to determine, with special reference to suprasternal cross-sectional echocardiography, whether two-dimensional imaging from multiple transducer positions could be used to localize various diseases of the thoracic aorta.

2. PROCEDURE

2.1. Material and methods

2.1.1. Patients

Cross-sectional echocardiographic studies were performed in a group of 38 patients. There were 21 males and 17 females, mean age being 44 ± 9 years. The underlying aortic disease was confirmed in all patients by aortography and in 31 cases at surgery (see Table I).

Table 1. Aortographic and echocardiographic (2DE) features.

Exact localization		Aortography	2DE
I.	Aortic aneurysms		
	1 ascending aorta only	12	10
	2 ascending aorta + aortic arch	5	5
	3 ascending aorta + aortic arch + descending aorta	2	0
	4 aortic arch only	1	0
	5 descending aorta only	2	1
II.	Dissecting aortic aneurysms	4	4
III.	Aortic coarctation	12	12

56

22 patients (group I) had true aortic aneurysms: 12 were confined to the ascending aorta; 5 extended to the aortic arch; 2 extended to the descending aorta; 1 was confined to the aortic arch; 2 were confined to the descending aorta. A further four patients (group II) had aortic root dissection with Marfan's syndrome. The remaining 12 patients (group III) had coarctation of the aorta.

2.1.2. Echocardiographic methods

A phased-array imaging system was used for cross-sectional examination. * Images of the ascending and descending aortic region were obtained in the standard parasternal and apical transducer positions [2, 3].

The transducer, with a diameter of 24 mm, was then placed in the suprasternal notch. The sector-scan was aligned parallel to the long-axis plane of the aortic arch. Thus the ascending aorta, aortic arch, origin of the brachiocephalic vessels, and proximal descending aorta were visualized [2]. A normal suprasternal cross-section of the aorta is depicted in Figure 1.

Correlative echocardiographic/anatomic studies made in our laboratory showed that the ascending aorta and descending aorta are not always in the same plane in adult patients. Using the aortic arch as reference, the transducer must be rotated to the right and tilted superiorly when recording the ascending aorta. This manoeuver must be performed in reverse in order to image the proximal descending aorta fully. The latter examination technique is particularly informative in aortic coarctation [4, 5].

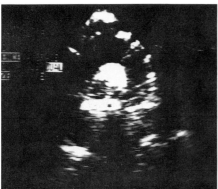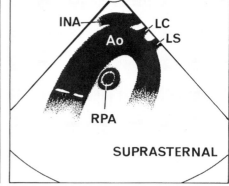

Figure 1. Suprasternal cross-sectional image of a normal person (left: original recording). The ascending aorta is on the left. The origin of the innominate artery (INA), the left common carotid artery (LC) and the left subclavian artery (LS) are clearly visualized. The proximal parts of the descending aorta are also imaged. A cross-section of the right pulmonary artery (RPA) can be seen.

---

* Varian V3000, V3400; Varian Ass. Palo Alto, USA.

3. RESULTS

The results of a comparison of two-dimensional echocardiography with angiography are summarized in Table I.

3.1. Group I

Abnormal aneurysmatic enlargement of the thoracic aorta could be visualized with two-dimensional echocardiography in all patients. The diagnosis of an aneurysm depended on the demonstration of an obvious increase in the diameter of the aortic segment relative to surrounding segments (cross-sectional values of 30 normal persons: ascending aorta 39 ± 6 mm; aortic arch 33 ± 6 mm; descending aorta 27 ± 7 mm).

Furthermore, the precise configuration of the aneurysm and its exact localization could be recorded in 16 out of 22 patients (73%). An example of a cross-sectional echocardiogram obtained in this study is given in Figure 2.

The discrepancies in the true extent of the thoracic aortic abnormality were due to poor echocardiographic visualization of one or two anatomic segments of the aorta. The cross-section of the descending aorta was particularly susceptible to misinterpretation as this section can only be imaged in one anatomic plane from the suprasternal notch position. A small

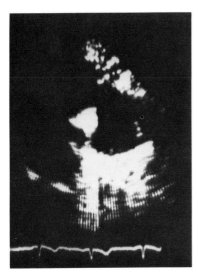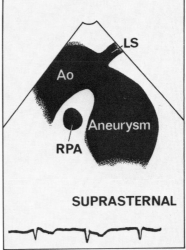

Figure 2. Suprasternal cross-section in aortic aneurysm: the fusiform aneurysm, which is confined to the descending aorta, distal to the origin of the left subclavian artery (LS), is delineated. (RPA = right pulmonary artery).

58

section of the descending aorta is also accessible from the parasternal transducer position [6]. The ascending aorta, which is accessible from a range of transducer positions, showed much better agreement.

3.2. Group II

Four patients had acute or subacute proximal dissecting aneurysms with Marfan's syndrome. In three patients the dissection was confined to the ascending aorta and in one patient the dissection extended beyond the ascending aorta and the aortic arch. In all four patients an exact two-dimensional echocardiographic diagnosis, confirmed at surgery, was possible.

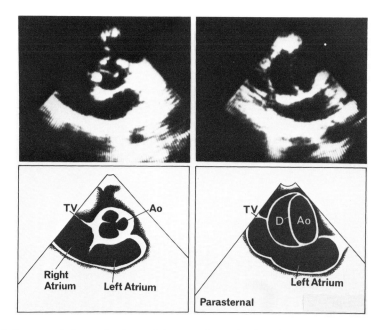

Figure 3. Parasternal short-axis views of the aorta in aortic dissection. Left: aortic root (Ao) at the level of the aortic valve. Right: the scan now transsects the aorta above the level of the aortic valve. Echo-dense line (D), which separates the two aortic lumens (TV = tricuspid valve).

The parasternal long-axis and short-axis views were superior to the suprasternal sections in delineating the thin dissected inner wall, which separated the true aortic lumen and the false channel (Figure 3). In the one case with dissection beyond the aortic arch, suprasternal echocardiography was also useful.

3.3. Group III

12 patients had significant aortic coarctation, confirmed with angiography and at surgery. Two-dimensional suprasternal echocardiography demonstrated the presence of the focal narrowing of the aortic lumen (situated distal to the subclavian artery in all cases).

The post-stenotic dilatation of the aortic root, distal to the constructed segment could be clearly visualized (see Figure 4). The augmented pulsation of the pre-stenotic area was an additional sign.

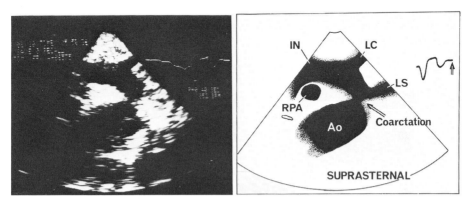

Figure 4. Suprasternal cross-section in aortic coarctation. Focal narrowing of the aortic lumen (arrow) distal to the innominate artery (IN), left carotid artery (LC) and subclavian artery (LS). Post-stenotic dilatation of the descending aorta. (RPA = right pulmonary artery in cross-section).

4. DISCUSSION

Suprasternal echocardiography, in combination with the conventional parasternal and apical views, appears to be a promising technique for the detection of thoracic aortic aneurysms. Exact localization was possible in 73% of cases. Aneurysms of the ascending thoracic aorta (7), of the aortic arch and of the descending aorta could all be detected (group I). In all cases with aortic coarctation (group III), it was possible to visualize the anatomic abnormality, situated beyond the origin of the left subclavian artery, using the suprasternal approach.

It should be noted that the patients in groups I and III were partly selected on the basis of a previously established diagnosis. Further prospective studies are therefore necessary to define the true sensitivity and specificity of this technique.

In the four patients with aortic root dissection secondary to Marfan's syndrome, two-dimensional echocardiography allowed a sensitive emergency diagnosis.

In conclusion, though aortic angiography is clearly the definitive diagnostic procedure, two-dimensional echocardiography – especially the suprasternal approach – allows a fast and dynamic assessment of various aortic disorders. The information provided by this technique is of importance for planning invasive and therapeutic procedures.

REFERENCES

1. Brown OR, RL Popp, FE Kloster: Echocardiographic criteria for aortic root dissection. Chest 67:441, 1975.
2. Tajik AJ, JB Seward, DJ Hagler, DD Mair, JT Lie: Two-dimensional ultrasonic imaging of the heart and great vessels. Mayo Clin Proc 53:271, 1978.
3. Bubenheimer P, M Schmuziger, R Roskamm: Ein- und zweidimensionale Echographie bei Aneurysmen und Dissektionen der Aorta. Herz 5:226, 1980.
4. Sahn DJ, HD Allen, G McDonald, SJ Goldberg: Real-time cross-sectional echocardiographic diagnosis of coarctation of the aorta: a prospective study of echocardiographic-angiographic correlation. Circulation 56:762, 1977.
5. Weyman AE, RL Caldwell, RA Hurwitz, DA Girod, JC Dillon, H Feigenbaum, D Green: Cross-sectional echocardiographic detection of aortic obstruction: 2. coarctation of the aorta. Circulation 57:498, 1978.
6. Mintz GS, MN Kotler, BL Segal, WR Parry: Two-dimensional echocardiographic recognition of the descending thoracic aorta. Am J Cardiol 44:232, 1979.
7. DeMaria AN, W Bommer, A Neumann, L Weinert, H Bogren, DT Mason: Identification and localization of aneurysms of the ascending aorta by cross-sectional echocardiography. Circulation 59:755, 1979.

7. VISUALIZATION OF THE CORONARY ARTERIES BY TWO-DIMENSIONAL ECHOCARDIOGRAPHY

HARVEY FEIGENBAUM

Several investigators have now demonstrated the ability to use two-dimensional echocardiography to visualize the proximal coronary arteries [1, 2, 3, 4, 5]. The ability to recognize and record the coronary arteries has required many technical advances [6]. One important advance was the use of higher frequency transducers. Merely using a 3 MHz transducer rather than the usual 2.25 MHz transducer used in adult cardiology permits better resolution in examining small structures such as the coronary arteries. A second major advance was the development of a strobe freeze-frame capability [6]. This feature is present on most instruments which use digital scan conversion. With the recordings in a digital form it is possible to use a freeze-frame capability which is gated to the R-wave of the electrocardiogram. Thus, one records only during a selected portion of the cardiac cycle. The recorded image is constantly updated with each subsequent beat. This particular feature is important in examining the coronary arteries because the vessels are constantly moving in and out of the examining plane. One could not hope to track the coronary arteries by rapidly moving the plane of the examination. What in fact happens is that the examiner holds the probe in a stationary fashion in the vicinity of the coronary arteries and the vessels move through the ultrasonic plane. Any given part of the coronary arteries may be recorded only for a very brief period of time with any given transducer position. During the real-time examination it is almost impossible to clearly identify the coronary arteries unless the cardiac motion is extremely poor, as might occur with a cardiomyopathy. It should be recognized, however, that, even with severe coronary artery disease, the base of the heart to which the coronary arteries are attached usually moves vigorously. Thus, the examiner usually adjusts the strobe indicator on the electrocardiogram so as to record only that portion of the cardiac cycle when the coronary arteries are clearly seen. For example, in Figure 1A, the strobe indicator is in mid-diastole. The left main coronary artery is usually recorded best in either mid or late diastole.

Another important development in using two-dimensional echocardiography to examine the coronary arteries was the introduction of new videotape and videodisc analyzing systems. We have been using a combined videotape-videodisc system developed by Micro Sonics Incorporated. A ten second

Rijsterborgh H, ed: Echocardiology, p 61-72. All rights reserved.

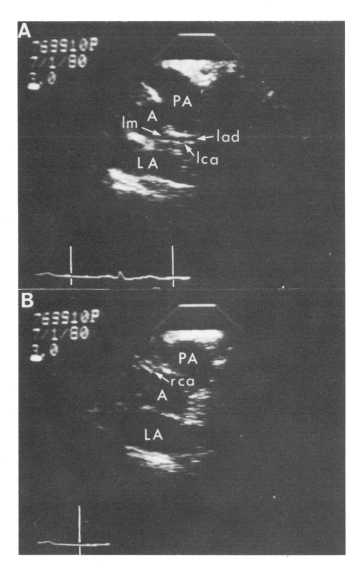

Figure 1. Short-axis, two-dimensional echocardiogram of the aorta (A), pulmonary artery (PA) and left atrium (LA). A: The left main coronary artery (lm) can be seen originating from the aorta and dividing into the left anterior descending (lad) and the left circumflex (lca) coronary arteries. B: The right coronary artery (rca) originates from the right upper hand corner of the aorta.

videodisc analyzer is coupled to the videotape recorder and functions as a memory loop. This system provides the capability of detecting fine details within the coronary arteries, utilizing frame-by-frame, slow motion, forward and reverse analysis. For example, it is almost impossible to identify the bifurcation of the left main coronary artery without such a videodisc system.

The development which is proving to be critical in analyzing pathology within the coronary arteries is gray scale present in the newer two-dimensional echocardiographic systems. As will be discussed later, the detection of atherosclerotic disease depends upon the identification of high intensity echoes within the coronary arteries and requires good gray scale characteristics in the instrument [7, 8].

NORMAL CORONARY ANATOMY

Although a technique has been described whereby the transducer is placed over the cardiac apex when examining the coronary arteries [2, 4], most investigators examine the coronary arteries with the transducer in the parasternal position [1, 3]. When obtaining a short-axis examination of the root of the aorta, one can direct the examining plane so as to record both the left and right coronary arteries (Figure 1) [5]. In Figure 1A one can see the

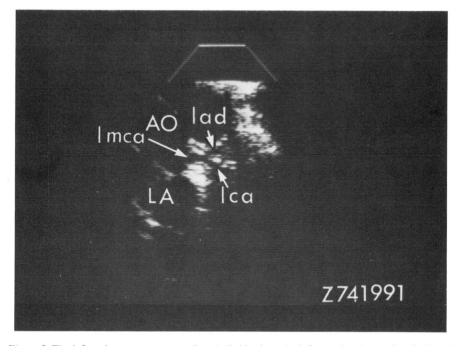

Figure 2. The left main coronary artery (lmca) divides into the left anterior descending (lad) and the left circumflex (lca) coronary arteries. In this patient the bifurcation is easily visualized in this two-dimensional echocardiogram. AO = aorta; LA = left atrium. (From Feigenbaum, H: Echocardiography. Third edition, Lea & Febiger, 1981).

left main coronary artery (lm) originating from the aorta (A). The left main coronary artery is just posterior to the pulmonary artery (PA) and is identified as two parallel, horizontal echoes to the left of the aorta. Just posterior to the left main coronary artery is the left atrium (LA). The right coronary artery (Figure 1B) originates from the upper right portion of the aorta and can be seen as two linear echoes for a distance of a centimeter or two.

The left main coronary artery bifurcates into the left anterior descending (lad, Figure 1A) and the left circumflex coronary artery (lca). Usually very little of the left circumflex artery is seen and its origin is fairly subtle (Figure 1A). Figure 2 demonstrates an unusual patient in whom a longer portion of the left circumflex coronary artery is recorded. The bifurcation of the left main coronary artery into its two major branches is readily apparent in Figure 2. Figure 3 illustrates another common example of the left main coronary artery bifurcation. In this patient one records a left main coronary artery (lm) which abruptly expands as it divides. The individual walls of the left anterior descending and left circumflex arteries are not visualized.

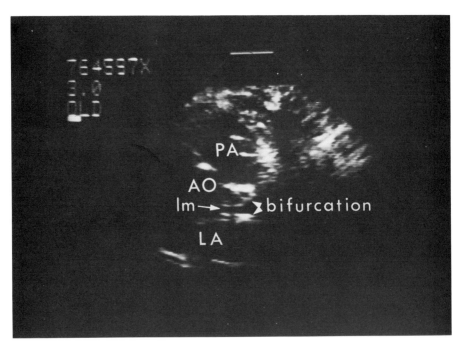

Figure 3. Frequently the bifurcation of the left main coronary artery (lm) is recorded as an abrupt widening of the artery. Individual echoes from the walls of the left anterior descending and left circumflex coronary arteries may not be seen. PA = pulmonary artery; AO = aorta; LA = left atrium.

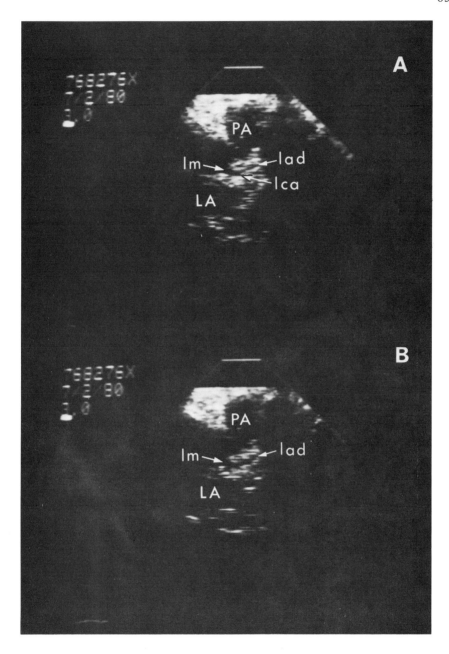

Figure 4. A: The left anterior descending (lad) and left circumflex (lca) arteries can faintly be seen originating from the left main coronary artery (lm). B: With a slightly different view of the coronary arteries a much longer and clearer segment of the left anterior descending coronary artery can be seen. PA = pulmonary artery; LA = left atrium.

Figure 3 also illustrates the common situation whereby the left main coronary artery appears as two parallel echoes between the left atrium and the pulmonary artery. There is usually an echo-free space between the anterior wall of the left main coronary artery and the posterior wall of the pulmonary artery. It is somewhat unusual for the anterior wall of the left main coronary artery to blend into the posterior wall of the pulmonary artery as noted in Figure 1A. However, it is not unusual for the posterior wall of the left main coronary artery to blend into the anterior wall of the left atrium.

Figure 4 demonstrates a better example of the left anterior descending coronary artery. The left main coronary artery is recorded well in Figure 4A. One faintly sees the origin of the left circumflex coronary artery (lca) and a somewhat better but still faint recording of the left anterior descending (lad) artery. With a slightly different view of the coronary arteries (Figure 4B) a much better examination of the left anterior descending coronary artery can be seen. One must remember that the two-dimensional examination represents slices or tomograms and that it is unusual for both the left main coronary artery and the left anterior descending coronary artery to be in the same examining plane. Even the left main coronary artery may be sufficiently curved for it to be impossible to record the entire length with one examining plane.

ATHEROSCLEROTIC OBSTRUCTION OF THE CORONARY ARTERIES

Figure 5 demonstrates an atherosclerotic lesion within the left main coronary artery. One can appreciate a thick mass of high intensity echoes which almost completely obstructs the lumen of the left main coronary artery. Looking for these high intensity echoes has greatly improved the practical use of echocardiography for detecting obstructive lesions within the coronary arteries [7, 8].

The basis for the high intensity echoes is probably calcium or other dense substances within the atherosclerotic plaque [7]. Thus, echocardiography should be as good as fluoroscopy in the detection of calcium within the coronary arteries. Our experience indicates that echocardiography is probably a more sensitive calcium indicator than fluoroscopy, since many of our patients who had high intensity echoes within the left coronary artery had atherosclerotic disease but no calcium was noted on fluoroscopy [7].

Thus far our greatest experience has been in examining patients with obstructions within the left main coronary artery. The criteria which have been developed for detecting such obstruction require the identification of high intensity echoes within the walls of the left main coronary artery and partial or complete obstruction of the lumen [6]. Utilizing these criteria we

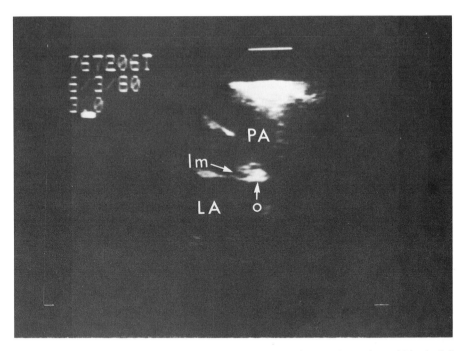

Figure 5. Two-dimensional echocardiogram from a patient with an obstruction within the left main coronary artery (lm). The obstructing lesion (o) is noted as a mass of high intensity echoes within the lumen of the left main coronary artery. PA = pulmonary artery; LA = left atrium.

have examined several series of patients to determine the reliability of this technique in detecting patients who have obstructed left main coronary arteries.

Our initial pleasant surprise was that we were able to identify the left main coronary artery in seventy-one out of seventy-two consecutive patients [6]. After we established our criteria for the existence of left main coronary artery obstruction, we had a 'blinded' observer interpret the echocardiograms from twenty-eight randomly selected patients. Four of the patients had left main coronary artery obstruction. The investigator was able to identify all four of these patients. There was only one false-positive and two questionable false-positives. All three patients had obstructions within the proximal left anterior descending coronary artery. In a follow-up study, thirty-one consecutive patients were prospectively examined by two independent investigators. Three of the thirty-one patients had left main coronary artery obstruction. Both investigators identified the three patient with obstructed left main coronary arteries. One investigator had no false-positives and the other had one false-positive, again in a patient with a lesion within the proximal left anterior descending coronary artery.

This experience has made us extremely optimistic that two-dimensional echocardiography is a practical means of identifying patients with left main coronary artery obstructions. These findings are clearly the most optimistic to date with regard to using echocardiography for this purpose. Previous investigators have not had this high degree of success. We believe that our success rate is based upon several factors. First of all, our laboratory has been interested in examining the coronary arteries for over five years and we have developed a fair amount of experience and expertise. In addition, the other investigators have not used all of the technical advances, such as the strobe freeze-frame and the offline videotape-videodisc analyzer.

We have preliminary experience using two-dimensional echocardiography to detect atherosclerotic obstruction of the proximal left anterior descending coronary artery [9] and the right coronary artery. Figure 6 demonstrates a two-dimensional echogram from a patient with an obstruction within the left anterior descending coronary artery. The obstructing lesion (lado) is identified as a mass of bright, high intensity echoes within the distribution of the left anterior descending coronary artery. These high intensity echoes can be seen moving in and out of the examining plane in real-time. The lesions are best seen when analyzed with the videodisc system. Our experience to date

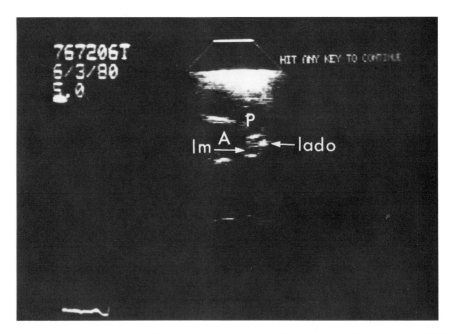

Figure 6. An echocardiogram of a patient with an obstructing lesion within the proximal left anterior descending coronary artery. The obstructing lesion (lado) is noted as a mass of high intensity echoes in the distribution of the left anterior descending coronary artery. lm = left main coronary artery; P = pulmonary artery; A = aorta.

with detecting left anterior coronary artery obstructions is not as extensive as with the left main coronary artery obstruction. We are able to identify the left anterior descending coronary artery in about seventy-five percent of the cases [9]. There are also still several false-positives and false-negatives. However, the preliminary experience is certainly encouraging.

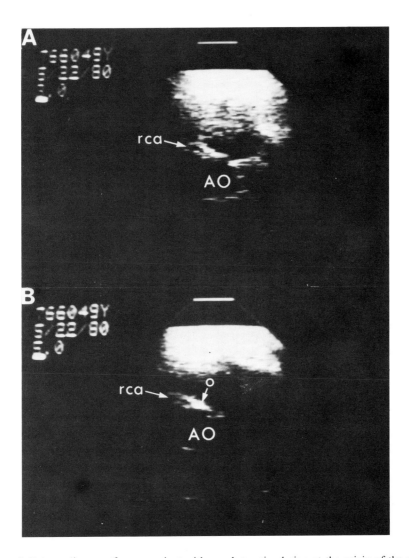

Figure 7. Echocardiograms from a patient with an obstructing lesion at the origin of the right coronary artery. A: The right coronary artery originates from the upper right hand corner of the aorta (AO). In this recording the right coronary artery cannot be seen communicating with the aorta. B: In another view of the same patient a mass of bright echoes (o) can be seen originating from an atherosclerotic lesion at the origin of the right coronary artery.

We have an even smaller experience with regard to obstructions of the right coronary artery. Figure 7A shows one echocardiogram of the right coronary artery whereby there is no continuity between that vessel and the aorta. In another view of the same patient (Figure 7B) one can see high intensity echoes at the origin of the right coronary artery. These echoes correspond with an obstruction near the ostium of the right coronary artery. There are too little data thus far with regard to right coronary obstructions to estimate the accuracy and usefulness of this examination. Solid criteria as to the identity of such obstructive lesions have yet to be established.

OTHER CORONARY ARTERY ABNORMALITIES

Atherosclerotic disease is not the only pathology within the coronary arteries which can be detected with echocardiography. Several investigators have noted aneurysmal dilatation of the coronary arteries in patients with muco-cutaneous lymph node disease [10, 11]. Figure 7 is an echocardiogram of a patient with such an aneurysm. The markedly dilated coronary vessel is striking and readily identified.

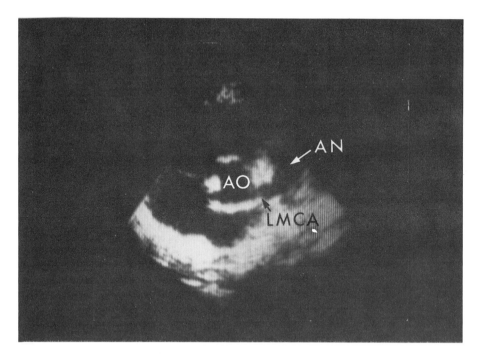

Figure 8. Two-dimensional echocardiogram of a patient with coronary artery aneurysm in a child with a mucocutaneous lymph node disease. The aneurysm (AN) can be seen communicating with the left main coronary artery (LMCA). AO = aorta. (From Feigenbaum, H.: Echocardiography. Third edition, Lea & Febiger, 1981)

There have been reports demonstrating that two-dimensional echocardiography can be used to identify congenital anomalies of the coronary arteries [12, 13]. For example, one may be able to record the right coronary artery originating from the left coronary sinus. One might also see failure of the left main coronary artery to communicate with the aorta.

SUMMARY

It is now established that two-dimensional echocardiography offers an opportunity to record the proximal coronary arteries. With experience the left main coronary artery can be recorded in almost all patients. The bifurcation of the left main coronary artery is able to be seen in approximately seventy-five percent of patients using the newer techniques now available. Hopefully, with increasing experience this percentage may become higher. As yet, the frequency with which the right coronary artery can be accurately recorded has not been evaluated. Preliminary data indicate that two-dimensional echocardiography may be a practical means of detecting obstructions within the left main coronary artery. Technical difficulties still remain and the examination is not easy. Training and experience is obviously necessary to make this type of examination reliable.

The clinical role for this ultrasonic examination depends upon one's management of patients with coronary artery disease. It is quite possible that echocardiography could be a reasonable substitute for coronary angiography in patients in whom only the question of left main coronary artery obstruction need be answered. It is also possible that the finding of atherosclerotic disease in the proximal coronary arteries could prove to be an independent risk factor for the presence of obstructive disease. The absence of high intensity echoes within the proximal coronary arteries may be a reliable way of excluding the possibility of atherosclerotic obstruction anywhere in the coronary system. This possibility, of course, remains to be proven.

Thus, two-dimensional echocardiography is a very promising means of helping to manage patients with known or suspected coronary artery disease.

REFERENCES

1. Weyman AE, H Feigenbaum, JC Dillon, KW Johnston: Noninvasive visualization of the left main coronary artery by cross-sectional echocardiography. Circulation 54:169, 1976.
2. Ogawa S, CC Chen, FE Hubbard, TJ Mardelli, J Morganroth, LS Dreifus, M Akaishi, Y Nakamura: A new approach to visualize the left main coronary artery using apical cross-sectional echocardiography. Am J Cardiol 45:301, 1980.

3. Chandraratna PAN, WS Aronow, K Murdock, H Milholland: Left main coronary arterial patency assessed with cross-sectional echocardiography. Am J Cardiol 46:91, 1980.

4. Chen CC, J Morganroth, S Ogawa, TJ Mardelli, LL Meixell: Detecting left main coronary artery disease by apical, cross-sectional echocardiography. Circulation 62:288, 1980.

5. Rogers EW, RW Godley, AE Weyman, ST Vakili, H Feigenbaum: Evaluation of left coronary artery anatomy in vitro using cross-sectional echocardiography. Circulation 62:782, 1980.

6. Rink LD, H Feigenbaum, JE Marshall, RW Godley, D Doty, JC Dillon, AE Weyman: Improved echocardiographic technique for examining the left main coronary artery.Am J Cardiol 45:II–435, 1980.

7. Rogers EW, H Feigenbaum, AE Weyman, RW Godley, KW Johnston, RC Eggleton: Possible detection of atherosclerotic coronary calcification by two-dimensional echocardiography. Circulation 62:1046, 1980.

8. Friedman MJ, DJ Sahn, S Goldman, DR Eisner, NC Gittinger, FL Lederman, CM Puckette, JJ Tiemann: High frequency, high resolution cross-sectional (2D) echo for evaluation of left main coronary artery disease (LMCAD): Is resolution alone enough? Circulation 60:II–153, 1979.

9. Rink LD, H Feigenbaum, JE Marshall, RW Godley, JF Phillips, JC Dillon, AE Weyman: Detection of proximal left anterior descending coronary artery obstruction with two-dimensional echocardiography. Circulation 62:III–333, 1980.

10. Yanagihara K, H Kato, T Owaki, Y Takagi, J Yoshikawa, T Fukaya, Y Tomita, K Baba: Ultrasonic features of coronary artery dilatation and aneurysm. J Cardiogr 8:401, 1978.

11. Hiraishi S, K Yashiro, S Kusano: Noninvasive visualization of coronary arterial aneurysm in infants and young children with mucocutaneous lymph node syndrome with two-dimensional echocardiography. Am J Cardiol 43:1225, 1979.

12. Caldwell RL, A Weyman, RA Hurwitz, DA Girod, H Feigenbaum: Cross-sectional echocardiographic evaluation of coronary artery abnormalities in children. Am J Cardiol 45:II–467, 1980.

13. Caldwell RL, AE Weyman, DA Girod, RA Hurwitz, H Feigenbaum: Cross-sectional echocardiographic differentiation of anomalous left coronary artery from primary myocardiopathy. Circulation 58:II–786, 1978.

8. TWO-DIMENSIONAL ECHOCARDIOGRAPHY AND INDIUM-111 PLATELET SCINTIGRAPHY IN THE DIAGNOSIS OF LEFT VENTRICULAR THROMBI – COMPETITIVE OR COMPLEMENTARY

M.D. Ezekowitz, D.A. Wilson, E.O. Smith, P.J. Kanaly, and D.E. Parker

1. INTRODUCTION

Between 6% and 12% of patients with left ventricular aneurysms will have a clinically manifest, often catastrophic and unsuspected, systemic embolus during the course of their disease [1, 2, 3]. It is presumed that the major source of these emboli are the mural thrombi which form within the left ventricle. Therefore, critical evaluation of currently available and, particularly, newer diagnostic tests for the identification of mural thrombi is urgently required.

At the present time, the most exciting diagnostic techniques for the identification of left ventricular thrombi are two-dimensional echocardiography and Indium-111 labeled platelet scintigraphy. Several recent reports have pointed out the potential value of two-dimensional echocardiography in the diagnosis of left ventricular thrombi [4, 5, 6]. However, the diagnostic accuracy of this technique has not been well defined. Indium-111 platelet scintigraphy employs both the favorable physical properties of Indium, which enable scintigraphic study, and the fact that when it combines with 8-hydroxyquinoline a lipid-soluble complex is formed which is suitable for platelet labelling and results in very little attenuation of platelet function [7, 8, 9, 10]. Platelets labelled in this way are thus suitable for the identification of thrombi in the body. In a preliminary paper, we reported the identification of left ventricular thrombi using this technique [11]. The purpose of this paper is to compare the techniques of platelet scintigraphy with two-dimensional echocardiography in the diagnosis of left ventricular thrombi. Patients with left ventricular aneurysms were selected for this study because between 30% and 70% develop mural thrombi [12, 13] and a significant number undergo aneurysmectomy, providing a unique opportunity of validating the preoperative diagnosis at surgery.

Rijsterborgh H, ed: Echocardiology, p 73-79. All rights reserved.
Copyright © 1981 Martinus Nijhoff Publishers, The Hague/Boston/London.

2. PROCEDURE

2.1. Material and methods

2.1.1. Patient population

A total of 19 patients were studied. Each patient underwent coronary angiography with left ventriculography because symptoms of angina and/or shortness of breath necessitated their evaluation for surgery. Each patient had a discrete aneurysm exhibiting paradoxical wall motion located in the apical or antero-apical area of the left ventricle. The time interval from the last myocardial infarction to the beginning of the scintigraphic study and the echo study varied from 2 days to 10 years. In 4 patients, this time interval could not be clearly determined. Clinical evidence for possible systemic emboli in the form of transient cerebral ischemic episodes and/or clear cut peripheral emboli was found in 4 patients. Of the 19 patients studied, 18 had two-dimensional echocardiography and all had platelet scintigraphy.

2.1.2. Radionuclide imaging

Platelets were labelled according to a method described elsewhere [14, 15, 11]. Images were obtained daily, or at least on alternate days including the day of injection, for a minimum of 5 days and a maximum of 8 days in the anterior, left lateral, LAO and RAO views. Altogether, in all patients, 200,000 count images were obtained. Imaging was performed on a wide field of view gamma scintillation camera (fitted with a medium energy collimator) set on both photopeaks of Indium-111, with a 20% window. All images were interpreted by two observers blinded to the clinical and laboratory data. The criterion for positivity was an obvious area of increased activity in the region of the left ventricle which increased with time against a decreasing blood pool.

2.1.3. Echocardiographic studies

All patients were specifically evaluated for the presence of a left ventricular aneurysm, mural thrombi and left ventricular function. In all cases, a two-dimensional echocardiogram was obtained using a Varian Model V3000 phased-array 80° sector-scanner. All examinations were performed supine with the patient in the 30° to 45° left lateral position. The transducer was initially placed in the parasternal area and manipulated until a sector-scan parallel to the long axis of the left ventricle was obtained. A short-axis view was then obtained by rotating the transducer at right angles. The transducer was then placed at the apex of the heart (point of maximum impulse) with the notch on the transducer facing upwards and the ultrasonic beam directed towards the right scapula. An apical four-chamber view was recorded in this way. With the transducer in the same position, counter-clockwise rotation directed the ultrasonic beam parallel to the interventricular septum producing a right anterior oblique equivalent view. All views were recorded on video tape for later detailed studies. The cross-sectional echocardiographic illustrations were taken from single frame, stop action television images using Polaroid film. There was significant degradation of image quality when compared with motion images because only one-half of a 2-part video frame is displayed with each photograph.

Each study was reviewed from video tape in real-time, slow motion and stop action modes. These studies were read by two observers prior to surgery. Each observer analyzed the echo with respect to the quality of the echo and the probability of thrombus. Echo quality was divided into three grades: (1) excellent, (2) adequate, and (3) poor. Excellent was defined as sharply defined left ventricular endocardium and mitral valve from all views. Adequate was defined as poor interface definition between blood and endocardium with a lower signal to noise ratio, but of sufficient quality to confidently identify thrombus. Poor was defined as a failure to clearly define the left ventricular endocardium. Only studies from the first two categories were used for diagnostic purposes. Diagnosis of probability of a left ventricular thrombus was also divided into three categories: positive (+), possible (+/−), and negative (−). Positive was defined as an area of persistent echo, often of increased intensity, adjacent to, but clearly distinct from the left ventricular myocardium. Care was taken not to confuse echoes arising from the area of papillary muscles with those due to thrombi. Possible was defined as intermittent, usually lower intensity, echoes which were suspiciously different from the endocardium but could not be clearly defined. When echoes from the endocardium were clearly visualized as a single interface, the reading was negative for mural thrombi. Following surgery, a retrospective analysis was performed and compared to the preoperative assessment.

3. RESULTS

3.1. Isotopic studies

In all patients, well defined images of the cardiac blood pool and great vessels were seen on day 1. In none of the patients were positive images clearly seen until 60 hours following injection of the platelet suspension. In all positive patients, images were positive by 96 hours. Positive images remained positive at least up to and including the 120 hour image. Positive images varied in appearance. Most commonly, a homogeneous area of increased activity was evident (Figure 1). In one patient, two separate thrombi were seen on the scintiphoto and confirmed at surgery. Two patients had doughnut-shaped images in the LAO view reflecting a thrombus lining

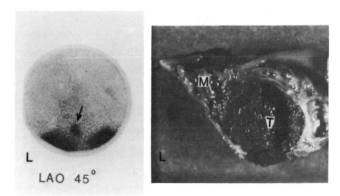

LAO 45°

Figure 1. The left hand frame represents an Indium-111 scintiphoto obtained 96 hours following the injection of the platelet suspension. The right hand frame represents the corresponding surgical specimen. The orientation of the scintiphoto is with the top of the figure cephalad. The increased activity in the right lower quadrant is due to the spleen and that in the left lower quadrant due to the liver. The arrow points to a rounded homogeneous area of increased activity. This represents an active thrombus within a large antero-apical left ventricular aneurysm. The corresponding surgical specimen indicates a large fresh thrombus 2 cm × 1 cm contained within a sacular component of the aneurysm. M = myocardium, T = thrombus, L = left.

the entire endocardial surface of the aneurysm. The sensitivity and specificity of platelet scintigraphy was 80% and 100%, respectively (both observers).

3.2. Two-dimensional echocardiography

Considering both groups together, both observers concurred with respect to the quality of the images obtained. Four out of 19 were regarded as excellent, 15 adequate, 0 poor. Both observers noted focal areas of dyskinesis in all patients. The sensitivity of the technique for identifying thrombi by both observers was 90%. The specificity was 50% and 67%, respectively, for observers 1 and 2. In 3 patients, at least one observer recorded the probability of thrombus as "possible". All three studies were negative at surgery. The overall observer agreement for the whole group was 16 out of 19 (84%). An example of a typical positive study is shown in Figure 2. A retrospective analysis of falsely interpreted studies revealed that artifacts arising from the junction between aneurysmal tissue and normal tissue, as well as from the maladjustment of the near gain setting, resulted in extraneous echoes and thus in the false interpretation. In two patients, echoes indistinguishable from those derived from surgically verified thrombi were seen. These patients proved to be free of thrombi at surgery. We would like to speculate that this is probably due to the somewhat irregular motion of the aneurysm itself during the cardiac cycle causing the echo artifact.

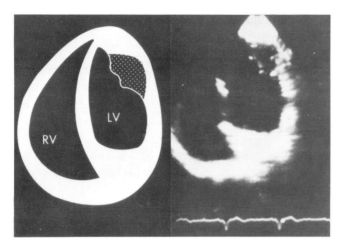

Figure 2. A two-dimensional echocardiogram from a patient with a large antero-apical aneurysm. The oblique apical four-chamber view defines the right ventricle (RV) and left ventricle (LV). The stippled area in the adjacent and corresponding diagram reveals a large thrombus protruding significantly into the left ventricular chamber

3.3. Findings at surgery

Most patients had discrete aneurysms consisting of a thin fibrous wall which moved paradoxically during systole in the beating heart and following insertion of the left ventricular vent collapsed inward thereby demarcating the edges of the infarct fairly precisely. Occasionally, the aneurysmal tissue consisted of patchy scarring interspersed with viable but ischemic myocardium. In these instances, greater difficulty was found in demarcating the edge of the aneurysm. The ventriculotomy incision was made between traction sutures at what was thought to be the center of the aneurysm and was extended to within 5 mm of the margin of the aneurysm. In this way, complete visualization of the interior of the left ventricular chamber was possible. The entire septum was visualized from apex to base and the aortic and mitral valves were inspected for thrombus. The papillary muscles were also inspected.

4. DISCUSSION

The main finding of this paper is that both the techniques of Indium-111 platelet scintigraphy and two-dimensional echocardiography have a significant role in the diagnosis of left ventricular thrombi. Platelet scintigraphy utilizes the dynamic nature of the blood/thrombus interface and would

78

detect only thrombi that are actively incorporating platelets. It, therefore, represents a surface phenomenon and the positivity of the study does not reflect the mass of the thrombus. By contrast, echocardiography identifies mass lesions and does not reflect surface activity. It appears that echocardiography is a more sensitive technique than platelet scintigraphy, which is more specific. Therefore, the two techniques appear to complement each other.

Since the two techniques reflect different pathological processes, it is possible to obtain positive two-dimensional echocardiographic studies which do not incorporate platelets. Two such cases were encountered. It is interesting to postulate that in these patients the thrombi might be inactive and the use of anticoagulants or antiplatelet agents would be of little benefit. It is not clear at the present time whether platelet avarice thrombi have a greater propensity to embolization than do those that are non-active thrombi. This determination would have to be made in a larger series.

REFERENCES

1. Grabar JD, CM Oakley, BN Pickering et al.: Ventricular aneurysm: an apparaisal of diagnosis and surgical treatment. Br Heart J 34:830–838, 1972.
2. Cooley DA, GL Hallman: Surgical treatment of left ventricular aneurysm: Experience with excision of post-infarction lesions in 80 patients. Prog Cardiovasc Dis 11:222–228, 1968.
3. Favaloro RG, DB Efler, LK Groves et al.: Surgical treatment of ventricular aneurysms – clinical experience. Ann Thorac Surg 6:227–245, 1968.
4. DeMaria AN, W Bommer, A Newman et al.: Left ventricular thrombi identified by cross-sectional echocardiography. Ann Intern Med 90:14–18, 1979.
5. Ports TA, J Cogan, NB Schiller et al.: Echocardiography of left ventricular masses. Circulation 58:528–536, 1978.
6. Meltzer RS, D Guthaner, H Rakowski et al.: Diagnosis of left ventricular thrombi by two-dimensional echocardiography. Br Heart J 42:261–265, 1979.
7. Goodwin PA, JT Bushbert, PW Doherty et al.: Indium-111 labelled autologous platelets for location of vascular thrombi in humans. J Nucl Med 19:626–623, 1978.
8. Riba AL, ML Thakur, A Gottschalk et al.: Imaging experimental coronary artery thrombosis with Indium-111 platelets. Circulation 60:767–775, 1979.
9. Davis HH, WA Heaton, BA Siegel et al.: Scintigraphic detection of atherosclerotic lesions and venous thrombi in man by Indium-111 labelled autologous platelets. Lancet 1:1185–1187, 1978.
10. Dewanjee MK, V Fuster, MP Kaye et al.: Imaging platelet deposition with ^{111}In-labelled platelets in coronary artery bypass grafts in dogs. Mayo Clin Proc 53:327–331, 1978.
11. Ezekowitz MD, JC Leonard, EO Smith et al.: The identification of left ventricular thrombi in man using Indium-111 labelled autologous platelets – A preliminary report. Circulation (in press).
12. Moran JN, PJ Scanlon, R Nemickas et al.: Surgical treatment of postinfarction ventricular aneurysm. Ann Thorac Surg 21: 107–113, 1976.

13. Loop FD, DB Efler, JA Navia et al.: Aneurysms of the left ventricle. Survival and results of a ten-year surgical experience. Ann Surg 178:399–405, 1973.
14. Thakur NL, JJ Welch, JH Joist et al.: Indium-111 labelled platelets: Studies in preparation and evaluation of in vitro function. Throm Res 9: 345–357, 1976.
15. Heaton WA, HH Davis, MJ Welch et al.: Indium-111: A new radionuclide label for studying human platelet kinetics. Br J Haematol 43:613, 1979.

I. ECHOCARDIOLOGY IN ADULTS

B. APPLICATIONS IN LEFT VENTRICULAR FUNCTION ANALYSIS

9. QUANTITATIVE TWO-DIMENSIONAL ECHOCARDIOGRAPHY IN CORONARY ARTERY DISEASE

JAMES L. WEISS

1. INTRODUCTION

Because the functional and structural hallmarks of ischemic heart disease are abnormal regional wall motion and shape, two-dimensional echocardiography seems ideally suited for the noninvasive evaluation of this entity. It should be possible with this technique to assess the extent and location, as well as the presence, of regional left ventricular dysfunction. The purpose of this presentation is twofold. First, the utility of quantitative two-dimensional echocardiography in acute myocardial infarction will be exemplified by examining regional cardiac dilatation in acute myocardial infarction. Second, we will address the accuracy of quantitative two-dimensional echocardiography in identifying, localizing, and sizing myocardial infarction in patients and in the intact canine heart.

2. QUANTITATIVE TWO-DIMENSIONAL ECHOCARDIOGRAPHY IN ACUTE MYOCARDIAL INFARCTION: THE IDENTIFICATION OF REGIONAL CARDIAC DILATATION

Perhaps the commonest example of the structural change in ventricular shape is the infarcted left ventricle. Studies in patients with chronic ischemic heart disease have demonstrated a good correlation between cross-sectional echocardiographic and cineangiographic detection of both ventricular aneurysm and areas of regional asynergy [1, 2, 3]. The importance of *acute* changes in topography has recently been illustrated. In its capability for repeated noninvasive examination, two-dimensional echocardiography raised the attractive possibility of serial evaluation of the left ventricle in acute myocardial infarction. The initial impetus for using two-dimensional echocardiography in this way was provided by the pathologists. Post-mortem studies of patients dying within 30 days after acute myocardial infarction had shown that up to two-thirds of such patients had some thinning and dilatation of the infarcted area within one week of acute infarction [4] and that in approximately one-third of patients' hearts with transmural infarcts there was marked expansion of the infarcted zone, resulting in obvious

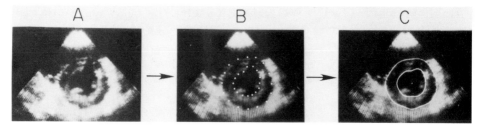

Figure 1. Computer-aided contouring system for echocardiographic analysis. A) Cross-sectional image at level of papillary muscles. B) Process for dividing same image into 16 equally spaced myocardial segments. Each of two sets of 16 points is superimposed on the endocardial and epicardial margins. C) Points are smoothed by the computer and are repositioned every 16–32 ms.

cardiac dilatation. This process occurred with little or no histologic evidence of infarct extension or further necrosis after the initial acute event.

Two-dimensional echocardiography made it feasible to look for such acute alterations in cardiac topography by serial examination of patients with acute myocardial infarction, and make the ante-mortem diagnosis noninvasively [5]. For quantitative evaluation of these serial echocardiograms, we utilized a computer-aided system for contouring myocardial borders and evaluating regional wall thickness and segment lengths (Figure 1) [6]. This

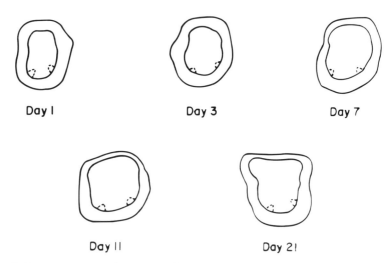

Figure 2. Computer-generated contours of transverse end-diastolic views of the left ventricle from serial echocardiographic studies of a patient with infarct expansion, who had an anterior transmural infarction on day 1 with serial studies through day 21. Papillary muscle locations are represented here by dotted lines. Progressive development of regional dilatation and thinning in the infarcted area is apparent by day 7.

type of evaluation could not be achieved by subjective visual impression. We calculated regional segment lengths and wall thicknesses serially throughout a cross-sectional view of the left ventricle in patients with acute transmural myocardial infarction. Approximately one-third of patients with anterior transmural myocardial infarction showed infarct expansion, with disproportionate dilatation and transmural thinning of the infarcted zones, and this occurred during the first few days after admission (Figure 2). Although the patients with regional expansion did not have significantly higher peak creatine kinase or Killip classification, they had a significantly greater 8 week mortality (4 out of 8 versus 0 out of 20, P<0.004). Thus, a selective topographic change in myocardial structure within the area of necrotic myocardium was responsible for a major alteration in left ventricular topography. The mortality data suggest functional, and possibly prognostic, implications. The development of regional dilatation probably increases overall wall stress and may thus be deleterious to overall left ventricular function.

3. TWO-DIMENSIONAL ECHOCARDIOGRAPHY AND INFARCT SIZE: DETECTION, LOCALIZATION AND QUANTIFICATION

Because of its unique ability to provide cross-sectional information on regional wall motion, two-dimensional echocardiography holds promise for noninvasive detection of myocardial injury in patients with ischemic heart disease. Until recently, however, it was unknown to what extent wall motion abnormalities on two-dimensional echocardiography could predict the presence and extent of infarcted tissue in man. We have had the opportunity to evaluate this in man by using post-mortem studies as the standard for comparison [7]. From 800 two-dimensional echocardiograms at the Johns Hopkins Hospital, we found twenty patients with post-mortem examinations. Eleven of these had coronary artery disease, four valvular disease, two primary myocardial disease, and three had normal hearts. Two-dimensional echocardiograms were subjected to independent visual segmental wall motion analysis (Figure 3). The hearts were cut with specific reference to the echocardiographic sectors. The transmural extent of infarction (normal, subendocardial, or transmural) was compared with the degree of regional wall motion abnormality (normal, regional hypokinesis, or akinesis/dyskinesis).

Infarct was almost always associated with regional wall motion abnormalities, which were present in 90% of the pathologically infarcted segments. However, although infarct meant regional wall motion abnormality, regional wall motion abnormality signified myocardial infarction far less frequently. Forty-six percent of morphologically normal segments demonstrated seg-

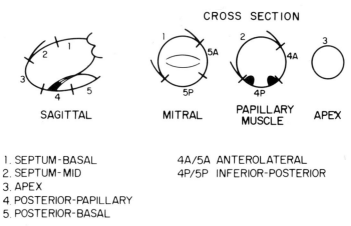

1. SEPTUM-BASAL   4A/5A ANTEROLATERAL
2. SEPTUM-MID   4P/5P INFERIOR-POSTERIOR
3. APEX
4. POSTERIOR-PAPILLARY
5. POSTERIOR-BASAL

Figure 3. Format for segmental wall motion analysis of two-dimensional echocardiograms. When technically feasible, three cross-sectional views were obtained.

mental wall motion abnormalities. It is of interest that 66% of these segments were directly adjacent to scar. These wall motion abnormalities may in part explain the overestimation of infarct by two-dimensional echocardiography and may be the result of chronic ischemia within the occluded coronary bed or of the direct proximity of scar to the majority of spuriously abnormal echocardiographic areas.

The degree of wall motion abnormality usually corresponded to the degree of thickness of the infarct. If we compare the presence of normal, hypokinetic, and akinetic/dyskinetic wall motion with muscle histology (normal, subendocardial or transmural infarction), all transmurally infarcted segments were akinetic or dyskinetic; subendocardially infarcted segments were unpredictable in their wall motion. From the echocardiographic standpoint, the majority of akinetic or dyskinetic segments were transmurally infarcted; hypokinesis could not distinguish subendocardial infarction from uninjured myocardium. Most importantly, normal wall motion excluded transmural infarction. Thus, while one cannot diagnose with certainty the presence of infarction in a given segment, one can identify with confidence the absence of transmurally infarcted tissue.

Because two-dimensional echocardiography gives information on the wall motion of the entire left ventricular circumference, it should be possible to determine the circumferential extent of infarction if a relationship exists between wall motion abnormalities and the presence of infarct. To assess this, we examined the relationship of the extent of left ventricular circumference demonstrating akinesis or dyskinesis to the circumferential extent of transmurally infarcted left ventricle by post-mortem examination. Circumferential extent of akinesis or dyskinesis was examined by light-pen analysis.

Superimposing stop-frame end-diastolic and end-systolic circumferences, extent of circumference showing either absent or dyskinetic motion was calculated as a percent of the entire end-diastolic circumference. The extent of segmental wall motion abnormalities (akinesis/dyskinesis) correlates well with the percentage of left ventricular circumference demonstrating morphologic infarction (Figure 4). Echocardiographic wall motion abnormalities tended to exceed, by approximately 14%, the amount of myocardial circumference involved by injury.

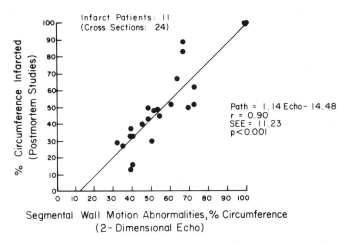

Figure 4. Comparison of the extent of left ventricular circumference demonstrating akinesis/dyskinesis and the percent of transmurally infarcted left ventricular circumference by post-mortem examination from 11 patients with post-mortem evidence of transmural infarction. Where technically feasible, cross-sections included the apex, papillary muscle and mitral valve tips. Each point represents an individual echocardiographic cross-section and the corresponding slice examined pathologically.

We can conclude from these human data that 1) normal segmental wall motion excludes transmural infarction, but is occasionally associated with subendocardial injury; 2) regional akinesis or dyskinesis usually signifies, but is not entirely predictive of, transmural infarction; 3) circumferential extent of akinesis/dyskinesis and circumferential extent of scar correlate closely; and 4) circumferential and regional scar are overestimated, possibly because most pathologically normal segments seen by echocardiography as akinetic or dyskinetic are either adjacent to scar or in the perfusion area of a critically stenosed coronary artery.

4. QUANTITATIVE TWO-DIMENSIONAL ECHOCARDIOGRAPHY AND INFARCT-
SIZE: STUDIES IN THE INTACT, INFARCTED CANINE HEART

The above studies in man, as well as prior studies in animals, suggest that the extent of two-dimensional echocardiographic wall motion abnormalities exceeds pathologic infarct size, though the reason remains unclear. Recent investigations have pointed to wall thickening as a possibly more accurate measure for evaluating infarction, but these investigations have not clarified the relationship between extent of thickening and infarct size or the degree of transmurality of the infarction.

To address these issues, we have studied regional systolic thickening in the intact, infarcted canine heart [8], have compared this functional index with tissue histology, and asked (1) can thickening accurately separate non-infarcted from infarcted myocardium and, if so, (2) can we delineate the transmural extent of infarcted myocardium, as an initial approach to the use of this technique in quantifying infarct size? The study protocol is illustrated in Figure 5. In open-chested dogs, we obtained cross-sectional views. Three anatomic regions were assessed individually: grossly infarcted regions; the normal zones directly adjacent to and within 1 cm of the infarct but not themselves grossly infarcted; and the distant, non-infarcted regions. A castor oil filled standoff device with a polyurethane membrane was attached to the transducer head to offset it from the epicardial surface and minimize cardiac distortion. A tricoordinate system of calibrated steel rods allowed accurate distance measurement and transducer location. Echocardiographic images

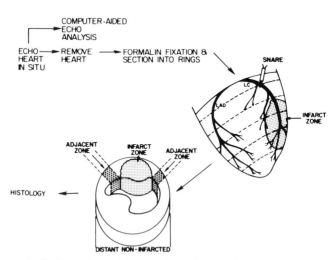

Figure 5. Protocol of echocardiographic and histologic analysis. A snare is placed around the coronary artery. Ten days later, ligation is performed. 48-hours later, echocardiographic study is performed epicardially. Following this, the heart is removed, fixed, and sectioned into rings corresponding to the echocardiographic section.

were obtained at 1 cm intervals from apex to base, and the ventricle was later sliced at the same intervals, beginning at the same landmark. We were able to superimpose the echocardiographic images in their proper anatomic locations over transparancies of the pathologic specimens. Histologic sections verified gross pathologic examination in every case.

For evaluation of the echo data, we utilized the computer-aided contouring system described previously, to measure regional systolic thickening in 16 equally spaced segments per slice. Percent systolic thickening showed a clear separation between normal, adjacent, and infarcted tissue, and by analysis of variance this separation was significant between all three groups ($P<0.001$). Only 3 of 41 infarcted zones demonstrated any systolic thickening (to a maximum of 9%). The rest revealed systolic thinning of varying degrees, to a mean value of 12.5%. All distant normal zones showed some degree of systolic thickening, with a mean value of 37.4%. However, the extent of dysfunction exceeded the boundaries of the infarcted tissue itself to include that immediately adjacent to infarct. Reductions in adjacent zone thickening were intermediate between distant normal and infarcted regions, but almost all adjacent zones thickened. Though grossly non-infarcted, two-thirds of these adjacent zones contained microscopic islands of infarct (mean infarct content = 3.9% at $<1/2$ cm from the infarct border). Dysfunction of adjacent regions might then be attributable to small islands of infarct, adjacent local ischemia, or mechanical tethering to more profoundly infarcted regions.

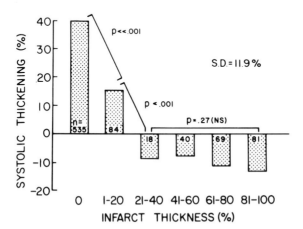

Figure 6. Relationship between transmural extent of infarct thickness and percent systolic thickening. Systolic thickening is plotted as a function of infarct thickness measured histologically, in 20% increments. Positive values = thickening, negative values = thinning. One way analysis of variance with contrasts. SD = overall standard deviation.

90

We then attempted to answer the important question of the accuracy of percent systolic thickening in determining the extent of transmural involvement of the infarct (Figure 6). For each individual segment within each slice, we plotted segmental percent thickening against percent infarct thickness measured histologically. A "threshold" effect is evident here: infarct-free segments show significantly greater degrees of systolic thickening than segments with small amounts of infarction (1-20%). Likewise, segments containing greater than 20% transmural extent of infarct thin during systole. Beyond this degree of infarct thickness (21-100%), segments manifest similar degrees of systolic thinning.

Thus, there is no gradual decrease in percent systolic thickening from normal regions to zones containing transmural infarction. Rather, there is an abrupt deterioration in systolic function when more than 20% of the transmural thickness of a segment is infarcted. This threshold effect would limit absolute infarct size determination with two-dimensional echocardiography.

Conversely, however, the presence of any systolic thickening is indicative of less than 20% transmural extent of infarction. This latter finding has significant clinical implications. If in the future it can be shown in man that the presence of systolic thickening excludes significant transmural infarction, this technique could have substantial potential for the identification of non-infarcted or "salvaged" myocardium. The use of quantitative two-dimensional echocardiography should provide a means to realize this potential.

REFERENCES

1. Kisslo JA, D Robertson, BW Gilbert, O Von Ramm, VS Behar: A comparison of real-time, two-dimensional echocardiography and cineangiography in detecting left ventricular asynergy. Circulation 55:135, 1977.
2. Heger JJ, AE Weyman, LS Wann, JC Dillon, H Feigenbaum: Cross-sectional echocardiography in myocardial infarction: Detection and localization of regional left ventricular asynergy. Circulation 60:531, 1979.
3. Weyman AE, SM Peskow, ES Williams, JC Dillon, H Feigenbaum: Detection of left ventricular aneurysms by cross-sectional echocardiography. Circulation 54:936, 1976.
4. Hutchins GM, BH Bulkley: Infarct expansion vs extention: Two different complications of acute myocardial infarction. Am J Cardiol 41:1127, 1978.
5. Eaton LW, JL Weiss, BH Bulkley, JB Garrison, ML Weisfeldt: Regional cardiac dilatation after acute myocardial infarction: Recognition by two-dimensional echocardiography. N Engl J Med 300:57, 1979.
6. Garrison JB, JL Weiss, WL Maughan, OM Tuck, WH Guier, NJ Fortuin: Quantifying regional wall motion and thickening in two-dimensional echocardiography with a computer-aided contouring system. Proceedings of Computers in Cardiology 1977, Ed. by H, Ostrow, K Ripley. Long Beach, California, Institute of Electrical and Electronics Engineers, 1977, 25.

7. Weiss JL, BH Bulkley, GM Hutchins, SJ Mason: Two-dimensional echocardio-graphic recognition of myocardial injury in man: Comparison with postmortem studies. Circulation 63:401, 1981.
8. Lieberman AN, JL Weiss, BI Jugdutt, LC Becker, BH Bulkley, JB Garrison, GM Hutchins, CA Kallman, ML Weisfeldt: Two-dimensional echocardiography and infarct size: Relationship of regional wall motion and thickening to the extent of myocardial infarction in the dog. Circulation 63:739, 1981.

10. EARLY DETECTION OF ACUTE MYOCARDIAL ISCHAEMIA AND INFARCTION BY CROSS-SECTIONAL ECHOCARDIOGRAPHY

M.J. MONAGHAN, K. DALY, G. JACKSON, and D.E. JEWITT

INTRODUCTION

Early detection of acute myocardial infarction may help to reduce cardiovascular morbidity and mortality. Traditional diagnostic techniques have relied upon standard 12-lead electrocardiographic patterns and elevated serum cardiac enzymes. The results of these investigations may be inconclusive or unavailable during the early hours following infarction.

Several experimental and human studies have demonstrated the ability of M-mode echocardiography to record the alteration in left ventricular (LV) wall movement patterns that immediately follow acute myocardial ischaemia or infarction [1, 2]. Cross-sectional echocardiography may be used in a similar way [3, 4] and affords improved spatial orientation and visualisation of the left ventricular wall.

This study was undertaken in order to evaluate the sensitivity and specificity of cross-sectional echocardiography in the early detection of acute myocardial infarction and ischaemia.

MATERIAL AND METHODS

Patients

Fifty consecutive patients (38 male and 12 female, mean age 58 years) admitted to the coronary care unit with a provisional diagnosis of acute myocardial infarction were examined by cross-sectional echocardiography. Patients were excluded from the study if more than 12 hours had elapsed from the onset of pain or if they had a history of previous infarction, hypertension or conduction defects as evidenced on the 12-lead electrocardiogram.

CPK and ECG

12-lead electrocardiograms and blood samples for creatinine-phosphokinase analysis were taken on admission and subsequently every 24 hours.

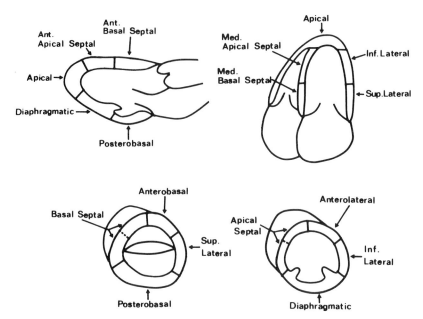

Figure 1. Segmental division of long-axis, apical four-chamber and short-axis cross-sectional echo views.

Echocardiography

Cross-sectional echocardiographic studies were performed at the time of admission and 48 hours later, using a Smith Kline Ekosector III with an 82° mechanical scanning probe. The echocardiograms were recorded using a Sanyo VTC-7100 video cassette recorder, enabling re-examination in real-time and slow motion.

Recordings were made of the 4 views illustrated in Figure 1 with the patients in a 35° left lateral position. Using these 4 views the left ventricular wall was divided into 9 segments, with the basal and apical septal segments further subdivided into anterior and medial. Ventricular wall motion in the 11 segments was then analysed by 2 independent observers, neither of whom had prior knowledge of CPK or ECG findings. Each segment was awarded a score which depended on the presence and degree of asynergy, a normal segment was scored 0, hypokinetic 1, akinetic 2, dyskinetic 3. The total score for all eleven segments was then summed and expressed as a percentage of the maximum possible score 33. Therefore a normal ventricle would achieve a score of 0% and a theoretical totally dyskinetic ventricle would be scored 100%. Patients were excluded from the study if satisfactory recordings of all 4 views were not obtained.

To distinguish chronic abnormalities from those seen in acute myocardial infarction, we examined 20 patients with angiographically proven coronary artery disease and no previous history of myocardial infarction using the same echocardiographic technique described above. The results were compared with those found in the acute infarction group.

RESULTS

Forty out of fifty patients were diagnosed as having greater than twice normal CPK (n = 150 i.u./l) and a typical ECG pattern as defined by WHO criteria [6]. Elevated percentage asynergy was present in 39 of these patients on admission (mean 32.5%) and in all at 48 hours (mean 29%). Ten patients did not suffer myocardial infarction. Eight had normal echocardiograms (asynergy 0%). The remaining two whose ECG's showed acute ischaemic patterns had LV asynergy (% score 15) on admission; these echocardiograms reverted to normal after the acute ischaemic episode. The control group of 20 patients with ischaemic heart disease also had evidence of LV wall asynergy, however the mean percentage score was 7%. Figure 2 illustrates a comparison of the asynergy scores in three groups, namely, those admitted to the coronary care unit with acute myocardial infarction, those in this study who did not suffer myocardial infarction, and the control group of patients with ischaemic heart disease.

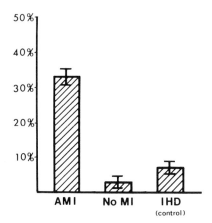

Figure 2. Percentage asynergy in 3 groups of patients on admission (see text). AMI = Acute myocardial infarction, NoMI = No myocardial infarction, IHD = Ischaemic heart disease.

In 17 patients, myocardial infarction could not be diagnosed on admission but was subsequently confirmed at 48 hours. Eight patients had normal CPK (mean 134 i.u./l) rising to 1012 at 48 hours (Figure 3) and 9 had non diagnostic ECG patterns.

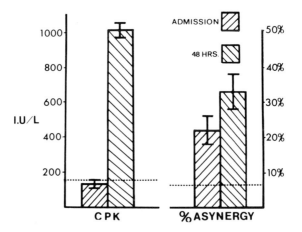

Figure 3. Comparison of CPK and asynergy score in patients with acute myocardial infarction on admission and at 48 hours.

All had evidence of LV wall motion abnormality (mean percentage asynergy score 23 on admission rising to 33 at 48 hours). CPK and asynergy values are compared in Figure 3, with dotted lines indicating normal CPK value and the asynergy score of the control group.

DISCUSSION

The ability of cross-sectional echocardiography to detect regional left ventricular wall asynergy in patients with myocardial infarction is well documented [4, 7]. In addition it has been used to assess prognosis in this condition [8]. However, the potential of the technique in the early detection of myocardial infarction and in the monitoring of therapeutic intervention has yet to be fully evaluated. The purpose of this study was to assess the sensitivity and specificity of cross-sectional echocardiography in the early detection of acute myocardial infarction.

The results of the study demonstrate the high sensitivity (97.5%) of the technique, in that 39 out of 40 patients with acute myocardial infarction had elevated asynergy scores on admission (mean 32.5%). This score is considerably higher than that seen in the control group of patients with ischaemic heart disease but no previous infarction (mean 7%). The significance of this finding lies in the fact that, although asynergy has been described in stable ischaemic heart disease [9], its incidence is higher in patients with myocardial infarction [10], whether acute or long-standing. To evaluate the specificity of the technique in the acute situation, patients with a history of myocardial infarction were excluded from this study.

Serial echocardiographic studies have demonstrated improvement in wall motion in some segments after acute myocardial infarction [11], suggesting that a reversible process is partly responsible for the high degree of asynergy (32.5%). This is supported by the demonstration of reversible asynergy in stress-induced ischaemia [12] and also by the presence of transient asynergy (15%) in two patients in our study with acute ischaemic episodes which did not progress to myocardial infarction. The inclusion of these two patients resulted in a specificity of 80%. Further studies will be necessary to determine whether this technique will allow separation of acute myocardial infarction from acute ischaemia, as suggested by the difference in asynergy seen in this study.

The value of the technique is demonstrated by the fact that 17 patients in whom ECG patterns and CPK values were not diagnostic on admission had markedly elevated asynergy scores. Both 12 lead ECG and CPK values are known to be unreliable in the early stages of infarction.

In conclusion, cross-sectional echocardiography has been shown to be a highly sensitive technique for the early detection of myocardial infarction and acute ischaemia. It is particularly of value when initial CPK values and ECG patterns are not diagnostic. The technique will undoubtedly play an important role in the early assessment and continuing management of patients admitted to the coronary care unit with a provisional diagnosis of acute myocardial infarction.

ACKNOWLEDGEMENTS

We would like to thank Dr. Richard Popp (Stanford University Medical Centre, California) for his advice in the setting up of this project.

REFERENCES

1. Stefan G, RJ Bing: Echocardiographic findings in experimental myocardial infarction of the posterior left ventricular wall. Am J Cardiol 30:629–639, 1972.
2. Heikkila J, M Nieman: Echoventriculographic detection localization and quantification of left ventricular asynergy in acute myocardial infarction. A correlative echo and electrocardiographic study. Br Heart J 37:46, 1975.
3. Meltzer R, G Jang, J Woythaler, E Alderman, R Popp, D Harrison: Circulation (abstr) 60,4: 11–152, 1975.
4. Heger J, A Weyman, S Wann, E Rogers, J Dillon, H Feigenbaum: Cross-sectional echocardiographic analysis of the extent of left ventricular asynergy in acute myocardial infarction. Circulation 61,6:1113, 1980.
5. Nelson J, M Quinones, W Winters, D Kenon, A Waggoner, R Miller: Circulation (Abstr) 62,4:No. 1268, 1980.

6. World Health Organisation: Hypertension and coronary heart disease: Classification and criteria for epidemiological studies. Technical report of the World Health Organisation, series No. 168, 1959.
7. Visser C, R Lie, J Durrer, F van Capelle, D Durrer: Quantification and localisation of uncomplicated acute myocardial infarction by cross-sectional echocardiography (abstr), Circulation 60,4:11–152, 1979.
8. Rogers E, A Weyman, H Feigenbaum, J Heger, J Dillon: Predicting survival after myocardial infarction by cross-sectional echo (abst) Circulation 57, 58:Suppl II:II–907, 1978.
9. Corya B: Echocardiography in ischaemic heart disease. Am J Medicine 63:10–20, 1977.
10. Jacobs J, H Feigenbaum, B Corya: Detection of left ventricular asynergy by echocardiography. Circulation 48:263, 1973.
11. Wynne J, J Birnholz, H Finberg, J Alpert: Regional left ventricular wall motion in acute myocardial infarction as assessed by two-dimensional echocardiography (abstr). Circulation 56 (Suppl III):III–152, 1977.
12. Corya B: Applications of echocardiography in acute myocardial infarction. Cardiovasc Clin II:113, 1975.

11. DYNAMIC EXERCISE CROSS-SECTIONAL ECHOCARDIOGRAPHY: COMPARISON WITH CORONARY ARTERIOGRAPHY AND RADIONUCLIDE ANGIOGRAPHY

C. A. VISSER, L. R. VAN DER WIEKEN, G. KAN, and D. DURRER

INTRODUCTION

Since regional left ventricular dysfunction is the principal consequence of acute ischaemia [1], this study was designed to determine the value of cross-sectional echocardiography in detecting exercise-induced asynergy.

MATERIALS AND METHODS

Thirty-four consecutive patients were included in the study. They were referred to our hospital because of suspected coronary artery disease. Their mean age was 55 years (range 34–70 years). There were 8 females and 26 males. Patients with unstable angina or evidence of a prior myocardial infarction were not admitted to this study.

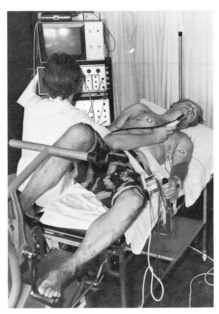

Figure 1. Apparatus and patient position for cross-sectional echocardiography during supine bicycle exercise.

Rijsterborgh H, ed: Echocardiology, p 99-102. All rights reserved.
Copyright © 1981 Martinus Nijhoff Publishers, The Hague/Boston/London.

Supine bicycle exercise was performed in the left lateral decubitus position on a table with a bicycle ergometer mounted on the lower end. Two sturdy belts around the abdomen and hips of the patient and handgrips on both sides of the table prevented sliding upwards during exercise (Figure 1).

Cross-sectional echocardiograms were obtained using a commercially available mechanical sector-scanner (EkoSector I, Smith Kline Instruments) with a 30° sector arc. The images obtained were stored on videotape for independent analysis by two observers who had no knowledge of other clinical data. Discrepancies were resolved by consensus. The bipolar standard electrocardiographic leads and the unipolar lead V1 and V6 were continuously monitored during exercise and the recovery period.

Cross-sectional echocardiograms were performed at rest and continuously during supine bicycle exercise and the recovery period. From each standard acoustic window, multiple views were used to obtain enough images of nine segments of the left ventricle (Figure 2).

Exercise was performed at an increasing workload of 15 or 20 Watt increments at an interval of two minutes, culminating in loads that produced symptoms of angina or dyspnea, or fatigue of sufficient severity to limit further exercise.

Cross-sectional echocardiographic data were compared to the coronary arteriogram at rest and the radionuclide cineangiograms at rest and during supine bicycle exercise. The same exercise protocol was used for both techniques. Cardiac catheterization and radionuclide cineangiography were performed within two weeks of exercise cross-sectional echocardiography.

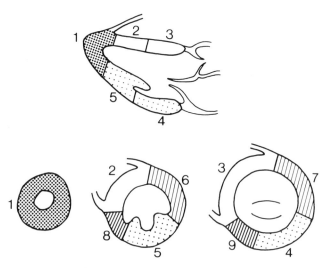

Figure 2. Schematic diagram of the nine segments of the left ventricle examined in this study. 1 = apex; 2 and 3 = septum low and high; 4 and 5 = posterolateral high and low; 6 and 7 = anterolateral low and high; 8 and 9 = inferior low and high.

RESULTS

Adequate cross-sectional echocardiograms during exercise could be obtained in 27 (80%) of the 34 patients studied. Fifteen of these 27 patients had significant (>50% luminal stenosis) coronary artery disease. Two of these 15 patients demonstrated asynergy at rest on their cross-sectional echocardiograms and 14 patients showed exercise-induced or increased asynergy (Figure 3).

There was one false positive and one false negative exercise echocardiographic study. Thirteen patients demonstrated asynergy during exercise by both techniques. In 11 of these 13 patients there was a close correspondence of the site of asynergy between the echocardiographic and radionuclide studies.

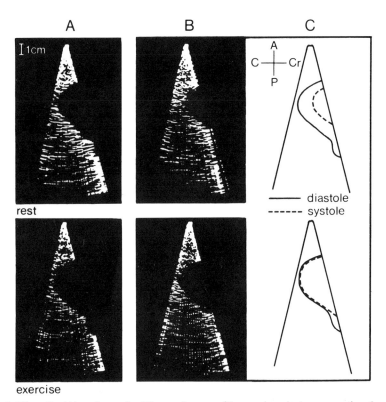

Figure 3. Diastolic (A) and systolic (B) stop-frames of long-axis apical cross-sectional echocardiograms of a patient with a subtotal stenosis of the left anterior descending artery. At rest (above) motion of the cardiac apex is normal (C); during exercise (below) the cardiac apex becomes akinetic. Abbreviations: A: anterior, P: posterior, C: caudal, Cr: cranial.

CONCLUSIONS

1. Cross-sectional echocardiographic examination of the left ventricle during dynamic exercise is feasible in the majority of patients studied.
2. Dynamic exercise-induced asynergy as determined by cross-sectional echocardiography is a fairly sensitive and specific sign of significant coronary artery disease.
3. The site of asynergy as determined by cross-sectional echocardiography correlated well with radionuclide cineangiography.

REFERENCE

1. Tennant R, C Wiggers: The effect of coronary occlusion on myocardial contraction. Am J Physiol 112:351, 1935.

12. COMPARISON OF REGIONAL WALL MOTION DETERMINED BY TWO–DIMENSIONAL ECHOCARDIOGRAPHY, RADIONUCLIDE ANGIOGRAPHY, AND LEFT VENTRICULOGRAPHY

R. Brad Stamm, Blase Carabello, Denny Watson, George Taylor, George Beller, and Randolph P. Martin

Considerable recent interest has been focused on the use of noninvasive methods for assessing left ventricular wall motion. Two-dimensional echocardiography (2DE) and gated radionuclide angiography (RNA) have been shown to accurately assess left ventricular segmental wall motion [1, 2, 3, 4]. The current investigation compared both noninvasive techniques with contrast left ventriculography (LVG) in the same patients. When significant discrepancies existed between techniques, coronary artery and valvular anatomy were examined to determine the basis of the discrepancy.

METHODS

The initial study population consisted of 53 consecutive patients who underwent 2DE, RNA, and LVG within an average of 7.5 days. Six patients were eliminated due to inadequate studies: 3 2DE, 1 RNA, 2 LVG. Twenty-two of the patients had coronary artery disease and 25 had valvular disease.

Equilibrium ECG gated scans were obtained by labeling patients' blood with 21 mCi technetium-99m pertechnetate [3, 4]. Patients were imaged for 8 minutes in both the anterior and 45° left anterior oblique views. After background subtraction, images were viewed in real-time and in slow motion using a Digital Equipment Corporation computer.

All patients had routine 2DE performed using commercially available equipment. Views were obtained in the parasternal long and short-axis, apical two and four-chamber, and subcostal long and short-axis.

Contrast left ventriculography and coronary artery angiography were performed using standard techniques. All patients had right anterior oblique views and 23 had additional left anterior oblique images.

All studies were interpreted by two or more independent observers who had no knowledge of the patient's history or results of the other tests. Wall motion was graded: 0 = normal, 1 = hypokinetic, 2 = akinetic and 3 = dyskinetic. The ventricle was divided into 7 segments: anterior base, anterior mid, apex, inferior base, inferior mid, septum and lateral. The 2DE segments are shown in Figure 1.

Rijsterborgh H, ed: Echocardiology, p 103-107. All rights reserved.

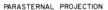

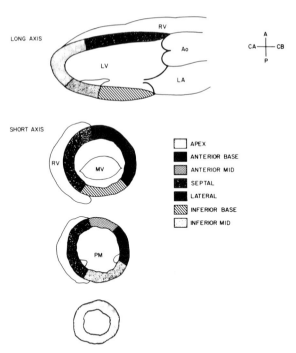

Figure 1. Left ventricular segments as visualized on the parasternal long and short-axis two-dimensional echo. Contrast ventriculographic and radionuclide angiographic anterior and right anterior views are divided as in the 2D echo long-axis projection. In the parasternal long axis projection A =anterior, P = posterior, CA = cardiac apex and CB = cardiac base.

Agreement between techniques was defined as follows: 1) precise agreement was the same wall motion score, 2) agreement on the presence of kinetic motion (normal or hypokinetic) versus akinetic motion (akinetic or dyskinetic), and 3) agreement on akinetic motion in segments graded akinetic on LVG. A significant discrepancy was considered to exist when techniques disagreed on kinetic versus akinetic motion.

Table 1. Two-dimensional echocardiographic (2DE) and radionuclide angiographic (RNA) determined wall motion agreement with contrast ventriculography at three levels of agreement: 1) precise agreement on wall motion grade, 2) agreement on kinetic versus akinetic motion, and 3) agreement on akinesis in segments graded akinetic on contrast ventriculogram.

	Precise Agreement		Kinetic vs Akinetic Motion		Detection of Akinetic Segs.	
2DE	214/279	77%	261/279	94%	40/43	93%
RNA	209/279	75%	243/279	87%*	23/43	53%**

* p = 0.01, ** p = 0.001 for probability of difference in rate of agreement with contrast ventriculogram.

RESULTS

Table 1 presents the agreement of 2DE and RNA determined wall motion with wall motion as assessed by LVG. The 2DE and LVG were in precise agreement (same wall motion score) for 77% of the segments while RNA and LVG agreed for 75%. When distinguishing kinetic from akinetic segments the techniques agree even more closely: 2DE and LVG agreed for 94% of the segments while RNA and LVG agreed for 87% (p = 0.01). The difference in rates of agreement is predominantly due to poor RNA and LVG agreement for segments scored akinetic/dyskinetic on LVG. Of the 43 segments graded akinetic/dyskinetic on LVG, the 2DE scored 93% as either akinetic or dyskinetic while RNA agreement was 53% (p = 0.001).

The segment with the greatest discrepancies between techniques was the apex. The 2DE and LVG precise agreement at the apex was 67%, anterior base 72%, inferior mid 74%, septum 74%, lateral 83%, anterior mid 83%, and inferior base 87%. Precise agreement between RNA and LVG at the apex was 62%, inferior mid 62%, lateral 74%, inferior base 78%, anterior mid 81%, anterior base 83%, and septum 87%.

Seventeen segments were significantly discrepant, comparing 2DE and LVG for gauging kinetic versus akinetic wall motion. Three segments scored kinetic on 2DE, but were graded akinetic on LVG: 2 apical and 1 inferior mid segment. The apical discrepancies occurred in a patient with normal coronary arteries and a cardiomyopathy due to aortic insufficiency, and in a patient with 100% occlusion of the right coronary artery. The discrepant inferior mid segment was in a patient with normal coronary arteries and a severe cardiomyopathy following mitral valve replacement.

Fourteen segments were graded akinetic on 2DE, but were scored kinetic on LVG. The discrepancies occurred most frequently at the anterior base (4), mid inferior (4), and inferior base (3). Eleven of the fourteen discrepant segments were perfused by coronary arteries with 90% or greater stenosis. In 8 of the 11 segments, the perfusing coronary artery was 100% occluded. One additional inferior base segment was akinetic on 2DE in a patient with 100% occlusion of the proximal circumflex artery. Twice segments with normal coronary arteries were scored akinetic on 2DE. Two patients had significant aortic valve disease.

DISCUSSION

Two-dimensional echocardiography and radionuclide angiography are non-invasive techniques that allow accurate assessment of ventricular wall motion. Our results agree with previous reports comparing 2DE and RNA with contrast left ventriculography (LVG) [1, 3, 4]. 2DE and LVG agreement on precise grade of wall motion was 77 % while agreement between RNA and LVG was 75%. The techniques agreed even more closely when distinguishing kinetic segments from akinetic segments: 2DE/LVG concurred 94 % and RNA/LVG agreed 87 %. Overall congruence between techniques was good.

There was a significant difference between noninvasive techniques when evaluating segments with severely depressed wall motion. Forty-three segments were scored akinetic or dyskinetic on LVG. The 2DE graded 93 % of these segments akinetic or dyskinetic while RNA scored 53 % akinetic or dyskinetic. 2DE appears to be more sensitive than RNA for grading severely depressed wall motion. The lower RNA/LVG agreement for severely depressed wall motion has been reported by others [3, 4]. The difference between 2DE and RNA detection of akinetic segments is clinically important. The number and location of akinetic segments have been associated with patient mortality, congestive heart failure, coronary artery anatomy, and complex ventricular arrhythmias [5, 6, 7]. 2DE and LVG are in substantially better agreement in detecting significantly abnormal segments than are RNA and LVG.

The technical quality of a 2DE study is critically important if accurate results are to be obtained. Previous reports have obtained adequate studies in 82–84 % of patients or segments [1, 2]. The current investigation obtained adequate results in 94 % of the patients. An important difference is that the current report utilized all possible transducer positions: parasternal, apical, and subcostal. Endocardial definition is best when the incident sound beam is perpendicular to the endocardium. The use of multiple transducer positions enabled the visualization of most segments from two or more incident angles with improved endocardial definition. The subcostal position was especially important in patients with respiratory as well as cardiac disease. The use of multiple transducer positions produces a higher percentage of interpretable studies.

In this study 14 segments were scored akinetic on 2DE while the same segments were graded as kinetic on LVG. The majority of the discrepant segments were perfused by significantly stenosed coronary arteries. A stenosis of 90 % or greater was present in the perfusing vessel of 78 % of the segments; 57 % of the perfusing arteries were 100 % occluded. These segments may be considered as false-negative contrast ventriculograms. Kisslo [1] has demonstrated that a significant number of 2DE and LVG discrepancies are due to false-negative LVG. Contrast ventriculography utilizes a silhouette of the blood pool to infer wall motion. 2DE has the advantage of assessing systolic wall thickening as well as endocardial motion, enabling more accurate determination of wall motion in some patients.

Contrast ventriculography has been considered the gold standard for assessing ventricular wall motion, but recent studies have questioned the implications of wall motion as determined by LVG. Using post-mortem pathology [8] or intraoperative biopsy [9], it has been found that as many as 43% of segments graded hypokinetic or akinetic by LVG appear histologically normal, while normal or near normal motion can occur in segments with as much as 35% myocardial fibrosis. Wall motion abnormalities exist in varying clinical and pathological states, and it is not surprising that different techniques at times yield different results.

Our study demonstrates that significant discrepancies between 2DE and LVG in scoring wall motion may involve false-negative LVG results. This is not to imply that either technique is the better standard. Rather, it is important to recognize that when discrepancies do occur, they usually involve segments perfused by critically stenosed coronary arteries.

REFERENCES

1. Kisslo JA, D Robertson, BW Gilbert, O von Ramm, VS Behar: A comparison of real-time, two-dimensional echocardiography and cineangiography in detecting left ventricular asynergy. Circulation 55:134, 1977.
2. Heger JJ, AE Weyman, LS Wann, JC Dillon, H Feigenbaum: Cross- sectional echocardiography in acute myocardial infarction: detection and localization of asynergy. Circulation 60:531, 1979.
3. Federman J, M Brown, RG Tancredi, H Smith, DB Wilson, GP Becker: Multiple gated acquisition cardiac blood pool isotope imaging evaluation of left ventricular function correlated with contrast ventriculography. Mayo Clin Proc 53:625, 1978.
4. Okada RD, GM Pohost, AB Nichols, KA McKusick, HW Strauss, CA Boucher, PC Block, SV Rosenthal, RE Dinsmore: Left ventricular regional wall motion assessment by multigated and end-diastolic, end-systolic gated radionuclide left ventriculography. Am J Cardiol 45:1211, 1980.
5. Herman MW, R Gorlin: Implications of left ventricular asynergy. Am J Cardiol 23:538, 1969.
6. Friesinger GC, EE Page, RS Ross: Prognostic significance of coronary arteriography. Trans Assoc Am Phys 83:78, 1970.
7. Schulze RA, J Humphries, LS Griffith, H Ducci, S Achuff, MG Baird, ED Wellits, B Pitt: Left ventricular and coronary angiographic anatomy: relationship to ventricular irritability in the late hospital phase of acute myocardial infarction. Circulation 55:389, 1977.
8. Baltaxe HA, DR Alonso, JG Lee, J Prat, JW Husted, JW Stakes: Impaired left ventricular contractility in ischemic heart disease: angiographic and histopathologic correlations. Radiology 113:581, 1974.
9. Bodenheimer MM, VS Banka, GA Hermann, RC Trout, H Pasdar, RH Helfant: Reversible asynergy, histopathologic and electrographic correlations in patients with coronary artery disease. Circulation 53:792, 1976.

13. DETECTION OF TRANSIENT MYOCARDIAL ISCHEMIA BY M-MODE ECHOCARDIOGRAPHY IN MAN

A. DISTANTE, A. L'ABBATE, D. ROVAI, C. PALOMBO, and A. MASERI

1. INTRODUCTION

The diagnosis of acute transient myocardial ischemia may be difficult because of the absence of a gold standard against which currently used techniques may be compared.

The sensitivity and specificity of tests for detection of acute myocardial ischemia are currently evaluated against the findings of coronary arteriography. However, recently, various data indicate that the presence or absence of transient acute myocardial ischemia may not necessarily be related to the presence of organic coronary obstruction. Acute myocardial ischemia may occur, indeed, in the absence of appreciable stenosis and, conversely, even severe stenosis may not result in ischemia when adequately compensated by collateral circulation [1].

Moreover, the diagnosis of ischemia is complicated by the demonstrated occurrence of transient ischemic episodes unaccompanied by chest pain and by the occurrence of chest pain without typical electrocardiographic changes [2].

Since acute myocardial ischemia has been shown to be associated with transient impairment of left ventricular (LV) function [3], it seems reasonable to try to assess the presence of ischemia from the evaluation of changes in cardiac mechanics.

The purpose of this study was, therefore, to assess the possibility offered by echocardiography for the detection of changes caused by transient myocardial ischemia in man, with a view to a possible diagnostic application of this technique.

2. MATERIAL AND METHODS

Among patients admitted with frequent episodes of chest pain at rest, fourteen were selected on the basis of unequivocal evidence of transient myocardial ischemia at rest, as documented by one or more of the following procedures: continuous monitoring of the ECG, ergonovine maleate test [4], [201]Thallium perfusion scintigraphy [5], hemodynamic monitoring [2], coronary arteriography showing vasospasm [6]. In these patients continuous M-mode echocardiographic studies were performed one or more times during: a) spontaneous ischemic episodes with typical ECG changes, with or without chest pain; b) ergonovine tests which reproduced cardiac changes similar to those observed during spontaneous ischemic episodes [7].

These studies were performed with an Echocardiovisor 03 (Organon Teknika), linear array, and an Aloka SSD 800, phased-array, from which a line could be selected for appropriate M-mode signals. During the study, which could last up to several minutes, the operator held the transducer as stable as possible in the acoustic window, aiming at the LV area just below the mitral valve and obtaining paper recordings at a speed of 2.5 or 5.0 cm/sec. All M-mode recordings of acceptable quality were analyzed semi-automatically by a minicomputer system from groups of at least four to five cycles taken every 10–20 seconds (during rapid changes) or every 1–2 minutes (during phases of steady state) [8].

For this study we analyzed the right and left septal endocardium, the endocardium of the posterior wall, the onset of the R-wave on the ECG and, when available, LV pressure, peak contraction dP/dt and relaxation dP/dt. The data were processed to obtain the following parameters for each of the three phases (basal, ischemia and post ischemia) considered:

1. Septal wall thickness and amplitude of motion.
2. Posterior wall motion amplitude.
3. LV diameter at end-systole and end-diastole.
4. LV percentual fractional shortening.
5. Systolic percentual wall thickening.
6. Heart rate.
7. LV systolic and end-diastolic pressure.
8. Peak contraction and relaxation dP/dt.

In each digitized set of data, minimum and maximum values for each parameter in the different cycles were automatically calculated together with mean values, standard deviation and coefficient of variation, and subsequently presented on a printer-plotter.

3. RESULTS

In fourteen patients we recorded 25 ischemic attacks (13 spontaneous and 12 induced by ergonovine). Both the manual and the computerized analysis of the M-mode recordings of the ischemic episodes demonstrated a consistent type of change in cardiac mechanics, both in the ischemic wall and in the overall ventricular dynamics (see Figures 1, 2, 3, 4 and 5):

a) Ischemic wall showed a marked reduction in amplitude of motion (even paradoxical in some cases), reduction in systolic thickening and in diastolic thickness.

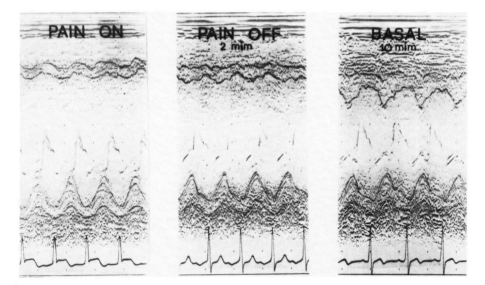

Figure 1. M-mode and ECG findings during a spontaneous ischemic attack at rest, studied at the onset of chest pain. PAIN ON: in the presence of both ST elevation in V_3 and pain there is already a pronounced reduction in systolic and diastolic thickness, with paradoxical septal motion, absence of systolic thickening and increase in LV dimensions. PAIN OFF: ECG shows a pseudo-normalization of a basally negative T wave, whereas a partial restoration of septal contraction is seen and LV dimensions appear less enlarged. BASAL: these findings were obtained 10 minutes after onset of pain and closely resemble the pre-ischemic ones, but diastolic septal thickness and systolic percentual thickening show a reactive increase (the sequence of this attack is reported in Figure 3). In this patient, coronary angiography performed during one of these episodes showed a proximal, complete but temporary occlusion of left anterior descending coronary artery on top of a critical stenosis (80%) constantly present in basal conditions.

b) LV diameter increased; such a change was more pronounced and earlier during systole than during diastole, causing a marked reduction in percentual fractional shortening.

c) Chest pain occurred 1 to 3 minutes after the onset of definite changes in the ischemic wall, usually only when the increase in diastolic dimensions over the control values became considerable.

d) Ischemic alterations on the ECG, defined by ST elevation or by pseudo-normalization of a basally negative T-wave, appeared a few seconds after the mechanical changes as in a).

112

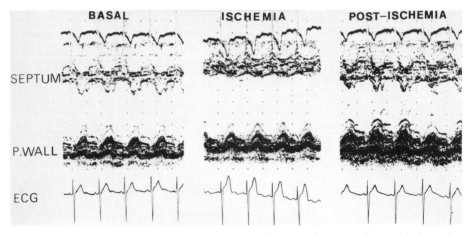

Figure 2. Three M-Mode recordings with the ECG during a transient ischemic attack induced by ergonovine, not accompanied by pain. BASAL: LV dimensions are normal, septal and posterior walls have a normal thickness and contract regularly. ISCHEMIA: in the presence of ST elevation in V_2, septal wall motion and systolic % thickening appear heavily compromised, as a direct expression of ischemic changes. POST-ISCHEMIA: septal motion and systolic thickening appear to be "exaggerated" as an expression of a "rebound effect"; a decrease in LV dimensions and an increase in LV fractional shortening are also evident.

e) LV end-diastolic pressure increases after the onset of the ischemic changes on the echocardiogram; LV systolic pressure does not increase until the onset of pain (when present). Conversely, contraction and relaxation dP/dt were also early indicators of ischemia, although they are an expression of global LV function, rather than regional.

f) An increase in wall thickness, LV fractional shortening and contraction dP/dt above basal values was often observed after the ischemic attack; such a "rebound effect" was noted both in attacks which spontaneously subsided and in attacks interrupted by nitrates.

g) The sequence of events showed that chest pain, the most common symptom suggestive of ischemia, occurs rather late when compared to direct ischemic changes in the involved wall, in dP/dt and even in the continuously monitored ECG.

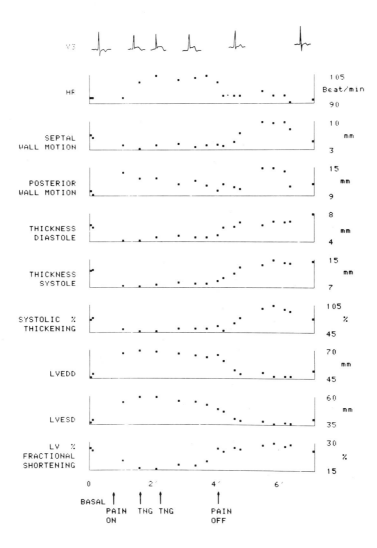

Figure 3. Computer printout of the full sequence of the spontaneous ischemic attack (antero-septal ischemia) seen in Figure 1. The most common parameters obtainable by single M-mode recording of LV are reported. The first two small squares were obtained half an hour before the onset of pain under basal conditions which were characterized by negative T-waves on ECG. When chest pain appeared (PAIN ON) ST segment was elevated, HR was unchanged, while motion, thickness in diastole and in systole, and systolic % thickening of septal wall were markedly reduced due to ischemia; moreover, LV end-diastolic and end-systolic diameter were greatly increased with a reduction in LV % fractional shortening. These changes became more pronounced over the following four minutes during which tachycardia was also present. Two minutes after trinitroglycerine (TNG) s.l. anginal pain disappeared (PAIN OFF) while all the parameters were returning towards basal values, going through a "rebound effect" which is particularly evident at six minutes.

114

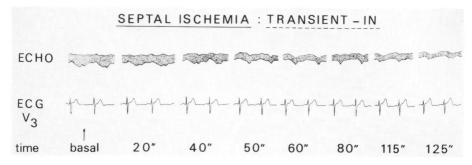

SEPTAL ISCHEMIA : TRANSIENT – IN

ECHO

ECG
V₃

time   basal   20″   40″   50″   60″   80″   115″   125″

Figure 4. Schematic re-drawing of M-mode and ECG findings in the first phase of a transient ischemic attack induced by ergonovine maleate (0.05 mg i.v.). Myocardial ischemia is detected earlier by echocardiographic changes than by ECG changes. TRANSIENT-IN = transient from basal state to ischemic attack.

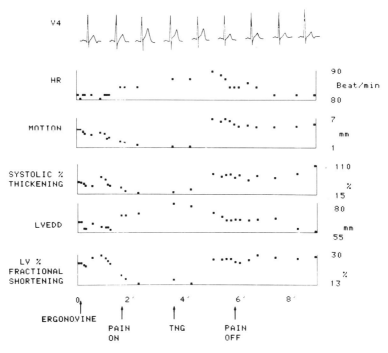

Figure 5. Computer printout of the full sequence of an ischemic attack with antero-septal ischemia induced by an injection of ergonovine maleate (0.05 mg i.v.). Note that when ST segment elevation is evident (4 minutes after the injection of the drug), M-mode echocardiographic alterations of the ischemic wall are already pronounced and easily appreciable.

4. DISCUSSION

Our results indicate that M-mode echocardiography allows the detection of obvious abnormalities of LV function in all episodes of acute myocardial ischemia, whether spontaneous or induced by ergonovine and whether with or without chest pain.

Under appropriate conditions, therefore, this technique may be applied in the diagnosis of transient ECG changes without chest pain or of anginal pain with atypical ECG changes. This is often the case during angina at rest and during provocative tests. These results should be extended to patients with angina and ST depression because ischemia associated with ST segment elevation, as in our population, is usually associated with greater severity of regional perfusion alterations [5] and of global LV function [2, 3] than angina with ST depression.

Our experience indicates that, in patients with atypical angina, the response to provocative tests such as ergonovine, cold pressor, hyperventilation, is often difficult to interpret, because they may elicit chest pain similar to that occurring during spontaneous episodes but without diagnostic ECG changes or they may elicit "ischemic" ECG changes without pain. Since in patients in whom angina is not caused by increased myocardial metabolic demand, coronary arteriography cannot be used to evaluate the sensitivity and specificity of techniques for detecting ischemia, independent means for assessing the presence of transient myocardial ischemia become necessary.

Studies of regional myocardial perfusion by ^{201}Tl present the disadvantage of high cost and may not be sensitive if ischemia is not severe enough [9]. Radionuclide studies of LV function by blood pool gating also appear promising and a comparison of their sensitivity with that of echocardiography would be desirable [10].

ACKNOWLEDGEMENTS

We express our thanks to Mr. Franco Cerri and Mr. Gianni Sesto for their secretarial help, and to Mr. Antonio Benassi, Mr. Claudio Michelassi and Mr. Paolo Pisani for their valuable technical advices.

This study was partially supported by C.N.R. Project Biomedical Technology, Subproject BIOI 4, Grants 102060/86/8002397, 212310/86/8002395 and 104520/86/8002396.

REFERENCES

1. Maseri A, S Severi, MD De Nes, A L'Abbate, S Chierchia, M Marzilli, AM Ballestra, O Parodi, A Biagini, A Distante: "Variant" angina: one aspect of a

continuous spectrum of vasospastic myocardial ischemia. Am J Cardiol 42:1019, 1978.

2. Chierchia S, C Brunelli, I Simonetti, M Lazzari, A Maseri: Sequence of events in angina at rest: primary reduction in coronary flow. Circulation 61:759, 1980.

3. Maseri A, R Mimmo, S Chierchia, C Marchesi, A Pesola, A L'Abbate: Coronary artery spasm as a cause of acute myocardial ischemia in man. Chest 68:625, 1975.

4. Schroeder JS, JL Bolen, RA Quint, DA Clark, WG Hyden, CB Higgins, L Wesler: Provocation of coronary spasm with ergonovine maleate. Am J Cardiol 40:487, 1977.

5. Maseri A, O Parodi, S Severi, A Pesola: Transient transmural reduction of myocardial blood flow, demonstrated by thallium-201 scintigraphy, as a cause of variant angina. Circulation 54:280, 1976.

6. Maseri A, A L'Abbate, A Pesola, AM Ballestra, M Marzilli, G Maltinti, S Severi, M De Nes, O Parodi, A Biagini: Coronary vasospasm in angina pectoris. Lancet 1:713, 1977.

7. Tavazzi L, JA Salerno, M Ray, G Specchia, M Chimenti, L Angoli, S De Servi, A Mussini, P Bobba: Acute myocardial ischemia induced by ergonovine maleate in patients with "primary angina". Primary and Secondary Angina Pectoris (A Maseri, GA Klassen, M Lesch, eds.). New York, Grune & Stratton, 1978.

8. Distante A, C Michelassi, D Rovai, A Benassi, L Landini, A L'Abbate: Computerized analysis of continuous echocardiographic recordings: study of trends in transient myocardial ischemia. Computers in cardiology, Williamsburg, Virginia USA, IEEE Computers Soc., Long Beach, 1980.

9. Jengo JA, R Freeman, RN Brizendine, M Ismael: Detection of coronary artery disease: comparison of exercise stress radionuclide angiocardiography and thallium stress perfusion scanning. Am J Cardiol 45:535, 1980.

10. Davies GJ, W Bencivelli, O Parodi, P. Pisani, E Falchi, A L'Abbate, A Maseri: ECG gated blood pool imaging tailored to study transient changes in left ventricular contractility. Computers in Cardiology, Williamsburg, Virginia USA, IEEE Computers Soc., Long Beach, 1980.

14. ECHOCARDIOGRAPHIC DIFFERENTIAL DIAGNOSIS OF CONGESTIVE CARDIOMYOPATHY AND ADVANCED CORONARY HEART DISEASE

A. Bloch, Ch. Mayor, and G. Merier

INTRODUCTION

Clinical discovery of a cardiomegaly, with severe decrease of left ventricular function, is not an uncommon finding in patients without valvular disease. The two main diseases which may be responsible for such an association are advanced coronary heart disease and congestive cardiomyopathy. In other words, the myocardial disease is either due to coronary artery disease, or is a primary form of cardiomyopathy whose origin usually remains unknown, except for the probable role of chronic alcoholism.

In typical cases, the diagnosis of advanced coronary heart disease can be made by means of (1) the past clinical history which reveals one or more myocardial infarctions and/or angina, (2) the ECG which shows signs of old infarctions. Actually, the differential diagnosis between coronary heart disease and congestive cardiomyopathy can be clinically difficult because angina is not unusual in congestive cardiomyopathy and because silent coronary artery disease can lead to severe myocardial dysfunction without chest pain. This differential diagnosis can also be electrocardiographically difficult, because congestive cardiomyopathy can produce pathological Q-waves which simulate those of myocardial infarction. Another problem is related to the frequent presence in both diseases of left bundle branch block which prevents the diagnosis of old myocardial infarction from being made from the ECG.

When faced with such a patient with severe heart failure of unknown origin, the question of coronary arteriography is raised, particularly if the patient is young. It would be useful therefore to have a simple noninvasive method available in order to define the origin of the heart diease. This diagnosis is not entirely academic. In the case of a congestive cardiomyopathy, complete abstinence from alcohol is indeed mandatory and can produce impressive improvements. In the case of coronary disease, surgery can be considered even in severe cases, especially when a left ventricular aneurysm is present. The purpose of the present study was to determine how efficient echocardiography is for the differential diagnosis between congestive cardiomyopathy and advanced coronary heart disease.

MATERIAL AND METHODS

The study population consisted of a consecutive series of 55 patients under 62 years old who presented signs of severe left ventricular dysfunction on M-mode echocardiogram. Patients with valvular disease other than slight mitral regurgitation, with prior cardiac surgery or with poor quality echocardiograms had been excluded. M-mode selection criteria were dilatation of the left ventricle, defined as an end-diastolic diameter greater than or equal to 32 mm/m^2 (indexed by body surface area, BSA) and severe decrease of left ventricular function, defined as a percent shortening of less than 20% and/or a mitral-septal separation of more than 10 mm. All patients had M-mode and two-dimensional echocardiograms (2DE), and either coronary arteriography with left cineventriculography, or autopsy. Three patients were subsequently excluded from the study because their final diagnosis remained unclear. Actually, in these cases cardiac catheterization showed the presence of significant coronary artery disease with disproportionately severe left ventricular dysfunction. The present study dealt, therefore, with 52 patients.

Of the many parameters which were studied on M-mode, only the excursion and systolic thickening of the interventricular septum and left ventricular posterior wall appeared to be useful for the differential diagnosis. The septum was considered normal if its excursion was more than 3 mm and its systolic thickening was more than 30%. The posterior wall was considered normal if its excursion was >9 mm and its systolic thickening was greater than 40%. Two-dimensional echocardiography was performed using a mechanical sector-scanner with a 30° angle or an 82° wide-angle transducer. They were recorded with the transducer in the parasternal and apical locations (long-axis, short-axis and four-chamber views). The left ventricle was divided into 5 main segments: septal, inferior, anterolateral, inferolateral and apical. Each segment was assessed as being normal, hyperkinetic, hypokinetic or dyskinetic. The diagnosis of segmental disease was made when one or more of the following features were present:
1) At least one normally moving segment.
2) A segment with increased echo density (due to myocardial scarring).
3) A severely dyskinetic segment, particularly an apical aneurysm.

Patients with diffuse and symmetrical left ventricular dysfunction on 2DE were diagnosed as having congestive cardiomyopathy. Patients with either one or more normal left ventricular segments, or the presence of one or more severely dyskinetic segments were diagnosed as having coronary heart disease; however, when the only normal segment on 2DE was the interventricular septum, diagnosis of coronary heart disease was made only if the systolic septal thickening on M-mode was also normal.

M-mode and 2DE were analyzed by two observers who did not know the clinical diagnosis of the patients nor the results of cardiac catheterization.

RESULTS

Cineventriculographies and autopsies confirmed the echocardiographic diagnosis of severe left ventricular dilatation and myocardial disease in all patients. Most catheterized patients had ejection fractions between 15% and 30%. There were 23 cases of congestive cardiomyopathy and 29 cases of advanced coronary heart disease. In two patients, the preliminary 2DE diagnosis was coronary disease because one segment, the interventricular septum, seemed to move normally. However M-mode showed in both cases that, despite a normal septal excursion, there was a marked decrease of systolic thickening; this allowed a correct prediction of the diagnosis of congestive cardiomyopahty.

The combined use of 2DE and M-mode led to the prospective diagnosis of congestive cardiomyopathy in 24 cases. One patient was wrongly diagnosed echocardiographically as having coronary heart disease. This was a 41 year old man who had diffuse hypokinesis of the left ventricle but whose lateral wall was moving better than the other segments. Echocardiography led to the prospective diagnosis of advanced coronary heart disease in 28 cases. Two patients were wrongly diagnosed echocardiographically as having congestive cardiomyopathy. The first one was a 62 year old man with diffuse myocardial disease due to severe coronary artery disease. The second one was a 60 year old man who also had diffuse left ventricular involvement. Looking back at his echocardiogram, it was seen, however, that the prospective diagnosis had been erroneous, because the increased echo density of the septum and the only slight hypokinesis of the posterior wall had been overlooked.

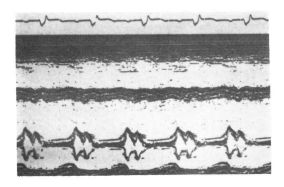

Figure 1. Typical case of congestive cardiomyopathy.

120

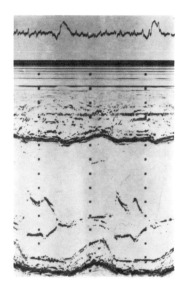 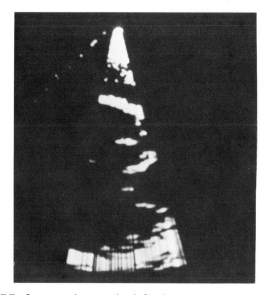

Figures 2 and 3. Typical M-mode and 2DE after extensive anterior infarction.

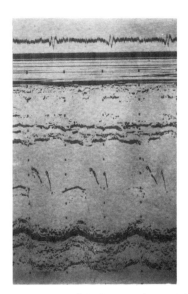 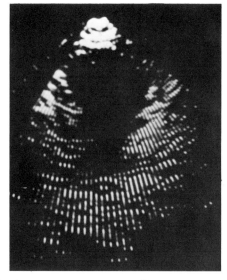

Figures 4 and 5. Old anterior and inferior infarctions. M-mode shows a diffuse hypokinesis consistent with a congestive cardiomyopathy but 2DE reveals a large apical aneurysm.

In summary, combined use of 2DE and M-mode allowed the correct prediction of the diagnosis of either congestive cardiomyopathy or advanced coronary heart disease in 49/52 patients, i.e. in 94% of the cases.

DISCUSSION

Echocardiographic differential diagnosis between congestive cardiomyopathy and coronary artery disease does not often represent a major problem. This is due to the fact that patients with cardiomyopathy have a grossly dilated left ventricle with diffuse hypokinesis. In contrast, patients with coronary artery disease usually have at least one normally moving wall. However this differential diagnosis can become very difficult if one includes cases of advanced coronary heart disease, sometimes called "ischemic cardiomyopathy".

A few useful M-mode signs have been described in the literature. Corya et al. [1] have shown that the total amplitude of the left septal and posterior endocardial wall motion is usually smaller in congestive cardiomyopathy than in coronary heart disease. The same group of investigators have shown [2] that abnormal changes in systolic wall thickening commonly occur in patients with coronary artery disease or congestive cardiomyopathy. Many factors can influence echocardiographic wall motion, whereas systolic thickening is more specifically related to contractility. However, decreased thickening does not allow one to differentiate coronary disease from congestive cardiomyopathy. Rasmussen et al. [3] have described that a wall on M-mode which is abnormally thin and more echo-producing than another left ventricular area, reflects myocardial scar tissue. This sign appears useful for diagnosing an old myocardial infarction. However Drobinski et al. [4] have recently stressed the difficulties in differentiating coronary disease from primary congestive cardiomyopathy with M-mode echocardiography.

In the present study we have combined 2DE and M-mode for the prospective differential diagnosis of congestive cardiomyopathy and advanced coronary heart disease. It is obvious that the echocardiographic differential diagnosis between these two diseases cannot be perfect. Coronary heart disease can indeed be entirely diffuse and symmetrical, whereas in rare cases congestive cardiomyopathy can produce myocardial infarctions [5]. However in the present study the correct diagnosis could be made prospectively by means of echocardiography in 94% of the patients with dilated left ventricle and severe decrease of left ventricular function. Combined use of 2DE and M-mode therefore appears to be an excellent noninvasive way of making the differential diagnosis between congestive cardiomyopathy and advanced coronary heart disease.

122

REFERENCES

1. Corya BC, H Feigenbaum, S Rasmussen, MJ Black: Echocardiographic features of congestive cardiomyopathy compared with normal subjects and patients with coronary artery disease. Circulation 49:1153, 1974.
2. Corya BC, S Rasmussen, H Feigenbaum, SB Knoebel, MJ Black: Systolic thickening and thinning of the septum and posterior wall in patients with coronary artery disease, congestive cardiomyopathy and atrial septal defect. Circulation 55:109, 1977.
3. Rasmussen S, BC Corya, H Feigenbaum, SB Knoebel: Detection of myocardial scar tissue by M-mode echocardiography. Circulation 57:230, 1978.
4. Drobinski G, JL Evans, P Borel, G Kin, Y Grosgogeat: Etude échocardiographique du ventricule gauche: possibilités et limites de l'échocardiographie TM à distinguer l'insuffisance ventriculaire gauche d'origine valvulaire, coronarienne ou myocardique. Cœur Méd Interne 43:15, 1979.
5. Isner JM, R Virmani, SB Itscoitz, WC Roberts: Left and right ventricular myocardial infarction in idiopathic dilated cardiomyopathy. Am Heart J 99:235, 1980.

15. DOES ECHOCARDIOGRAPHY AID IN THE MANAGEMENT OF ACUTE MYOCARDIAL INFARCTION?

JEFFREY A. WERNER, SARAH M. SPECK, H. LEON GREENE, CAROLYN L. JANKO, and BRIAN W. GROSS

INTRODUCTION

The development and refinement of echocardiographic techniques and the availability of reasonably portable equipment has made the use of cardiac ultrasound in the acute care setting feasible. In most parts of the world, acute manifestations of coronary artery disease, such as out-of-hospital ventricular fibrillation with unexpected collapse and acute myocardial infarction, represent the majority of admissions to a coronary care unit. While clinical information, including changes in the electrocardiogram and cardiac enzymes, frequently provide diagnostic and prognostic information, these tests and the clinical examination and history may be inconclusive or may not afford adequate specificity to discriminate among patients with a complicated clinical course. To attempt to explore the possible contribution of the echocardiographic examination in this clinical setting, we performed two-dimensional echocardiography on 48 patients admitted to the coronary care unit because of suspected acute myocardial infarction or following resuscitation for unexpected out-of-hospital cardiac arrest. Repeat examinations were performed during the hospitalization. The observations resulting from these studies and the relationship to other clinical information, hospital course and survival are reported.

MATERIALS AND METHODS

Standard M-mode and two-dimensional echocardiographic examinations were performed on 48 patients within 36 hours of admission to the Coronary Care Unit at Harborview Medical Center in Seattle, Washington. Thirteen patients underwent a second echocardiographic examination 24–36 hours after the initial study.

Criteria for inclusion in the study were: (1) strong suspicion of acute myocardial infarction (recent onset of prolonged typical ischemic chest pain with compatible initial electrocardiographic changes) or (2) resuscitation from out-of-hospital cardiac arrest requiring external chest compression, cardiovascular drugs and defibrillation. Patients excluded from the study included those with minor or atypical chest pain and those suffering unexpected collapse in whom a non-cardiac cause was likely. Patients otherwise satisfying the criteria were not included if studies were obtainable but not diagnostic or were refused.

Clinical examinations, serial cardiac enzymes, including CPK and LDH isoenzyme determinations, and electrocardiograms were performed for at least three days following admission. New Q-waves of equal to or greater than 0.04 sec. duration and/or elevated LDH isoenzyme levels with $LDH_1/LDH_2 > 1.0$ were considered diagnostic of acute infarction.

Echocardiographic examinations were performed in standard fashion using two acoustic windows (parasternal and apical) and multiple orthogonal positions at each window. Examinations were obtained using either an ATL Mark III wide-angle, mechanical sector-scanner with 3 MHz transducer or a Varian V-3400 wide-angle (80°) phased-array imaging system with 2.25 MHz transducer. Studies were recorded on videotape cassettes and later reviewed blind by two independent observers. Final diagnoses were made by consensus.

In addition to the conventional observations, global and segmental left ventricular wall function was analyzed and graded on a semiquantitative scale. Changes in segmental and global function, presence or absence of pericardial effusions and intracavitary thrombi were also evaluated on initial and follow-up studies.

The statistical methods employed were Chi-square analysis with Fisher's exact adaptation, and Student's t-test for upaired data.

RESULTS

Clinical characteristics

The clinical features of the study population are delineated in Table 1. There were 35 males and 13 females. Ages ranged from 23 to 86 years, mean 54.8 years. Twenty-five patients presented with typical chest pain and the remaining 23 patients were admitted to the Coronary Care Unit following resuscitation from out-of-hospital cardiac arrest. For purposes of analysis, patients were separated into three groups: acute anterior wall infarction (AMI), 24 patients; acute inferior wall infarction (IMI), 11 patients; and ventricular fibrillation without acute infarction (VF only), 13 patients. Of the 36 patients with acute infarction, 10 (30%) presented with out-of-hospital ventricular fibrillation (VF). Thirteen patients in the population died in hospital, 10 with acute MI and 3 with VF only, giving an in-hospital mortality rate of 27%.

Table 1. Clinical characteristics.

		n = 48		
		AMI	IMI	VF Only
n		24	11	13
Age	x̄	52.2	66.2	66.7
(yrs)	range	(23–86)	(36–92)	(28–70)
Sex	M	18	7	10
	F	6	4	3
Clinical	No VF	14	11	0
Presentation	VF	10	0	13
Deaths				
(In Hospital)		8	2	3

Laboratory data

Table 2 compares peak CPK and LDH values for the MI and VF only patients and also relates these values to hospital survival. While a peak LDH of more than 1200 units/dl occurred in significantly more patients with MI than with VF only ($p < 0.002$), there was no significant difference among these groups utilizing peak total CPK. Neither LDH nor CPK peak values were able to differentiate patients who would die in hospital. While mean peak CPK-MB was significantly higher in patients with MI compared to those with VF only (115 vs. 22, $p < 0.002$), these values did not distinguish survivors from those with in-hospital death (105 vs. 98, p = not significant).

Table 2. Enzyme characteristics of patients (n = 48).

	Peak LDH (IU)[1]		Peak CPK (IU)[2]		x̄ Peak CPK-MB (IU)[3]
Patient group	<1200	>1200	<1550	>1550	
	n (%)	n (%)	n(%)	n(%)	
MI	13 (37)	22 (63)	17 (48)	18 (52) ns	102.7 *
VF only	12 (92)	1 (8) *	7 (54)	6 (46)	22.1
Deaths	5 (38)	8 (62) ns	8 (62)	5 (38) ns	97.5 ns
Survivors	20 (57)	15 (43)	16 (46)	19 (54)	104.6

1 x̄ 1348 median 1200 range 127-4631

2 x̄ 2644 median 1548 range 98-18,800

3 range 3.0 - 276 IU

* p < .002

ns not significant

ECHOCARDIOGRAPHIC FINDINGS

Thrombus

Eight patients exhibited features compatible with left ventricular thrombus (7 with anterior MI, 1 with VF only). Six out of eight had thrombus on the first study, and two developed thrombus on the follow-up examination. All patients had thrombus in an area of apical akinesis.

Pericardial effusion

Pericardial effusion was demonstrated in 10 patients (9 with MI and 1 with VF only). No patient developed hemodynamic impairment or needed pericardiocentesis. Effusion persisted in 5 of the 6 patients with serial echo studies.

Right ventricular (RV) function

Of 12 patients with inferior wall infarction, 3 demonstrated RV dysfunction on the initial echo study and subsequent hemodynamic monitoring in all patients and autopsy in 1 patient were diagnostic of right ventricular infarction.

Table 3. Echocardiographic findings.

	n = 48		
	AMI	IMI	VF Only
LV thrombi	7	0	1
Pericardial effusion	7	2	1
RV dysfunction	0	3	0

Left ventricular (LV) function segmental wall analysis

Figure 1 illustrates the mean number and severity of abnormally contracting segments and their respective distribution among the three subgroups in the study population. There was no significant difference in the mean number of hypokinetic segments among the subgroups. In contrast, the mean number of akinetic or dyskinetic segments was significantly higher in the group with acute anterior infarction (2.5 segments) compared to patients with inferior infarction (1.0) or VF only (1.1 segments) ($p < 0.01$).

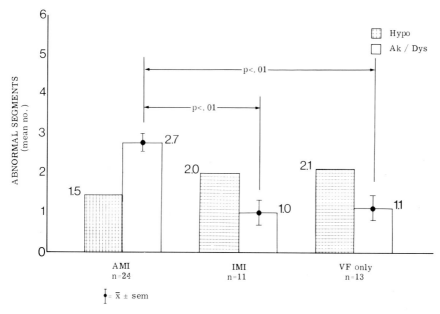

Figure 1. Segmental wall abnormalities (all patients).

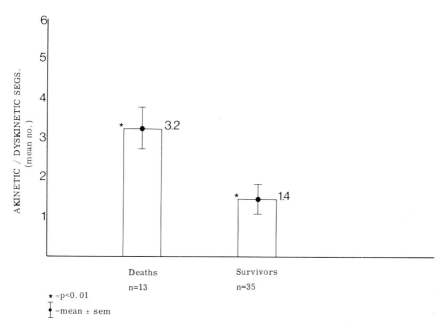

Figure 2. Segmental wall abnormalities (deaths vs. survivors).

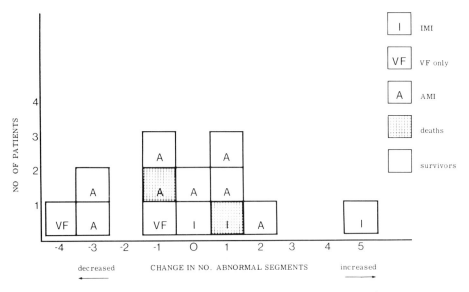

Figure 3. Segmental wall abnormalities (serial studies; n = 13).

Although the mean peak CPK-MB was not different, the mean number of segmental wall abnormalities was significantly greater in patients with in-hospital death than in survivors (mean 3.2 vs. 1.4, $p<0.01$) (Figure 2).

Thirteen patients underwent a second echo examination 24–48 hours following the initial study. Eleven of the thirteen demonstrated changes in segmental contractile function, as assessed semiquantitatively by severity and number of abnormal segments. Six patients had at least one improved segment and 2/6 showed a global improvement in LV function. In 5/13 patients, the number of abnormal segments increased and global LV function worsened in one of these 5. In this study population, a *change* in the number of abnormally contracting segments on a second study performed within two days of the initial study did not predict in-hospital mortality (Figure 3).

DISCUSSION

These data suggest that two-dimensional echocardiography is useful in the evaluation, and therefore presumably the management, of patients with suspected acute myocardial infarction. Several features of the study should be emphasized. The patient population studied was, on the whole, a group of very ill patients with a high likelihood of an acute coronary event. This explains the relatively high mortality rate of 27%, and, in part, explains the high median and mean enzyme values. An additional contribution to the elevated enzymes was cardiopulmonary resuscitation and low perfusion on initial presentation (out-of-hospital cardiac arrest) in 23 patients. However, if echo findings are likely to be helpful in the acute coronary setting, from the clinical standpoint, such information will be most useful in very ill or complicated patients, such as in this population. These data do not attempt to address the issues of sensitivity and specificity for diagnosis of acute infarction directly, but rather, primarily, the question of clinical utility in the acute care setting.

By establishing the feasibility of serially studying such patients using this noninvasive, repeatable and reasonably innocuous technique, it is likely that additional useful information will be obtained. Changes in tissue character of acutely infarcted muscle, the in vivo incidence and fate of intracavitary thrombus and the effects of pharmacological agents are important aspects of the management of acute infarction patients which are virtually unavailable by other means. Indeed in the application of two-dimensional echocardiography in a small prospective series of patients with acute transmural infarction, Eaton [1] et al. described pathophysiologic mechanisms of clinical deterioration in such patients caused by regional cardiac dilatation of acutely infarcted left ventricular segments. This concept of infarct expansion as an important, and otherwise undetectable, change in ventricular function and its relationship to hospital survival had previously only been appreciated at post mortem examination [2].

Kisslo [3], Schiller [4] and others [5] have analyzed left ventricular dimensions and wall motion by two-dimensional echocardiographic techniques and have demonstrated reasonable correlations with cineangiography in patients with and without left ventricular asymmetry. All have pointed out the inherent limitations of both the techniques and compared them. Although image quality improvement and quantitative methods for analysis are needed, the semiquantitative, subjective, wall motion assessment used here does probably identify real changes in wall motion, particularly in the same patient studied serially. Indeed, the abnormal segments seen on the echo study correlated well with the site of evolving infarction on the electrocardiogram in the infarct patients. Of the 13 patients admitted with ventricular fibrillation and not sustaining an acute infarction, 7/13 had known coronary disease and the wall motion abnormalities detected may have been due in part to prior infarction. In spite of this, when considering the entire study population, a higher mean number of left ventricular segments demonstrating akinesis or dyskinesis on the noninvasive study predicted hospital death (Figure 3), whereas clinical history, total and "cardiac specific" isoenzyme values and electrocardiogram were unable to predict hospital survival in these patients.

In summary, we believe that two-dimensional echocardiography will be a useful clinical tool in the management of patients who sustain an acute cardiac event and whose course is complicated. The greatest current limitations are the inability to obtain a diagnostic image in some patients and the lack of a validated, inexpensive method for quantitative analysis. Further investigations to demonstrate sensitivity, specificity and the reliability of pathophysiologic information available are warranted.

REFERENCES

1. Eaton LW, JL Weiss, BH Bulkley, JB Garrison, ML Weisfeldt: Regional cardiac dilatation after acute myocardial infarction – recognition by two-dimensional echocardiography. NEJM 300:57, 1979.
2. Hutchins GM, BH Bulkley: Infarct expansion versus extension: two different complications of acute myocardial infarction. Am J Cardiol 41:1127, 1978.
3. Kisslo JA, D Robertson, BW Gilbert, O vonRamm, VS Behar: A comparison of real-time, two-dimensional echocardiography and cineangiography in detecting left ventricular asynergy. Circulation 55:136, 1977.
4. Schiller NB, et al.: Left ventricular volume from paired biplane two-dimensional echocardiography. Circulation 60:547, 1979.
5. Wyatt HL, MK Hang, S Meerbaum, P Gueret, J Hestenes, E Dula, E Corday: Cross-sectional echocardiography. II Analysis of mathematic models for quantifying volume of the formalin-fixed left ventricle. Circulation 61:1119, 1980.

16. QUANTIFICATION FROM TWO-DIMENSIONAL ECHOCARDIOGRAPHIC IMAGES

O.L. Bastiaans, R.S. Meltzer, J. McGhie, P.W. Verbeek, and J. Roelandt

SUMMARY

An interactive image-processing computer system was used to extract quantitative information from two-dimensional echocardiographic images. Two short-axis views and three long-axis views were used to obtain an optimal overall representation of the left ventricle. Wall thickening was studied from the short-axis views and wall motion was studied from both short-axis and long-axis views. They were described using a radial coordinate system with a fixed origin. Average amplitudes for motion and thickening were obtained from a group of clinically normal subjects and were displayed graphically, showing the amplitudes in mm at each angle between 0° and 360°. The inter-observer variabilities for these measurements at each angle are displayed in similar graphs. The inter-observer variability in measuring cross-sectional surface area and long-axis length, which are used in volume calculations, was assessed by repeating measurements under equal or different conditions.

INTRODUCTION

In recent literature many reports can be found describing the possibility of extracting quantitative information on local and global parameters of left ventricular function from two-dimensional echocardiographic images. The local parameters of left ventricular function are local wall thickness, wall thickening and wall motion, whereas the global parameters are the instantaneous volume, stroke volume, cardiac output and ejection fraction.

Since two-dimensional echocardiography can only provide cross-sectional views of the ventricle, only local information can be extracted directly from the images. Usually this local information is extrapolated to regional or segmental information. Global parameters of left ventricular function are estimated by integrating local information from multiple cross-sectional views making use of mathematical models of the left ventricle.

With the aid of the Thoraxcentre image-processing system [1], a semi-automatic frame-by-frame analysis can be performed on time sequences of

Rijsterborgh H, ed: Echocardiology, p 131-143. All rights reserved.
Copyright © 1981 Martinus Nijhoff Publishers, The Hague/Boston/London.

132

routine two-dimensional echocardiographic images recorded on videotape (50 frames per second). With this system the local function can be studied throughout the complete cardiac cycle. The output of each analysis is presented as a number of graphs and functional images, thus offering a large amount of information. The complexity of this output, however, inhibits a clear insight in system accuracy.

In order to simplify the assessment of accuracy of quantitative left ventricular analysis, the amount of output data must be reduced. This can be accomplished by considering the maximum and minimum values of the parameters studied. Therefore, only end-diastolic and end-systolic values are measured and the absolute and/or relative changes of these parameters are computed.

A description of the computer programs developed for this purpose is given elsewhere [2]. This approach allows the study of the accuracy of most of the image-processing systems that are used for quantitative analysis of the left ventricle from echocardiographic images.

This paper reports on a set of twenty clinically normal subjects (normal history and physical examination) for determination of average amplitudes of the local parameters wall motion and wall thickening. Using the same group of subjects, the variability of the measurements was assessed and its influence on calculation of global parameters was determined.

EXAMINATION METHOD

The two-dimensional images, enabling optimal visualisation of the left ventricle, were obtained from the parasternal window and from the cardiac apex. Intracardiac anatomic landmarks were used to assure the reproducibility of the examination procedure, which is described below. Images from five

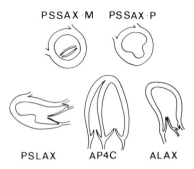

Figure 1. The two short-axis and three long-axis views studied in the clinical examination. (PSLAX = Parasternal long-axis view, PSSAX-M = Parasternal short-axis view at mitral level, PSSAX-P = Parasternal short-axis view at papillary level, AP4C = Apical four-chamber view, ALAX = Apical long-axis view).

cross-sectional views were recorded: two short-axis views and three long-axis views [3]. A diagrammatic illustration of these cross-sections is given in Figure 1.

First the parasternal long-axis view (PSLAX) was visualised. By rotating the transducer 90°, the parasternal short-axis views (PSSAX) were obtained; first the view at the level of the mitral valve (PSSAX-M) and second the view at the level of the papillary muscles (PSSAX-P). By shifting the transducer towards the cardiac apex, the apical four-chamber view (AP4C) was visualised and by rotating the transducer 90°, the apical long-axis view (ALAX) was found.

QUANTIFICATION METHOD

In order to quantify the local parameters from two-dimensional images, the outlines of the left ventricular wall had to be determined. Stop-frame video and lightpen techniques were used for interactive determination of muscular

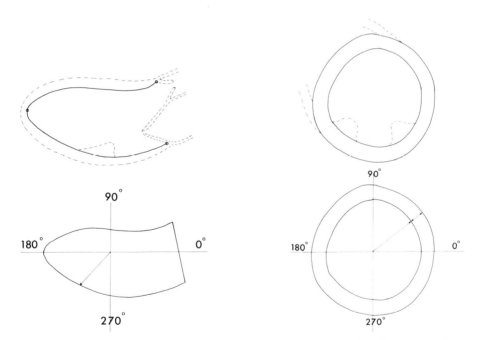

Figure 2. The radial coordinate system that is used for study of wall dynamics from cross-sectional images. In the long-axis views 0° is placed in the middle of the base and 180° is placed in the apex. The centre of the coordinate system is the middle of the long-axis. Wall motion is studied from the endocardial outline in end-diastole and end-systole. In the short-axis views the centre of the coordinate system is placed in the geometric centre of the endocardial outline in end-diastole. Wall motion and wall thickening are measured from the endocardial and epicardial outlines in end-diastole and end-systole.

outlines from end-diastolic and end-systolic images. For those regions in the image where the ventricular wall could not be visualised, e.g. the apical region in the parasternal long-axis view, the operator was requested to fill in an outline according to his interpretation.

A radial coordinate system was used for the measurements since the short-axis views normally show a circular outline of the ventricle. The centre of this coordinate system was fixed at the geometrical centre of the endocardial outline in end-diastole. In the short-axis views, 0° is in the lateral wall and the polar angle increases counter-clockwise. In the long-axis views 0° is the middle of the base, 180° is always the apex and the angle also increases counter-clockwise. These definitions are illustrated in Figure 2.

Wall thickness as function of the angle could be measured by sampling the endocardial and epicardial outline. Wall thickening could then be computed from wall thickness at end-diastole and end-systole. Since the wall thickening in long-axis views may be unrealistic due to components of ventricular motion perpendicular to the cross-sectional plane, wall thickness and thickening were only measured from the short-axis views. Wall motion was assessed by comparing the endocardial outlines at end-diastole and end-systole.

The endocardial outlines were also used for calculation of the cross-sectional surface areas of the ventricle. Together with the length of the ventricular long-axis which was measured from the endocardial outline in apical views, these areas are commonly used in estimations of end-diastolic and end-systolic volumes, stroke volumes and ejection fractions [4].

ASSESSMENT OF VARIABILITY

The accuracy of an echocardiographic measurement is limited by two main sources of error [5]. The first is a systematic error or bias, the second is random error.

The influence of bias in measurements can be estimated by comparing the measured with the true value. Usually in clinical measurements the true values are unknown and comparisons can only be made with values obtained from other quantitative methods, which are also subjected to bias. Thus only the difference in bias for both methods is shown. In most of the echocardiographic measurements this difference is a constant that can be eliminated by making use of regression equations obtained from in-vitro calibration experiments and/or from comparative angiographic or scintigraphic studies. The random error in measurements can be demonstrated by repeating the measurement. The outcome of the second measurement rarely equals that of the first. The standard deviation of the random error can be computed from paired measurments using the Grubbs estimator [6]. Random error can be eliminated by avering the results of multiple measurements.

An accurate separation of bias and random error can only be carried out if a sufficient amount of measurements is performed. In clinical research this requirement can not always be met. In the study described in this paper, the two sources of error could not be studied separately and therefore only variability was assessed.

Possible causes of this variability are:
— limitations in resolution for digitisation of outlines;
— limitations in operator accuracy in defining the outlines;
— changes in the operator's interpretation in defining the outlines;
— limitations of operator accuracy in finding the same plane;
— changes in the operator's interpretation in finding the same plane;
— differences of interpretation between different observers.

In order to study the causes of variability four experiments, described below, were performed. In each of these experiments a set of paired measurements (x_i, y_i) was obtained. From n paired measurements a standard deviation s was computed as:

$$s = \sqrt{\frac{1}{2n} \sum_{i=1}^{n} (x_i - y_i)^2} \tag{1}$$

this standard deviation s gives an indication of the accuracy of the measurments [7].

Experiment A: two observers performed the examination procedure independently on the same twenty subjects, both observers also carried out the computer-aided analysis. By computing the standard deviations s from these paires of measurements the inter-observer variability could be demonstrated.

Experiment B: one operator repeated the examination and analysis on the same group of subjects after three months. This delay was used to ascertain the independency between the measurements, making the assumption that cardiac anatomy did not change in this time interval. By computing s from these paires the intra-observer variability could be demonstrated.

Experiment C: one observer repeated the computer-aided analysis on the recording that was used in experiment B. In this way the variability caused by the examination was eliminated and by computing s, the variability caused by the analysis was demonstrated.

Experiment D: one observer performed the analysis on two consecutive beats from the tape that was used in experiment B. Although the pairs of measurements created in this way may not be regarded to be independent, computation of s gave an indication of the limitations in operator accuracy in defining outlines and system resolution in digitisation, since the changes in the operators interpretation in defining the outlines were eliminated.

NORMAL WALL MOTION

From the end-diastolic and end-systolic outlines that were digitised from the video-recordings of the group of normal subjects, the average amplitudes of wall motion at comparable sites in different subjects were computed. In each cross-sectional view, the average amplitude of wall motion at each angle between 0° and 360° was expressed in mm. The standard deviation in the group was also calculated for each angle. These average amplitudes of motion and standard deviations are graphically displayed in Figure 3 and are discussed for each cross-section separately. In the graphs of Figure 3 each horizontal axis corresponds to the polar angle and each vertical axis gives the wall motion amplitude in mm.

In the parasternal long-axis view the regions between 0° and 45° and between 315° and 360° correspond to the cardiac base. The inward motion of the cardiac base at 0° is shown to be about 13 mm. From Figure 2 it can be seen that the regions around 90° and 270° correspond to the septum and the posterior wall respectively. The average amplitude of wall motion in these two regions are 5 mm and 4 mm respectively. For the septum this is close to the normal range as obtained from M-mode echocardiography [8].

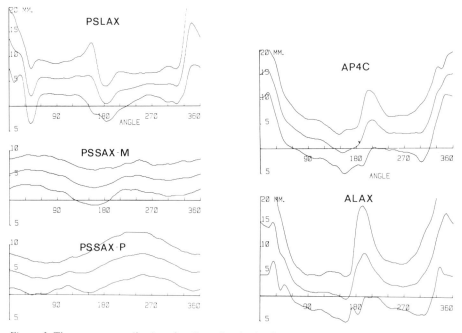

Figure 3. The average amplitudes of wall motion in the five cross sections expressed in mm for each angle in the radial coordinate system. For each cross-section the middle curve shows the average amplitude of wall motion for the group of twenty clinical normal subjects. The upper and lower curve delineate the range of plus or minus one standard deviation.

The region around 180° corresponding to the cardiac apex shows very little motion. This result may be misleading since in most recordings the wall in this region is not well visualised and outlines often result from the operators subjective interpretation only.

In the parasternal short-axis view at mitral level the region around 90° corresponds to the septum and the region at 270° corresponds to the posterior wall. As in the parasternal long-axis view the amplitude of motion in these regions is 5 and 4 mm respectively. The amplitude of motion is reasonably uniform around the ventricular circumference, apart from the region around 150°. In the parasternal short-axis view at papillary level the wall motion is not uniform around the circumference. It can be seen that the posterior wall (around 300°) has a larger amplitude of motion than the septum (around 120°). The average amplitude of wall motion at these sites is comparable to the normal range as measured from M-mode [8].

In the apical four-chamber view the motion of the cardiac base, (located around 0°), was found to be 15 mm. This amplitude is larger than the amplitude found in the parasternal long-axis view. The difference between them may be explained by the fact that the cardiac base is defined from the attachments of the aortic and mitral valve in the parasternal long-axis view and from the attachments of both mitral valve leaflets in the apical four-chamber view. The amplitude of septal motion (in the region around 270°) is about 3 mm and the amplitude for the lateral wall (90°) is small.

In the apical long-axis view the motion of the base is found to be 15 mm. In this cross-sectional view the septum (90°) shows little motion and the posterior wall (270°) has an only slightly higher amplitude.

NORMAL WALL THICKENING

The same display format as for the average amplitude of wall motion is used for the average amplitudes of wall thickening. In Figure 4 the amplitudes are displayed in mm as a function of the angle between 0° and 360°. Note the similarities between the curves of amplitudes of wall thickening and those of wall motion as shown in Figure 3.

In the parasternal short-axis view at mitral level, the aplitude of wall thickening is approximately uniform around the circumference, again apart from the region around 150°. The average amplitude of thickening for most angles is about 2 mm. Also in the view at papillary level the region around 150° shows little wall thickening. In this cross-sectional plane the posterior wall (around 270°) shows a larger thickening than the septum (around 90°). The amplitudes of wall thickening for these two regions are 2 mm and 4 mm respectively.

138

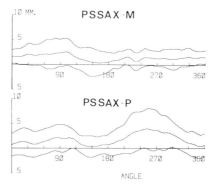

Figure 4. The average amplitudes of wall thickening in the two parasternal short-axis views expressed in mm for each angle.

VARIABILITY FOR WALL DYNAMICS

In previous paragraphs the average amplitudes of the dynamic parameters of the left ventricular wall (wall motion and thickening) were described. The variations in these parameters in normal subjects were indicated by the upper and lower curves on the graphs giving the range of plus or minus one standard deviation.

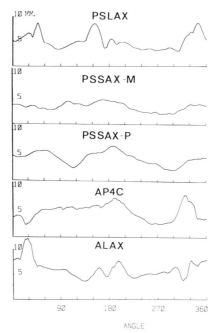

Figure 5. The inter-observer variations in measurement of wall motion expressed in mm for each angle. These values were calculated from the differences in wall motion as measured by two different observers.

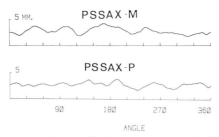

Figure 6. The standard deviation of variability in measurement of wall thickening expressed in mm. These values were calculated from the differences in wall thickening as found by two independent observers.

The inter-observer variations in measuring wall motion and thickening were assessed by computing standard deviations s according to equation (1) in experiment A. These measures for inter-observer variability are shown in Figure 5 for wall motion in all cross-sections, and in Figure 6 for wall thickening in both short-axis views. The standard deviations are calculated for each angle between 0° and 360° and they are expressed in mm.

In the long-axis views (PSLAX, AP4C and ALAX) the cardiac base areas are stongly subject to inter-observer variability for measured wall motion, as are the regions around the apex.

For measured wall motion of the septum s is 3 mm in PSLAX, 3 mm in PSSAX-M, 2½ mm in PSSAX-P and 2 mm in AP4C. The standard deviation s for wall motion measurements of the posterior wall is 3 mm in PSLAX, 2 mm in PSSAX-M, 2 mm in PSSAX-P and 5 mm in ALAX. For the lateral wall in AP4C the standard deviation in wall motion measurements is 5 mm.

Around the ventricular circumference in the parasternal short-axis view at mitral level, the standard deviation s for measurements of wall thickening is 2½ mm on average. This is the same as for the parasternal short-axis view at papillary level.

VARIABILITY IN AREA AND LENGTH

The surface area within the endocardial outline in end-diastole and end-systole is measured from the two parasternal short-axis views and from the two apical views. The length of the ventricular long-axis is measured from the apical four-chamber and the apical long-axis views. For each of the four experiments A-D the standard deviation s was calculated. These results are shown in Tables 1 and 2.

Since the number of measurements is small, the accuracy of these estimates is not high, which is illustrated by the fact that intra-observer

Table 1. The standard deviation of variability in measurement of long-axis length from the apical views in end-diastole (ED) and end-systole (ES). All values are in mm.

Experiment	AP4C		ALAX	
	ED (mm)	ES (mm)	ED (mm)	ES (mm)
A	8.3	5.0	7.8	13.0
B	7.1	7.3	5.8	7.8
C	3.4	5.1	5.1	8.0
D	2.2	1.9	4.0	3.5

Table 2. The standard deviation of variability in measurement of surface area within the endocardial outline in end-diastole and end-systole. All values in mm^2.

Experiment	PSSAX-M		PSSAX-P		AP4C		ALAX	
	ED mm^2	ES mm^2	ED mm^2	ES mm^2	ED mm^2	ES mm^2	ED mm^2	ES mm^2
A	520	380	320	290	620	350	480	670
B	200	190	250	190	420	420	550	390
C	220	210	180	200	260	280	370	480
D	150	80	110	120	190	110	220	130

variations were sometimes found to be higher than inter-observer-variations and therefore care must be taken in drawing conclusions from these data.

From Table 1 it can be seen that the standard deviations for measurements of length in the apical four-chamber view are lower than in the apical long-axis view. Therefore measurements of long-axis length should be performed in the apical four-chamber view.

For all views the differences in s between experiment C and D are large. This is an indication that beat-to-beat variations in measurements are large. From the differences in s between the experiments B and C it can be seen that reperforming the recording does not give rise to the value of s for the short-axis views and does give rise to a high value of s in the apical views. The differences between inter-observer and intra-observer variations can be seen from experiments A and B. In the apical views the inter-observer variations are not consistently higher than the intra-observer variations. In the short-axis views they are.

DISCUSSION

Since the five views that were used were all cross-sections of the same ventricle, one might expect that values for average amplitude of wall motion at equal sites but in different views would be equal. For instance the septum in PSLAX at 60° corresponds roughly to the septum in PSSAX-M at 120°. However, from the curves for average amplitude of motion in these two views different values for the amplitude of motion are found. This is explained by the fact that for each cross-section a specific coordinate system is defined. For wall motion at comparable sites in different views one can only compare the corresponding vectorial components. From this point of view, great care must be taken in comparing the results of this study to normal ranges obtained by other methods like M-mode and angiography. One comparison that actually can be made is the basal displacement which correlates very well with angio observations [9].

Since the plane for the apical long-axis view is roughly the same as for the parasternal long-axis view, the discrepancies for the amplitudes of wall motion for these two cross-sections are not easily understood. One explanation is that in the parasternal view a large portion of the ventricular wall is perpendicular to the ultrasound beam whereas in the apical view, for these areas the direction of the beam is along the endocardial surface. Thus the definition of echo targets differs for both planes resulting in drop-outs in one view versus good visualisation in the other. The problems in target definition also extend to research on fully automated outline definition. Although it may be expected that further automation will reduce random error in outline definition thus offering a more consistent measurement, this is not a guarantee for better measurements.

Although simple geometrical models can be used for estimation of left ventricular volume, the heart has a complex geometry. Due to this, the contraction of the cardiac wall is not uniform and wall motion is not understood completely at present. The complex motion of the entire ventricle during systole is illustrated by the differences in amplitudes for septum and posterior wall in both short-axis views. The findings in this study may contribute to a better understanding of left ventricular behavior in normal subjects.

In Tables 1 and 2 the results of assessment of variability in measurement of length and area are listed. The standard deviations are given in mm and mm^2 respectively. By dividing these values by the average values for length and area, the relative errors in measurements can be calculated as percentages. From these computations it was found that inter-observer variability for length measurements ranges from 5% to 15% and for area from 10% to 20%. If the volume is calculated from a mathematical model that employs one measurement of area and one of length, the variability in the computed volume may range from 15% to 35%. These findings provide an explanation for the poor correlation between the ejection fraction as estimated from two-dimensional echocardiography and that from other quantitative methods. Calculating volume from a mathematical model that uses measurements

142

in more than one view may result in even higher variability, unless a scan-arm is used to determine the spacial orientation of the different views.

CONCLUSIONS

Since the spread in measured wall motion and wall thickening between normal subjects is large, and since the inter-observer variability in these measurements is of the same magnitude as the measured values, it can be concluded that quantitative left ventricular analysis from two-dimensional echocardiography as performed in the way described in this paper, will not yield acceptable results for individual subjects. However, if the results of multiple measurements are averaged, more accurate results can be obtained. In the study on the group of healthy subjects, the measurements on twenty subjects were used to obtain average amplitudes of wall motion and wall thickening. In clinical practice averaging of measurements on one subject is nearly impossible. Therefore the usefulness of quantitative analysis is restricted to physiological studies on groups of subjects only.

Further automation in quantitative analysis may not be expected to reduce variability sufficiently. From the discussion on the contents of Tables 1 and 2 it is concluded that beat-to-beat variations are large. For the short-axis views the inter-observer variations are the most important source of variability and for the long-axis views the recording procedure.

Reduction of variability can therefore better be accomplished by improving standardisation in recording. Such standardisation however, would set aside the specific advantage of echo-techniques: the flexible way in which examinations can be made.

ACKNOWLEDGEMENTS

The research on quantitative left ventricular analysis from two-dimensional echocardiography is sponsored by the Dutch Heart Foundation. The authors wish to thank J. Lubsen, C. Slager, J. Vogel and N. Bom for their continuous interest and helpful discussions.

REFERENCES

1. Bastiaans OL, PW Verbeek, JA Vogel, FJ ten Cate: Interactive segmentation of video recorded echocardiographic images. Computers in Cardiology, IEEE Computer Society, Long Beach, California, 1979.
2. Bastiaans OL, RS Meltzer, JA Vogel, PW Verbeek, JRT Roelandt: Quantitative

left ventricular analysis from two-dimensional echoes. Computers in Cardiology, IEEE Computer Society, Long Beach, California, 1980.

3. Meltzer RS, C Meltzer, JRT Roelandt: Sector-scanning views in echocardiology: a systematic approach. Eur. Heart J (In press).
4. Folland ED, AF Parisi, PF Moynihan, DR Johnes, CL Feldman, DE Tow: Assessment of left ventricular ejection fraction and volumes by real-time two-dimensional echocardiography. Circulation 60, No. 4, 1979.
5. Lubsen J: Determination and consequences of bias and random error in echocardiographic measurements. In: Echocardiology (Lancée CT, ed.), Martinus Nijhoff, The Hague, 1979.
6. Grubbs FE: On estimating precision of measuring instruments and product variability. J Amer Statistics Ass 43, 1948.
7. Barnett RN: Clinical Laboratory Statistics. Little, Brown and Company, Boston.
8. Roelandt JRT: Practical echocardiology. In: Ultrasound in Biomedicine (White D, ed.), Vol. 1, Research Studies Press, Forest Grove, Oregon, 1977.
9. Slager CJ, TEH Hooghoudt, JHC Reiber, JCH Schuurbiers, F Booman, GT Meester: Left ventricular contour segmentation from anatomical landmark trajectories and its application to wall motion analysis. Computers in Cardiology, IEEE Computer Society, Long Beach, California, 1979.

17. QUANTITATIVE ANALYSIS OF THE ADULT LEFT HEART BY ECHOCARDIOGRAPHY

NELSON B. SCHILLER, THOMAS A. PORTS,
and NORMAN H. SILVERMAN

M-mode echocardiography provides linear measurements of the left ventricular cavity and walls and the left atrial cavity. These widely used variables provide important, usually reliable, information about the integrity and status of left ventricular function. It is common practice to derive volume estimations (three-dimensional information) from these linear dimensions. However, linear dimensions can provide only limited information and are a potential source of significant error. Many of the failings of M-mode echocardiography as a quantitative tool can be traced directly to its inability to examine the entire left heart and, thus, to its failure to insure against misrepresentation of an entire structure by unrepresentative samples. The development of two-dimensional echocardiographic techniques promised to partially circumvent this problem. Two-dimensional systems present left ventricular anatomy in a tomographic format and most permit simultaneous visualization of all parts of the left ventricle lying in a given projection. They also permit utilization of a variety of imaging windows, such as the subcostal or apical. With the introduction of apical two-dimensional imaging [1, 2, 3] our group, as well as others, demonstrated that this approach permitted

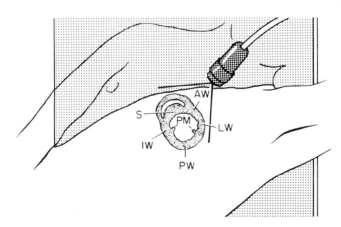

Figure 1a. Transducer position and beam plane for imaging the left ventricle in the short axis. PM = papillary muscles; S = septum; AW = anterior wall; PW = posterior wall; IW = inferior wall; LW = lateral wall. (Reprinted from Schiller, NB, et al. Circulation 60:547, 1979. By permission of the American Heart Association Inc.).

Rijsterborgh H, ed: Echocardiology, p 145-161. All rights reserved.

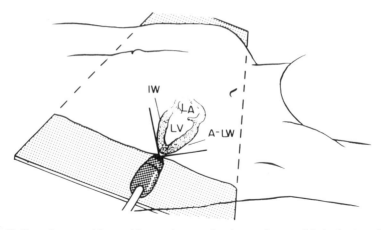

Figure 1b. Transducer position and beam plane used to image the ventricle in the two-chamber, long-axis apical view. LA = left atrium; LV = left ventricle; IW = inferior wall; A-LW = anterolateral wall. (Reprinted from Schiller, NB, et al. Circulation 60:547, 1979. By permission of the American Heart Association Inc.).

noninvasive measurement of left ventricular volumes. As we shall discuss, these methods, in contrast to M-mode echocardiography, are relatively uncompromised by the presence of segmental wall motion abnormalities and are thus applicable to patients with coronary artery disease.

The initial method for volume determination validated in our laboratory [2] utilized biplane methodology by employing the long-axis apical two-chamber view combined with a parasternal short-axis view through the level of the left ventricular minor axis (Figure 1). Subsequently, other groups have employed variations on this approach or a single plane method [4, 5, 6].

In our study, we prospectively performed M-mode and biplane two-dimensional echocardiograms of the left ventricles of forty-two patients, who also underwent biplane cineangiography (right anterior oblique and left anterior oblique). Of the forty-two patients, thirty had satisfactory studies with both techniques. In six patients, the echocardiograms were technically inadequate and in six, the angiograms. Of the thirty patients who remained, the majority (21) had coronary disease, six had valvular disease, two had atrial septal defects and one was normal. Of the twenty-one patients with coronary disease, sixteen had segmental wall motion abnormalities. The two patients with atrial defects also had a segmental abnormality of wall motion, in that septal motion was paradoxical.

Biplane diastolic and systolic tracings were performed from both the echocardiogram and the angiogram. In tracing the echocardiogram, it was necessary to affix exposed X-ray film to the video screen and, using a wax pencil, outline the ventricular cavity on the film. This particular approach was extremely difficult, owing to considerable parallax error introduced by the thick glass partitioning the observer from the video screen. In the course

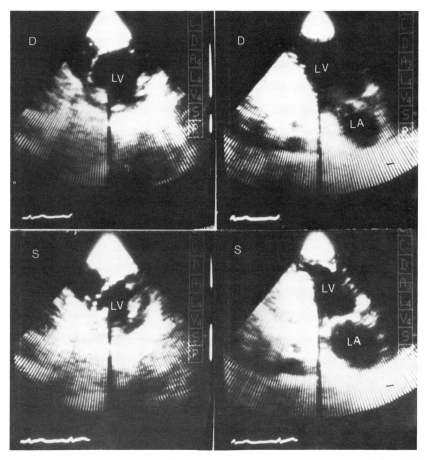

Figure 1c. Upper Left: Diastolic (D) frame of short-axis echogram recorded on Polaroid film. Lower Left: Systolic (S) frame of same beat. Upper Right: Diastolic frame of the long-axis, two-chamber view echogram, recorded on Polaroid film. Lower Right: Systolic frame from the same beat. LV = left ventricle; LA = left atrium.

of completing this study, inter- and intra-observer variation were also studied and both were 10% or less. By the time this phase of the study was performed, a lightpen computational system, developed commercially by Varian Associates, Palo Alto, California, was available [7]. This system allowed the operator to trace the outline of the left ventricle directly onto the video screen phosphor. From these tracings, the computer automatically calculated ventricular volume using a variety of algorithms. This latter feature bypassed the tedious calculations inherent in the execution of volume algorithms. As noted above, in our study, only the combination of precordial short-axis and apical two-chamber long-axis views was used. This choice of views was dictated by the fact that our biplane angiograms were performed in the right anterior oblique and left anterior oblique projections, which, in many ways, resemble short-axis and apical two-chamber echocardiographic views. All volume calculations in our study were performed according to the method of Georke and Carlsson [8]. In this method, computations are based on a modification of Simpson's Rule. The two orthogonal projections are oriented along their common axis and ventricular endocardial outlines are manually digitized. From the hand-traced outlines, the computer automatically divides each projection into twenty sections along a common axis and the volume is calculated according to the formula:

$$V = \frac{F\pi}{4} \sum_{i=1}^{20} a_i b_i$$

We found poor correlations between volumes and volume ejection fractions derived from M-mode echocardiographic measurements and those from angiography (Figure 2). However, the correlations between two-dimensional echocardiography and angiography ranged from acceptable to excellent (Figures 3, 4, 5). Of particular note was that the ejection fraction was accurately predicted noninvasively, suggesting that two-dimensional technique was sensitive to wall motion abnormalities. Correlations between diastolic volume by echocardiography and angiography were weakest. Both systolic volume and ejection fraction, on the other hand, correlated well with

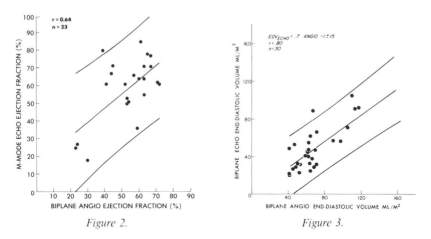

Figure 2.   Figure 3.

Figure 2. Biplane angiographic volumes and ejection fraction are plotted against volume and ejection fraction calculated from M-mode echocardiograms in twenty-three patients. Outer lines are the 95% confidence limits of the data. Angiographic ejection fraction vs. M-mode. (Reprinted from Schiller, NB, et al. Circulation 60:547, 1979. By permission of the American Heart Association, Inc.).

Figure 3. Biplane angiographic (ANGIO) end diastolic volumes are plotted against biplane echocardiographic end diastolic volume (EDV_{ECHO}) in thirty patients. Outer lines are the 95% confidence limits of the data. The standard error of the estimate is given at the end of the equation. (Reprinted from Schiller, NB, et al. Circulation 60:547, 1979. By permission of the American Heart Association, Inc.).

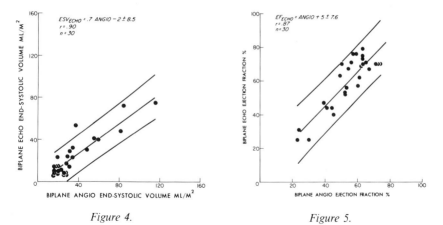

Figure 4.   *Figure 5.*

Figure 4. Biplane angiographic (ANGIO) end systolic volume plotted against biplane echocardiographic end systolic volume (ESV_{ECHO}) in thirty patients. Outer lines are the 95% confidence limits of the data. (Reprinted from Schiller, NB, et al. Circulation 60:547, 1979. By permission of the American Heart Association, Inc.).

Figure 5. Biplane angiographic (ANGIO) ejection fraction, plotted against biplane echocardiographic ejection fraction (EF_{ECHO}) in thirty patients. Outer lines are the 95% confidence limits of the data. (Reprinted from Schiller NB, et al. Circulation 60:547, 1979. By permission of the American Heart Association, Inc.).

angiography, but for both systole and diastole there was a bothersome systematic underestimation of volume which ranged between 20% and 30%. Furthermore, the scatter of the data which appeared when correlating echocardiographic diastolic volume with angiographic diastolic volume was of sufficient magnitude to make small, but important, changes in diastolic ventricular size somewhat difficult to detect with confidence. Thus, with two-dimensional echocardiography as with M-mode echocardiography, important technical limitations were present. However, it is probably more important that this technique can be used confidently in the setting of segmental disease and over the entire range of ventricular volumes. Thus, the two-dimensional technique has definite advantages over the M-mode approach in that it can be applied to ventricles which represent the entire spectrum of size and shape.

This chapter is primarily concerned with the development and application of quantitative two-dimensional echocardiography in adults. It is, however, relevant to summarize our studies in children because many of our findings in this population are likely to be applicable to adults.

In order to develop a two-dimensional method of measuring left ventricular volume in children, we evaluated a number of children undergoing cardiac catheterization for suspected congenital heart disease [9]. This population differed importantly from the adult population. In the children, biplane angiograms were performed in the postero-anterior and lateral

150

projections. Echocardiograms were performed from the apex impulse in orthogonal long-axis views (two- and four-chamber). Left ventricular volumes were obtained from these orthogonal views at end-systole and end-diastole by analyzing them separately by the single plane area-length and biplane Simpson's Rule methods. Left ventricular volumes derived from the various algorithms were compared to volumes from Simpson's Rule analysis of biplane angiograms in the same patients by regression analysis. When the results of these comparisons in pediatric patients were compared with our initial adult studies, the former provided a noninvasive prediction of angiographic systolic and diastolic volumes which was uniformly more accurate. Of the various algorithms tested in the pediatric study, biplane methods were slightly superior to the others, but the single plane approach was highly satisfactory (Figure 6) [9]. It is noteworthy that, even an ideal

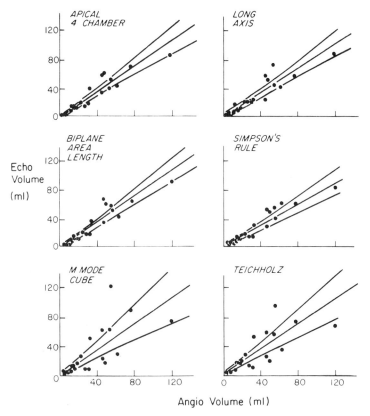

Figure 6. Comparison between various echocardiographic methods and angiography for calculating end diastolic volume. The regression line, and weighted 95% confidence limits for the line are displayed and data points are shown for each comparison. Note that the two-dimensional techniques are superior to M-mode methods (Cube and Teichholz correction). Among the two-dimensional methods, the biplane methods offered more effective prediction of angiographic measurements. (Reprinted from Silverman, NH, et al. Circulation 62:548, 1980. By permission of the American Heart Association, Inc.)

pediatric subject with high quality images in a geometrically uniform left ventricle, two-dimensional determinations were clearly superior to highly touted M-mode extrapolations. Furthermore, diastolic volumes were of sufficient accuracy to be clinically useful, and the systematic underestimation present in an adult study was not found. While these results may not be completely applicable to adult patients, they and another recent report [6] suggest that for routine applications, single plane analysis may be adequate. It should be cautioned, however, that in the setting of a a grossly deformed or misshapen ventricle, simple, single plane quantitative methods may be unreliable.

In the routine clinical application of the experimental work recounted above, we find that the selective use of quantitative two-dimensional techniques for estimating left ventricular volumes and ejection fraction is of considerable value. However, in the majority of patients, we are satisfied with a qualitative, visual estimation of left ventricular function. On the other hand, in patients with tachycardias, large segmental defects, or qualitatively borderline left ventricular function, a visual, qualitative assessment of left ventricular function is unreliable, and the ability to measure ejection fraction quantitatively is clinically useful. Since biplane measurements require meticulously executed technique and are time consuming, we almost always employ a single plane area-length analysis for calculating volume ejection fraction in relatively symmetrical ventricles. We have also found that a simple *area* ejection fraction closely approximates the value which would be obtained by measuring volume ejection fraction. In all echocardiographic volume determinations, particularly if one is to employ single plane analysis of a single projection, it is of utmost importance that the endocardium be accurately imaged (Figure 7). In ventricles that are not uniform, we rely almost exclusively on biplane Simpson's Rule, either combining the short-axis with the two-chamber view or using paired apical views. No matter what algorithm is employed, it is essential that the endocardium be visualized.

The left ventricle can be quantitatively imaged using radionuclides. This application of nuclear cardiology has grown very rapidly. The analysis of left ventricular function by radioisotopic methods has the advantage of being nearly automated and, thus, much less physician intensive. As shown in Figure 8, in fourteen of our patients (all with ischemic heart disease), the agreement between nuclear and echocardiographic methods was strong, suggesting that the methods were interchangeable [10]. Thus, if either method has yielded technically satisfactory images of the left ventricle, then the other method need not be repeated merely for the sake of obtaining another measurement of left ventricular ejection fraction. Close agreement between nuclear methods and echocardiography has also been demonstrated by Folland et al. [5].

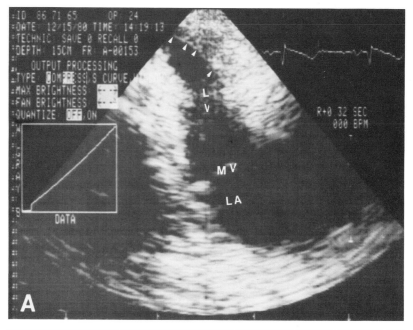

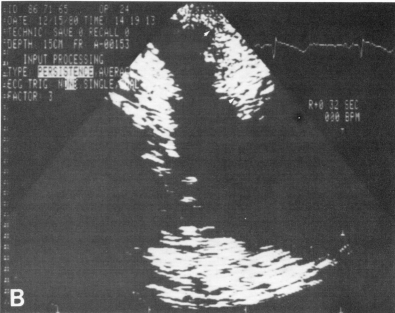

Figure 7. Two computer-processed, digitized, hard copies of an end-systolic apical two-chamber view freeze frame of the left ventricle (LV), showing the effect of two gray scale settings on endocardial visualization.

Panel A: Arrows point to the lateral apical endocardium which is well seen at nearly full gray scale. The gray scale is graphically shown in the middle left portion of the image.

Panel B: Arrow demonstrates artifactual border of the lateral apex caused by use of an abbreviated gray scale

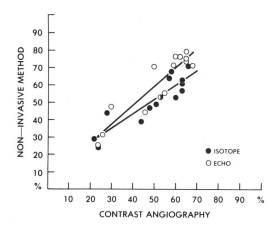

Figure 8. Fourteen patients with coronary disease underwent angiography, quantitative two-dimensional echocardiography, and blood-pool radioisotope ventriculography. Noninvasively calculated volume ejection fractions (ordinate) are plotted against angiography. Note that there was little, if any, difference between the relationship of either noninvasive technique to angiography, suggesting that in this study neither technique had any particular advantage over the other.

Another important way in which echocardiography can be used to evaluate left ventricular function is in the detection and evaluation of regional segmental wall motion abnormalities [11]. Two-dimensional echocardiography accurately identifies left ventricular aneurysms [12] both at the cardiac apex and the base. In addition to aneurysms, two-dimensional echocardiography has been found to be effective in the identification of most, if not all, segments which are hypokinetic, akinetic, or dyskinetic. In our own laboratory, agreement between angiographic and echocardiographic means of assessing regional wall motion ranged from 80% to 90%, depending on the habits of the individual reading the echocardiogram. To date, quantitative evaluation of wall motion has not been accomplished.

In the assessment of left ventricular function, we have found the evaluation of left atrial size by echocardiography extremely useful. In the presence of sinus rhythm and in the absence of significant mitral insufficiency, the left atrium can serve as a barometer of the diastolic properties of the left ventricle. In order to compare the traditional M-mode echocardiographic measurements of left atrial size with a two-dimensional method of measuring left atrial volume, we examined twelve patients by echocardiography. The results of volume analysis of the echocardiograms were compared with left atrial volumes obtained from levo-phase angiograms. The echocardiographic views used and the method of tracing the left atriums are demonstrated in Figures 9 and 10.

The algorithms used were biplane Simpson's Rule and single plane area-length. The lightpen computational system described above was used to

154

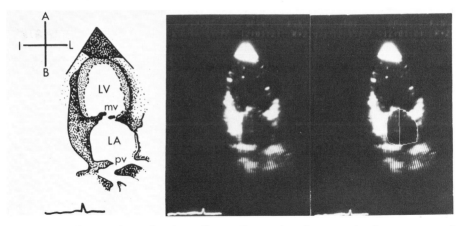

Figure 9. Stop-frame end-systolic echocardiogram from patient demonstrating the appearance of the left atrium (LA) in the two-chamber view. Of all the views used, this particular one appears to give the best definition of the atrial walls. Note that the pulmonary veins (pv) seen posteriorly are not included in the tracing. The atrial appendage, often seen in this view, is not seen in this particular patient. Where seen, it was excluded.

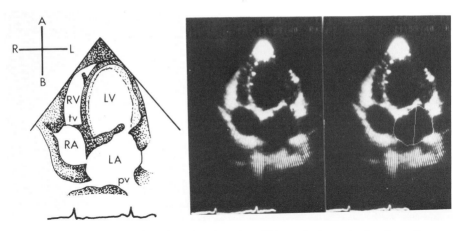

Figure 10. Echocardiogram of the four-chamber view. This particular patient's echocardiogram was chosen because it demonstrates the location and appearance of the pulmonary veins (PV). Note that the posterior wall of the left atrium (LA) is assumed to continue along a curvilinear course through the upper and middle portion of the confluence of these veins. The dropout of the inner atrial septum is exaggerated on this stop-frame image. A = apex; B = base; LA = left atrium; LV = left ventricle; pv = pulmonary veins; RA = right atrium; RV = right ventricle; tv = tricuspid valve.

trace the outlines and measure the chamber length. This instrument automatically combined the paired biplane views of the atrium from the long-axis apical two- and four-chamber views, as well as measuring each of these views singly with a simple area-length algorithm. M-mode estimations of left atrial volume correlated poorly with angiography in our study (Figures 11, 12), but

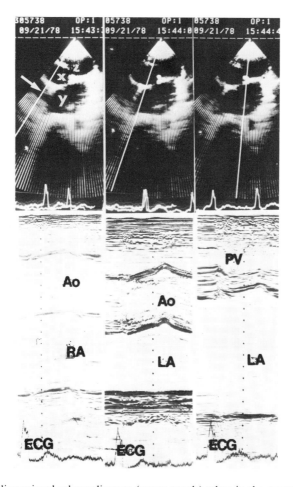

Figure 11. Two-dimensional echocardiogram (upper panels) taken in the parasternal short-axis through the base of the heart of a patient with an enlarged left atrium. While the two-dimensional image was displayed and recorded, an M-mode was performed. The bright line which runs the length of the fan-shaped display (arrows) represents the path of the M-mode beam. In the left upper panel, the beam passes through the aortic root (x), but misses the left atrium (y), passing instead through the right atrium. The M-mode display (lower left) shows what appears to be a normal-sized aorta and left atrium (distance between depth marks = 0.5 cm). In the upper middle panel, the beam now passes through the middle of the aortic root and a normal-sized left atrium. In the upper right panel, the beam is now to the left of the aorta, passing through the pulmonary valve and artery (z), left main coronary artery origin, and left atrium. The simultaneous M-mode (lower right panel) shows the pulmonary valve (PV) and the enlarged left atrium.

both single plane area-length and biplane Simpson's Rule measurements correlated well (Figures 13, 14) [13].

Clinically, left atrial volume determination has been consistently useful. Visually, it is often difficult to tell whether an atrium is enlarged. For example, in the apical four-chamber view, the perception of the size of any

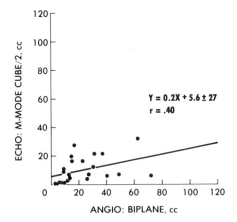

Figure 12. Left atrial volume obtained from biplane analysis of levo-phase left atrial angiograms was compared to linear M-mode dimensions by regression analysis.

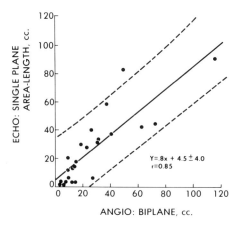

Figure 13. Left atrial volumes obtained from biplane analysis of levo-phase angiograms are compared to those volumes obtained from single plane analysis of the parasternal long axis view of the left atrium. The dashed lines are the 95% confidence limits.

given chamber often depends on the size of its neighbors; a large left ventricle can make an atrium appear smaller than it really is. Since the borders of the left atrium are usually fairly clear, we measure left atrial volume in the majority of our adult patients, in whom we consider 40 ml the upper limit of normal.

The thickness of the left ventricular septum and posterior wall has long been considered another important quantitative parameter which describes the state of the left ventricle. It is current practice in some laboratories to extrapolate left ventricular mass from M-mode measurements of wall thickness [14]. While correlation between these methods and post-mortem left ventricular weights has been satisfactory, these methods have the same

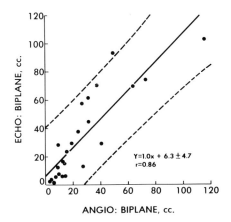

Figure 14. Left atrial volume obtained from biplane analysis of levo-phase left atrial angiograms is compared to volume information derived from biplane analysis of paired apical echocardiograms.

failings as the M-mode measurement of left ventricular volume in that a single beam technique, interrogating a small portion of the left ventricle, is used to make assumptions about quantitative global geometry. Two-dimensional echocardiography affords a noninvasive method of imaging most of the left ventricle. It is reasonable to assume that if the left ventricular cavity volume can be measured with reasonable accuracy, then left ventricular wall volume and, therefore, wall mass could similarly be measured accurately. In order to approach this problem, we sought to develop an anatomically logical algorithm based on a truncated ellipsoid as a model. This algorithm was derived by the method of concentric discs (Figure 15) and allowed calculation of the volume of concentric truncated ellipsoids, and, from their differences, wall volume. The product of wall volume and myocardial density (1.05 g/ml) provided an estimation of left ventricular mass. In the lower equation in the figure, the expression on the left is the volume of the shell or outer ellipsoid from which the expression on the right, the volume of

$$V = \pi \left\{ (b+t)^2 \int_0^{d+a+t} \left[1 - \frac{(x-d)^2}{(a+t)^2} \right] dx - b^2 \int_0^{d+a} \left[1 - \frac{(x-d)^2}{a^2} \right] dx \right\} =$$

$$\pi \left\{ (b+t)^2 \left[\tfrac{2}{3}(a+t) + d - \frac{d^3}{3(a+t)^2} \right] - b^2 \left[\tfrac{2}{3}a + d - \frac{d^3}{3a^2} \right] \right\}$$

MASS = 1.05 V

Figure 15. Formula derived from ellipse equation by integration – (Method of concentric cylindrical discs/washers). t = mean left ventricular wall thickness; b = minor axis radius inner ellipsoid; a = semi-major axis inner ellipsoid; d = truncated semi-major axis inner ellipsoid; V = volume.

158

the cavity or inner ellipsoid, is subtracted. To solve this problem, four echocardiographically available variables are required. These variables, depicted in Figure 16, are mean wall thickness (t), length of the semi-minor axis of the inner elipsoid (b), length of the semi-major axis of the inner ellipsoid (a), and length of the truncated semi-major axis of the inner ellipsoid (d). The first of these variables can be obtained from the short-axis view by measuring the total shell area which is bounded by the epicardial parameter. Each area is treated as the area of a circle from which the radius can be calculated. The difference between the radius of the total shell area and the radius of the total cavity area represents the mean wall thickness (Figure 17). This method is useful by itself to estimate mean mid wall thickness. The semi-minor axis was obtained from the short axis measured from the long-axis view. The location of the semi-minor axis was chosen as being just apical to the tip of the mitral valve. This location is considered the center of the inner and outer ellipsoids. The distance from the center of the ellipsoids to the apex is the semi-major axis, and the distance from the center to the middle of the mitral valve, the truncated semi-major axis. We tested this algorithm and the approach to the measurement of left ventricular mass by performing echocardiograms on ten litter-matched beagle dogs, five of whom underwent aortic banding 6–8 weeks prior to measurement and five of whom were unoperated controls. Following echocardiography of the left ventricle, the animals were sacrificed within one to two hours, and the isolated left ventricle was weighed. This weight was compared to the

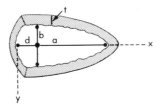

Figure 16. Variables of mass formula: t = mean left ventricular wall thickness; b = minor axis radius inner ellipsoid; a = semi-major axis inner ellipsoid; d = truncated semi-major axis inner ellipsoid.

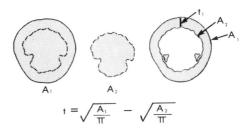

$$t = \sqrt{\frac{A_1}{\pi}} - \sqrt{\frac{A_2}{\pi}}$$

Figure 17. Using a light pen digitizing computer: Mean wall thickness (t) calculated from minor axis/short axis echocardiographic inner and outer areas.

calculated weight. The calculated weight was obtained by programming a programmable calculator with the previously mentioned algorithm and allowing it to solve the equation with the echocardiographic parameters from each dog. The linear relationship and correlation between post-mortem dog heart weights and calculated dog heart weights are shown on Figure 18. Note that the correlation coefficient was high with a good slope and a small standard error of the estimate. Intra-observer variation was 10% [15].

Thus, this study demonstrated that it was possible experimentally to obtain accurate noninvasive measurement of left ventricular mass from two-dimensional echocardiography. In patients in whom we have performed this calculation, we have been impressed by the apparent clinically relevant nature of a noninvasive determination of left ventricular mass. However, the accuracy of this technique is difficult to assess in a clinical setting in that no gold standard for mass, short of autopsy, exists.

In conclusion, we have presented a number of approaches to quantitative evaluation of the left heart by two-dimensional echocardiography. The use of a well designed lightpen digitizing computer system greatly facilitates these measurements can be justified by the relevance of the clinical information

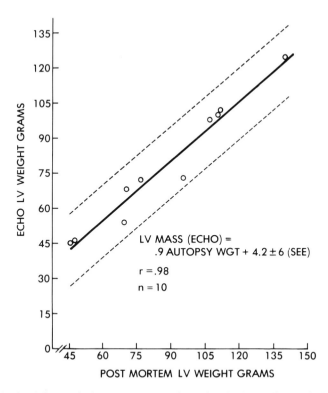

Figure 18. Canine left ventricular mass vs. two-dimensional echocardiographic left ventricular mass.

160

provided. As resolution of echocardiograms improves, it is to be expected that some of these measurements described in this chapter may be performed automatically. The development of automated quantitative echocardiography will greatly enhance the potency of this already indispensible noninvasive imaging technique.

ACKNOWLEDGEMENT

Many individuals have contributed to the work which is described in this study. Among them are Dr. Harry Acquatella, Dr. Dennis Drew, Dr. Claus Skioldebrand, Dr. John Cogan, Dr. Elias Botvinick, Ellen Schiller, Dr. Sergio Schabelman, Dr. Martin Lipton, Yin Yee, Jan Sundstrom and Cathy Cronkhite.

REFERENCES

1. Schiller NB, D Drew, H Acquatella, R Boswell, E Botvinick, B Greenberg, E Carlsson: Noninvasive, biplane quantitation of left ventricular volume and ejection fraction with a real-time two-dimensional echocardiography system. (Abstr) Circulation 54 (suppl II):II–234, 1976.
2. Silverman NH, NB Schiller: Apex echocardiography: a two-dimensional technique for evaluation of congenital heart disease. Circulation 57:503, 1978.
3. Schiller NB, H Acquatella, TA Ports, D Drew, J Goerke, H Ringertz, NH Silverman, B Brundage, EH Botvinick, R Boswell, E Carlsson, WW Parmley: Left ventricular volume from paired biplane two-dimensional echocardiography. Circulation 60:547, 1979.
4. Carr KW, RL Engler, JR Forsythe, AD Johnson, B Gosink: Measurement of left ventricular ejection fraction by mechanical cross-sectional echocardiography. Circulation 59:1196, 1979.
5. Folland D, AF Parisi, PF Moynihan, DR Jones, CL Feldman, DE Tow: Assessment of left ventricular ejection fraction and volumes by real-time two-dimensional echocardiography. Circulation 60:760, 1979.
6. Wyatt HL, MK Heng, S Meerbaum, P Gueret, J Hestenes, E Dula, E Corday: Cross-sectional echocardiography: II. Analysis of mathematic models for quantifying volume of the formalin-fixed left ventricle. Circulation 61:1119, 1980.
7. Daigle R, W Paineter, W Anderson, NB Schiller: A light pen measurement system for cross-sectional echocardiography. Ultrasound in Medicine 4:447–478, 1977.
8. Goerke RJ, E Carlsson: Calculation of right and left cardiac ventricular volumes: method using standard computer equipment and biplane angiograms. Invest Radiol 2:360, 1967.
9. Silverman NH, TA Ports, AR Snider, NB Schiller, E Carlsson, DC Heilbron: Determination of left ventricular volume in children: echocardiographic and angiographic comparisons. Circulation 62:548, 1980.
10. Cogan J, TA Ports, NB Schiller, E Rapaport: The assessment of segmental wall motion by sector echocardiography.Clinical Research 27:3A, 1979.

11. Kisslo JA, D Robertson, BW Gilbert, O vonRamm, VS Behar: A comparison of real-time, two-dimensional echocardiography and cineangiography in detecting left ventricular asynergy. Circulation 55:134, 1977.

12. Weyman AE, SM Peskoe, ES Williams, JC Dillon, H Feigenbaum: Detection of left ventricular aneurysms by cross-sectional echocardiography. Circulation 54:936, 1976.

13. Schabelman S, NB Schiller, TA Ports, NH Silverman, WW Parmley: Left atrial volume by two-dimensional echocardiography. (Abstr) Circulation 58 (suppl II):II–188, 1978.

14. Devereux RB, N Reichek: Echocardiographic determination of left ventricular mass in man. Anatomic validation of the method. Circulation 55:613, 1977.

15. Schiller NB, C Skioldebrand, E Schiller, C Mavroudis, HNS Silverman, S Rahimtoola, M Lipton: In vivo assessment of left ventricular mass by two-dimensional echocardiography. Circulation Publ II, 60:58, 1979.

18. DETERMINATION OF LEFT VENTRICULAR VOLUME FROM APICAL ORTHOGONAL TWO-DIMENSIONAL ECHOCARDIOGRAMS

R. Jenni, A. Vieli, J. Turina, M. Anliker, and H.P. Krayenbuehl

1. INTRODUCTION

Recently published evaluations of the left ventricular volume from two-dimensional echocardiographic images [1, 2, 3] showed that the technique resulted in underestimates when compared with cineangiographic measurements. An attempt has been made to reduce this systematic error by a judicious choice of the echographic planes from which the left ventricular volume is determined, assuming an ellipsoidal shape of the cavity.

2. METHOD

The study is based on data from 42 cardiac patients 14 of whom had coronary artery disease with wall motion abnormalities. Volumetric measurements were made first by means of biplane two-dimensional echocardiography and then by biplane angiography. A phased-array system (Varian V-3000) was used for the ultrasound determinations.

The two planes selected for echocardiographic recording were views from the same transducer position at the apex of the heart. One of these was the conventional apical four-chamber view. The other was the "RAO-equivalent" view, which is obtained by rotating the transducer through 90°, about the main axis. It includes the left ventricular outflow tract whose area is taken into account in defining the small axis of the ellipse corresponding to the entire left ventricular area in the "RAO-view".

The echocardiograms were recorded by means of a video tape recorder (Grundig BK 204) and played back in stop motion mode for volumetric evaluation. End-diastolic and end-systolic images were assumed to occur at the peak of the R-wave and at the end of the T-wave, respectively.

The raw data for the biplane volumetry were obtained by tracing the endocardial border of the two orthogonal silhouettes with the aid of a microprocessor-controlled lightpen system. The common axis of the two perpendicular views was defined by the distance from the midpoint of the mitral valve to the apex. The ventricular volume was estimated from the two orthogonal ellipses. Left ventricular volume (V) was calculated by the

Rijsterborgh H, ed: Echocardiology, p 163-166. All rights reserved.
Copyright © 1981 Martinus Nijhoff Publishers, The Hague/Boston/London.

164

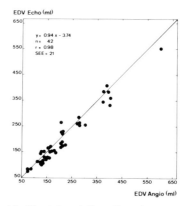

Figure 1a. Biplane angiographic (Angio) end-diastolic volumes (EDV) plotted against biplane echocardiographic (Echo) end-systolic volumes in 42 patients. The line of identity is shown.

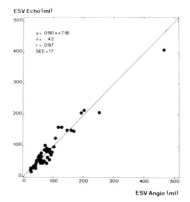

Figure 1b. Biplane angiographic (Angio) end-systolic volumes (ESV) plotted against biplane echocardiographic (Echo) endsystolic volumes in 42 patients. The line of identity is shown.

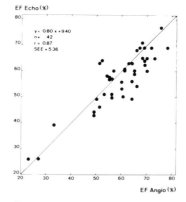

Figure 1c. Biplane angiographic (Angio) ejection fraction (EF) is plotted against the biplane echocardiographic (Echo) ejection fraction in 42 patients. The line of identity is shown.

area-length technique as follows

$$V = \frac{8 \cdot A1 \cdot A2}{3 \cdot \pi \cdot L} ;$$

V   Volume of the ellipsoid model

A1, A2   Areas of the ellipses

L   Length of common axis

Angiographic volumes were calculated from the RAO and LAO silhouettes using the area-length method.

3. RESULTS

Results of comparisons between echographic and angiographic measurements are given in Figure 1.

Correlation coefficients were found to be 0.98 and 0.97 for the end-diastolic and the end-systolic volumes respectively. In the case of the end-diastolic volumes, the small (8%) underestimate found using echocardiography is significant at $P<0.001$. The values of the end-systolic volumes however, showed no significant difference. The correlation coefficient for the ejection fraction is 0.87 but there is a small (3%), though significant, underestimate when using the echocardiographic method.

4. DISCUSSION AND CONCLUSION

Even though the two methods utilize different input data, the volumetric results obtained agree sufficiently well for clinical purposes. This conclusion is supported by the fact that the angiographic values themselves are not inherently accurate but are associated with an error, which is generally larger than 8%.

The lack of essential systematic differences indicates that the echographic sections chosen contain volumetric information from the left ventricle which is equivalent to that given by biplane cineangiography. The principal reasons for the scatter of the individual data may, in part, be associated with intra-observer variability in acquiring the raw data, with differences in the heart rate at the times the two procedures were employed and with the inter-patient variability of the shape and orientation of the heart.

REFERENCES

1. Carr KW, RL Engler, JR Forsythe, AD Johnson, B Gosink: Measurements of left ventricular ejection fraction by mechanical cross-sectional echocardiography. Circulation 59:1196–1206, 1979.
2. Schiller NB, H Acquatella, TA Ports et al.: Left ventricular volume from paired biplane two-dimensional echocardiography. Circulation 60:547–555, 1979

3. Folland ED, AF Parisi, PF Moynihan, DR Jones, CL Feldman, DE Tow: Assessment of left ventricular ejection fraction and volumes by real-time, two-dimensional echocardiography. A comparison of cineangiographic and radionuclide techniques. Circulation 60:760–766, 1979.

19. ECHOCARDIOGRAPHIC CHANGES DURING A ONE-YEAR EXERCISE PROGRAM IN PREVIOUSLY SEDENTARY NORMAL MIDDLE-AGED MEN

DENNIS M. DAVIDSON, RICHARD L. POPP, WILLIAM L. HASKELL, PETER D. WOOD, STEVEN BLAIR, and PING HO

INTRODUCTION

Previous echocardiographic studies of the effects of physical conditioning have focused primarily on persons aged 35 and younger who undergo exercise training for six months or less [1, 2, 3, 4]. In this study, 81 healthy but previously sedentary men, aged 35–55, were randomly assigned to exercise and control groups, to examine the effects on cardiac dimensions and plasma lipoproteins of a year-long running program.

METHODS

Selection of study population

Invitations to participate in the study were mailed to male Stanford University employees aged 35–55 who had previously participated in a cross-sectional study of plasma lipoproteins. Of those indicating a willingness to participate, 81 were chosen who met the eligibility criteria. These 81 men were randomly assigned (in 3:2 ratio) to exercise training (n = 48) and control (n = 33) groups. Those in the exercise group ran a mean distance of 14.3 km/wk. All men had M-mode echocardiograms done at baseline, and after three months and one year of the study. Without knowledge of patient identification or group assignment, all echocardiograms were reviewed for technical quality. In 35 men, all 3 records were technically excellent, and thus these 105 echocardiograms were selected for further analysis. Of these 35 men, 20 were in the exercise group. During the year, they ran 4.5–29.3 km (mean = 17.1 km) per week. Follow-up in both exercise and control groups was 100%.

Echocardiographic measurements

The following measurements were made according to the standards of the American Society of Echocardiography [5]. Left ventricular (LV) internal

Rijsterborgh H, ed: Echocardiology, p 167-170. All rights reserved.
Copyright © 1981 Martinus Nijhoff Publishers, The Hague/Boston/London.

diameter at end-diastole (ED) and at end-systole (ES), left atrial diameter (LA), thickness of intraventricular septum (S) and posterior LV wall (PW) at end-diastole and end-systole, as well as resting heart rate (HR) were measured. Percent fractional shortening was derived from these dimensions. Left ventricular volumes were calculated by the cube formula described by Popp [6]; stroke volume and ejection fraction were derived therefrom. Left ventricular mass was calculated as the product of density of cardiac muscle (1.05) and the difference in estimated external and internal volumes of the left ventricle. Estimated cardiac output was calculated from estimated stroke volume and resting heart rate. Absolute values of each parameter were compared on baseline, three month and twelve month echocardiograms. Each of these variables were divided by body surface area (BSA) and compared. In addition, percentage changes from baseline were calculated. Analysis of variance techniques were used to examine the changes.

RESULTS

Absolute changes

Table 1 lists the mean values for each variable which showed significant differences between baseline and twelve month examinations. There were no significant changes in percent fractional shortening, thickness or thickening of the intraventricular septum or posterior LV wall, or estimated cardiac output.

Table 1

	Exercise (X)			Control (C)			P for $\Delta(X-C)$	
	Base-line (B)	3 mos	12 mos	Base-line	3 mos	12 mos	B−3 mos	B−12 mos
LVED (mm)	50.4	51.5	52.7	50.3	50.8	50.4	0.20	0.005
LVES (mm)	31.4	32.2	32.5	31.6	31.3	31.4	0.20	0.05
SV (ml) *	96.8	103	112	96.9	101	98.5	−	0.02
LV mass (g)	210	221	242	215	215	219	−	0.01
LA (mm)	38.2	39.8	40.1	38.2	37.3	37.0	0.10	0.01
HR (bpm)	66.5	60.9	56.4	68.9	67.2	70.6	0.10	0.0001

* SV = stroke volume.

Thus, when compared to controls, progressive increases were seen in men exercising during the year in LVED, LVES, LA, SV and estimated heart mass, while resting heart rate decreased, resulting in no change in estimated cardiac output. The statistical significance values for each variable were identical for absolute, percentage and BSA-indexed changes.

Dose-response of exercise

When the exercise group was divided by total distance run per week, further discrimination was obtained. Men were arbitrarily divided into three groups, using the total exercise group (n = 48) mean of 14.3 km/wk and the mean of those exercisers with echocardiograms (n = 20) of 17.1 km/wk. Variables with significant differences are shown in Table 2; values represent mean changes from baseline to one year.

Table 2

	Group			
	A (n = 10)	B (n = 7)	C (n = 3)	Control (n = 15)
Distance run per week (km)	>17.1	14.3–17.1	<14.3	–
Δ Est. Heart Mass (g)	39.3	23.4	13.8	− 7.9
Δ Stroke Volume (ml)	21.1	13.6	−0.4	− 8.0
Δ Heart Rate (beats/min)	− 8.0	−13.0	−8.7	1.7
Δ HDL-cholesterol (mg/dl)	6.05	3.64	−1.83	1.0
Δ Body Density (10^{-4})	53.5	61.1	17.0	−20.0

DISCUSSION

Other investigators [1, 2, 3, 4] have found that ventricular volumes at end-diastole and end-systole enlarge in young persons undergoing short-term physical conditioning. Further, in competitive athletes and others undergoing vigorous training, intraventricular septum and left ventricular wall thickness increased as well as left ventricular mass [1, 3]. In none of the studies did ejection fraction increase. These factors suggest that exercise training induces adaptive changes similar to that of chronic volume overload.

Our investigation examined the long-term effects of moderate exercise training in an older group of previously sedentary men. Changes in estimated LV volume were progressive throughout the year, and varied inversely with resting heart rate, maintaining estimated resting cardiac output nearly constant. No significant changes in septal or LV wall thickness were seen at this intensity of exercise, suggesting that moderate exercise may increase LV mass as manifested primarily through increases in end-diastolic and end-systolic volumes. In contrast, in younger persons undergoing more strenuous exercise, concentric hypertrophy of the LV occurred.

We found that changes in LV mass, stroke volume and HDL-cholesterol were related to the amount of exercise done weekly. Some of the increase in resting LV dimensions may reflect the lower resting heartrate after training, but other studies have not provided adequate data in this lower heart rate range to correct for this assumption [7].

We conclude that middle-aged men who engage in regular moderate exercise can expect increases in left ventricular volumes and cardiac muscle mass which are related to the amount of exercise done weekly. These changes are accompanied by increases in body density and HDL-cholesterol.

REFERENCES

1. Ehsani AA, JM Hagberg, RC Hickson: Rapid changes in left ventricular dimensions and mass in response to physical conditioning and deconditioning. Am J Cardiol 42:52, 1978.
2. Wolfe LA, DA Cunningham, PA Rechnitzer, PM Nichol: Effects of endurance training on left ventricular dimensions in healthy men. J Appl Physiol 47:207, 1979.
3. Ikaheimo MJ, IJ Palatsi, JT Takkunen: Noninvasive evaluation of the athletic heart: Sprinters versus endurance runners. Am J Cardiol 44:24, 1979.
4. Stein RA, D Michielli, J Diamond, B Horwitz, N Krasnow: The cardiac response to exercise training: echocardiographic analysis at rest and during exercise. Am J Cardiol 46:219, 1980.
5. Sahn DJ, A DeMaria, J Kisslo, A Weyman: The Committee on M-mode Standardization of the American Society of Echocardiography: recommendations regarding quantitation in M-mode echocardiography: results of a survey of echocardiographic measurement. Circulation 58:1072, 1978.
6. Popp RL, DC Harrison: Ultrasonic cardiac echography for determining stroke volume and valvular regurgitation. Circulation 41:493, 1970.
7. DeMaria AN, A Neumann, PJ Schubart, G Lee, DT Mason: Systematic correlation of cardiac chamber size and ventricular performance determined with echocardiography and alterations in heart rate in normal persons. Am J Cardiol 43:1, 1979.

20. PREDICTION OF CORONARY ARTERY DISEASE IN HYPERTENSION

J.R. DAWSON and G.C. SUTTON

INTRODUCTION

If conventional M-mode echocardiography is combined with phonocardiography and processed using a simple digitizing technique, abnormalities reflecting incoordinate wall motion can be identified. Chen and Gibson [1] have shown that shortening of the time interval "aortic valve closure (A2) to minimum cavity dimension" is associated with incoordinate wall motion. Significant changes in dimension during the period of isovolumic relaxation (IVRT) also reflect incoordinate wall movement [2], irrespective of whether the part of the ventricle visualized by the echo beam is normal or abnormal.

Prolonged systemic arterial hypertension may result in left ventricular hypertrophy. The effect of hypertrophy on left ventricular performance is not clearly established. In an attempt to obtain further information on left ventricular performance in an unselected group of hypertensive patients, we studied patients using the digitizing technique paying particular attention to indices of coordinate wall motion. The results were compared to normal controls. The study findings were correlated with a retrospective clinical analysis and a further follow-up over a one-year period.

MATERIALS AND METHODS

Eighty-eight patients (60 men, 28 women, age range 24–73, mean 51) with hypertension (systemic arterial diastolic pressure persistently over 13.3 kPa (100 mmHg) before treatment) and 29 normotensive controls without evidence of cardiac disease (27 men, 2 women, age range 21–63, mean 38) were studied.

Simultaneous recordings of the electrocardiogram, phonocardiogram (identifying A2), and echocardiogram (identifying mitral valve opening and left ventricular thickness and dimension) were made (Figure 1). Plots were generated over one cardiac cycle to show the original data, the left ventricular cavity dimension, the rate of change of dimension and the rate of change of dimension normalised to refer to unit length of dimension. The timing of

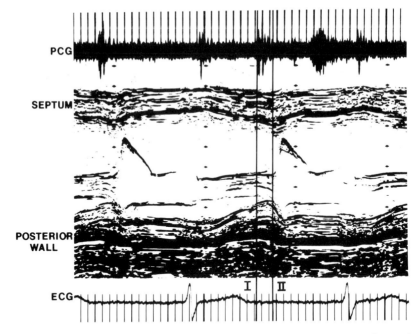

Figure 1. Echocardiogram from a normal control showing the septum and left ventricular posterior wall recorded with an electrocardiogram (ECG) and phonocardiogram (PCG). The vertical lines represent, from left to right, (I) aortic valve closure (II) mitral valve opening.

A2 and the timing of mitral valve opening (Figure 2) were superimposed on the plots.

Measurements were made of:

1. Septal and left ventricular posterior wall maximum and minimum thickness.
2. IVRT (A2 to mitral valve opening).
3. A2 to minimum cavity dimension (point where the derivative of cavity dimension alters from negative to positive).
4. Minimum cavity dimension to mitral valve opening.
5. Changes in left ventricular dimension during IVRT, expressed as a percentage of total change in dimension.

RESULTS

Normal subjects

Maximum septal and posterior wall thicknesses were 1.5 ± 0.2 cm and 1.7 ± 0.2 cm respectively. Minimum septal and posterior wall thicknesses were 1.0 ± 0.1 cm and 0.8 ± 0.1 cm respectively. IVRT was 65 ± 15 ms. A

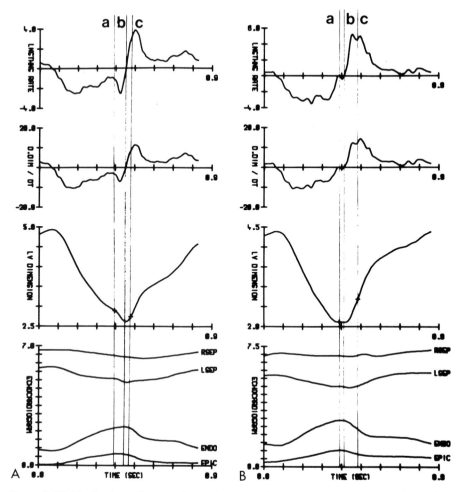

Figure 2. Digitized echocardiograms from (A) a normal control and (B) a hypertensive patient from Group II. Illustrated, from the bottom, are the original data, left ventricular dimension, rate of change of dimension and (top) normalized rate of change of dimension. The vertical lines represent, from left to right, (a) aortic valve closure, (b) minimum cavity dimension and (c) mitral valve opening.

constant relationship was observed in the timings of A2, minimum cavity dimension and mitral valve opening. A2 preceded minimum cavity dimension by 50 ± 15 ms and mitral valve opening followed minimum cavity dimension by 15 ± 20 ms. Only small changes were observed in left ventricular cavity dimension during IVRT ($-4 \pm 7\%$) (Figure 2A).

Hypertensive patients

Maximum septal and posterior wall thicknesses were significantly higher than in the normal population: 2.0 ± 0.3 cm and 1.9 ± 0.3 cm, respectively ($p < 0.001$). Minimum septal and posterior wall thicknesses were also signif-

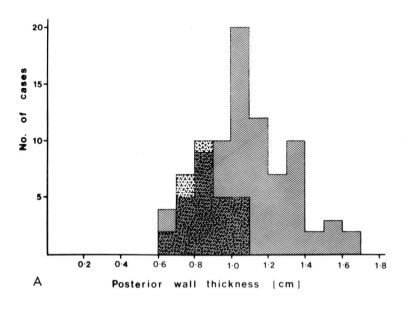

A   **Posterior wall thickness [cm]**

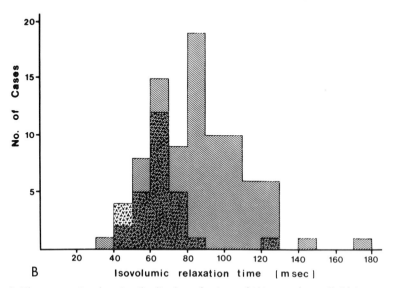

B   **Isovolumic relaxation time [msec]**

Figure 3. Histograms showing the distribution of values of (A) posterior wall thickness and (B) isovolumic relaxation time in hypertensive patients (hatched columns) and normal controls (dotted columns).

icantly higher than in the normal population: 1.2 ± 0.2 cm and 1.1 ± 0.2 cm, respectively ($p < 0.001$). IVRT was prolonged (85 ± 25 ms $p < 0.001$). The higher values of left ventricular wall thickness and prolongation of IVRT were unimodally distributed in the hypertensive population (Figure 3). When

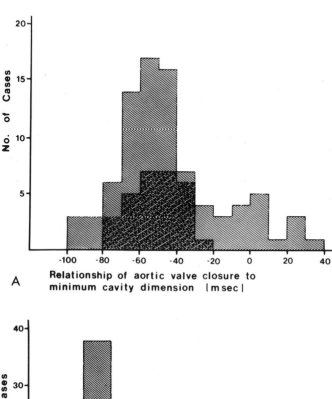

A   **Relationship of aortic valve closure to minimum cavity dimension [msec]**

B   **Dimension change during period of isovolumic relaxation [%]**

Figure 4. Histograms showing the distribution of values of (A) the time interval A2 to minimum cavity dimension and (B) dimension change during IVRT in hypertensive patients (hatched columns) and normal controls (dotted columns).

indices of coordinate wall motion were examined, a bimodal distribution was found (Figure 4) enabling the hypertensive patients to be separated into two well defined groups; those with coordinate (group I) and those with incoordinate (group II) wall motion.

Group I comprised 60 patients; 37 men, 23 women, age range 24–73, mean 49. A2 preceded minimum cavity dimension by 60 ± 15 ms and mitral valve opening followed minimum cavity dimension by 20 ± 15 ms, neither value significantly differing from normal. Dimension change during IVRT also remained within the normal range ($0 \pm 7\%$).

Group II comprised 28 patients; 23 men, 5 women, age range 39–70, mean 55. In contrast to group I the normal time relationship between A2, minimum cavity dimension and mitral valve opening were disturbed (Figure 2B). A2 preceded minimum cavity dimension by only 15 ± 30 ms ($p < 0.01$) and mitral valve opening followed it by 85 ± 30 ms ($p < 0.01$). Abnormal dimension changes occurred during IVRT ($28 \pm 18\%$ $p < 0.01$) (Figure 2B).

CLINICAL ANALYSIS

Group I

All patients in this group had normal electrocardiograms. Fifty-eight were asymptomatic, 2 had atypical chest pain with minor coronary artery disease (less than 50% narrowing) demonstrated at cardiac catheterization. No cardiac events occurred among the patients in this group during a one year follow-up.

Group II

At the time of study 10 had documented significant coronary artery disease, 5 by angiography (greater than 50% narrowing) and 5 by documented prior myocardial infarction. The remaining 18 patients all had abnormal electrocardiograms exhibiting T-wave inversion in the left ventricular leads. Seven of these 18 had a typical history of angina pectoris, while 11 were asymptomatic. In a one year follow-up, 7 of these 18 patients (3 with angina, 4 who were asymptomatic) had a major cardiac event (5 developed myocardial infarction while 2 died suddenly).

SUMMARY

These results show that hypertensive patients have increased left ventricular wall thickness and prolonged IVRT. Patients in group I had coordinate wall motion, and significant coronary artery disease was not evident. In contrast, the patients in group II had evidence of incoordinate wall motion and a high incidence of significant coronary artery disease. These findings indicate that in hypertensive patients the echocardiographic recognition of incoordinate wall motion distinguishes both retrospectively and prospectively those patients who have a high incidence of clinically significant coronary artery disease. We suggest that this group deserves further study to determine if any intervention could alter the prognosis.

REFERENCES

1. Chen W, DG Gibson: Relation of isovolumic relaxation to left ventricular wall movement in man. British Heart J 42:51–56, 1979.
2. Gibson DG, JH Doran, TA Traill, DJ Brown: Regional abnormalities of left ventricular wall movement during isovolumic relaxation in patients with ischaemic heart disease. Euro J Cardiol 7, suppl:251–264, 1978.

21. LEFT VENTRICULAR HYPERTROPHY IN PATIENTS ON CHRONIC HEMODIALYSIS

P.J. Voogd, I. Schicht, P.C.J. van Breda Vriesman,
and L.K. Monsjou

INTRODUCTION

Left ventricular hypertrophy (LVH) is defined as an increase in left ventricular muscle mass as a consequence of enhanced stroke work brought about by an increase in preload or an enhanced afterload or both [1]. Enhanced afterload will cause an increase in wall thickness [2] whereas an increase in preload will be accommodated by dilatation [3].

Patients on chronic hemodialysis are liable to develop left ventricular hypertrophy because an increase in preload due to anemia [4] and arterio-venous fistula [5], necessary to obtain vascular access for hemodialysis, is invariably present. Also, an excess in extracellular fluid volume, frequently noticed in this group of patients [6], will give rise to increased preload as well as afterload [7]. Sometimes there is increased afterload resulting from hypertension of renal origin. The purpose of this study was to establish the prevalence of left ventricular hypertrophy in patients on chronic hemodialysis, using electrographic (ECG) as well as echocardiographic techniques; we also investigated the relationship between blood pressure and degree of left ventricular hypertrophy, for which purpose a follow-up study was performed.

MATERIAL AND METHODS

Twenty-five patients on a chronic hemodialysis program, who were without spontaneous symptoms indicative of cardiac disease and without pedal edema, were examined by noninvasive techniques. Of the 25 patients, 2 showed ECG changes compatible with a previously sustained inferior wall myocardial infarction and one patient had a pericardial effusion on echocardiography. Thus 22 patients were available for follow-up. One anephric patient with severe hypertension excepted, all patients were considered "stable" by the nephrologists in charge and no change in dialysis regimen was indicated. The follow-up period lasted for 8 months. Of the 22 patients, 5 were lost to the follow-up, the reasons being development of pericardial effusion (1); symptomatic coronary heart disease resulting in acute myocardial infarction (1); bypass surgery (1); renal transplant (1); technically unsatisfactory echocardiogram (1).

Patients were hemodialyzed twice a week using regional heparinization. Access to the vasculature was by means of a fistula (23) or a Scribner shunt (2); fistula or shunt were not changed during the follow-up period. Dialysis ultra filtration was conducted in such a fashion that patients were either normotensive after dialysis or else close to their "ideal" or "minimal" weight. This weight was determined empirically by continuing dialysis ultra filtration of patients with hypertension before dialysis until hypotension (systolic blood pressure <90 mmHg), or orthostatic hypotension (30 mmHg difference in diastolic blood pressure between the upright and supine position) developed. Alternatively, in the absence of predialysis hypertension, the heart rate at the end of dialysis had to increase by over 25% of the initial rate. Hemoglobin concentration was maintained between 4 and 6 gm/100 ml of blood using infrequent transfusions of packed erythrocytes if necessary. Blood pressure was measured with a cuff applied either to the arm without the fistula or to the ankle. Phase IV was taken as diastolic blood pressure. At entry and during follow-up, blood pressures were averaged every two to three months; the mean blood pressure was calculated by adding one third of the pulse pressure to the diastolic blood pressure.

Standard 12 lead ECG's were read for the presence or absence of left ventricular hypertrophy by the criteria of Romhilt and Estes [8] using a point score system based on voltage (3 points), strain (3 points), P-wave changes (3 points), left axis deviation and prolongation of the QRS complex (3 points) and increased intrinsicoid deflection (1 point). ECG's were also read by means of a point score system used in computerized reading [9] for left ventricular hypertrophy, a system based primarily on voltage and ST-T changes.

Echocardiograms were taken in the left recumbent position using an Organon Technika 003 echocardiograph equipped with a multiscan and a 2.25 MHz single-element focussed transducer. After visualization of the cross-section through the long axis of the left ventricle, the transducer was positioned in the 3rd, 4th or 5th interspace, depending on the findings of the two-dimensional examination. Complete M-mode scans [10] were performed in such fashion that the anterior wall of the aorta was as far as possible on the same horizontal level as the right septal endocardium. Left ventricular dimensions were measured slightly caudal to the mitral valves [10]. Left ventricular end-diastolic diameter and septal as well as posterior wall thickness were measured at the onset of the QRS complex. The largest end-diastolic diameter and the smallest wall thickness were taken as the true dimensions [10]. Left ventricular end-systolic diameter was measured at the peak of the inward motion of the posterior endocardial echo. Measurements were made at the anterior edge of each echo. Great care was taken not to incorporate the septal tricuspid leaflet into septal thickness; when desired, the right septal endocardial echo was visualized by means of contrast echocardiography [14], using a forceful injection of a 10 ml bolus of saline into the fistula or shunt. The left posterior endocardial echo was differentiated from the chordae tendineae by taking the thinnest line with the highest motion velocity as the endocardial echo. The gain setting was such that visceral and parietal pericardial echoes were seen as separate lines. When desired, echocardiograms were read according to the "Philadelphia" convention and left ventricular mass calculated accordingly [12].

Echocardiograms were recorded on a Honeywell LS6 fiberoptic recorder at paper speeds of 25 and 50 mm/second. Measurements were made with a caliper with calibrations 0.05 mm apart. M-mode dimensions were read to 1 mm accuracy. Because left ventricular end-diastolic inner dimension varies with heart rate [15], care was taken to exclude an effect of heart rate on the measurements by always making the echocardiograms prior to dialysis and using patients who were thoroughly familiar with the procedure.

In order to determine the magnitude of variability of the relevant echo dimensions used in this study, 25 patients from the chronic hemodialysis program at that time (including 13 patients from the follow-up study) were each investigated, within a half hour, by two different echocardiographers who were unaware of each other's transducer position and of the degree of the patient's recumbency. Next, each echocardiographer measured the echo dimensions of his own investigation, independently. Variability of echo dimensions was expressed as twice the standard deviation of the difference between the measurements of the two observers.

RESULTS

Accuracy of echocardiographic measurements

In order to determine the reliability and reproducibility of the measurements made, the echocardiograms of the 25 patients were measured by two observers independently of each other. Each observer made his own echocardiograms. The variability of the left ventricular end-diastolic diameter was 3.4 mm, and of the septal and posterior wall thickness 2.6 mm (Table 1). No significant systematic differences were found between the two observers using the Student's t-test for paired data, so all differences between the measurements made by the two observers were random.

Table 1. Accuracy of echocardiographic measurements. Two independent observers measured left ventricular end-diastolic diameter, and septal and posterior wall thickness at the onset of the QRS complex.

	Variability[1] (mm)	Difference in bias (mm)
Left ventricular end-diastolic inner diameter	3.4	−0.48 (p = 0.18)
Septal width	2.6	0.14 (p = 0.6)
Posterior wall width	2.6	0.25 (p = 0.34)

[1] Expressed as twice the standard deviation (SD) of differences in measurements made by both observers as follows:

$$SD = \sqrt{\frac{\sum\limits_{i=1}^{n}(x_i - y_i)^2}{n-1}}$$

where x_i: measurements by observer I and
y_i: measurements by observer II
n: number of measurements

Prevalence of left ventricular hypertrophy on entry

Four of the twenty-five patients showed left ventricular hypertrophy on the electrocardiogram using both the Bonner and the Romhilt and Estes point scores. One of these patients also had ECG signs of an old inferior wall myocardial infarction. Two additional patients showed left ventricular hypertrophy according to the Bonner point score only. Of the 4 patients with a marked increased left ventricular wall thickness (combined width 35 mm or above) and no left ventricular dilatation, two showed left ventricular hypertrophy on the ECG using the Bonner point score; with the Romhilt and Estes point score only one patient showed LVH (Figure 1). Eight of the 25 patients had increased left ventricular end-diastolic diameter (>60 mm) by echocardiography and 4 of these 8 showed left ventricular hypertrophy on the ECG; this was associated with echocardiographically normal left ventricular combined wall thickness (<24 mm) in 2 of the 4 instances.

Clearcut concentric increased left ventricular wall thickness (combined width >30 mm) was associated with predialysis diastolic hypertension (>90 mmHg) in 4 out of 5 cases and with systolic hypertension (>160 mmHg) in all instances. None of the patients with a normal wall thickness proved to have diastolic or systolic hypertension prior to dialysis (Table 2). Of the four patients with septal hypertrophy (≥15 mm), 3 showed diastolic hypertension and one also had systolic hypertension before dialysis (Table 2).

After dialysis (Table 3), the blood pressure decreased in 4 of the 5 patients with a concentric increase in left ventricular wall diameter and became normal in three, indicating that fluid excess contributed to or mediated the predialysis hypertension in these patients. Blood pressure decreased in all of the 4 patients with septal hypertrophy after dialysis; two of these patients

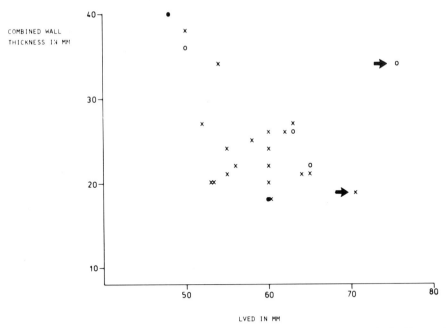

Figure 1. Effect of left ventricular wall thickness and end-diastolic diameter on the incidence of left ventricular hypertrophy by ECG in 25 patients on chronic hemodialysis. Left ventricular end-diastolic diameter (LVED) and posterior and septal wall thickness were measured echocardiographically. ECG were read according to the Bonner computer program [12] and according to Romhilt and Estes [11].○ left ventricular hypertrophy present by both Bonner and Romhilt and Estes, ● left ventricular hypertrophy present by Bonner only, × no left ventricular hypertrophy by ECG, → indicates two patients with an old myocardial infarction.

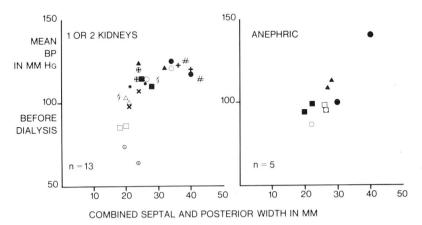

Figure 2. Relation between mean blood pressure before dialysis and left ventricular wall thickness in 18 patients on chronic hemodialysis. All patients had an A-V fistula. Systolic and diastolic blood pressures were averaged over a three month period prior to echocardiography. Mean blood pressure (diastolic BP + 1/3 the pulse pressure) was calculated from the average systolic and diastolic pressures. Combined wall thickness was calculated from the echocardiogram obtained at entry into the study and at the end of follow-up, at 7 to 13 months after entry. Symbols used (+, §, o, etc.) indicate individual patients at entry and at the end of follow-up.

Table 2. Effect of predialysis blood pressure[1], on left ventricular wall thickness in 25 patients on chronic hemodialysis.

Wall thickness at end-diastole in mm	No. patients	Mean bloodpressure[3]			Diastolic bloodpressure[2]			Systolic bloodpressure		
		<100	100≥ ≤110	>110	<90	90≥ ≤100	>100	<140	140≥ ≤160	>160
Septum 15	5	0	0	5	1	2	2	0	0	5
Posterior wall 15										
Septum 15	4	0	1	3	1	2	1	0	3	1
Posterior wall 15										
Septum 12–15	4	1	1	2	2	1	1	1	0	3
Posterior wall 12–15										
Septum 12	12	10	2	0	12	0	0	8	4	0
Posterior wall 11										

[1] Blood pressures were averaged over a three month period prior to echocardiography.
[2] Mean blood pressure: diastolic bloodpressure + $\frac{1}{3}$ the pulse pressure in mmHg.
[3] The switch from Korotkov III to IV was taken to indicate diastolic blood pressure.

Table 3. Effect of post dialysis blood pressure[1], on left ventricular wall thickness in 25 patients on chronic hemodialysis.

Wall thickness at end-diastole in mm	No. patients	Mean bloodpressure[3]			Diastolic bloodpressure[2]			Systolic bloodpressure		
		<100	100≥ ≤110	>110	<90	90≥ ≤100	>100	<140	140≥ ≤160	>160
Septum 15	5	1	3	1	3	2	0	1	2	2
Posterior wall 15										
Septum 15	4	1	2	1	2	1	1	1	2	1
Posterior wall 15										
Septum 12–15	4	2	1	1	4	0	0	2	1	1
Posterior wall 12–15										
Septum 12	12	11	1	0	12	0	0	11	1	0
Posterior wall 11										

[1] Blood pressures were averaged over a three month period prior to echocardiography.
[2] Mean blood pressure: diastolic bloodpressure + $\frac{1}{3}$ the pulse pressure in mmHg.
[3] The switch from Korotkov III to IV was taken to indicate diastolic blood pressure.

were normotensive after dialysis. In these patients, too, fluid excess appeared to contribute to or mediate the hypertension.

Left ventricular wall thickness during follow-up (Figure 2)

Of the 25 patients, 18 were followed up for at least 8 months without change in fistula or in dialysis regimen. Included in this series is one patient (patient 'o' in Figure 2) who had a subtotal parathyreoidectomy because of persistent hypercalcemia within two months after entry into the study; since his fistula and his dialysis regimen was not changed, he was not excluded from the follow-up. During the period of follow-up (Figure 2), significant (>5 mm) increases in combined left ventricular wall thickness occurred in 4 patients with one or two kidneys (patients ○, ▲, §, ● in Figure 2), which was associated with increases in mean blood pressure of 10 mmHg (§) and 5 mmHg (○), with no change in mean blood pressure (▲) and with a 8 mmHg decrease in blood pressure (●). A decrease in mean blood pressure of 10 mmHg (patient # in Figure 2), 8 mmHg (●) and 3 mmHg (+) was observed in those three patients with the greatest combined wall thickness at time of entry into the study. Among the anephric patients, a 10 mm decrease in combined left ventricular wall thickness was observed after treating the patient with malignant hypertension with prolonged dialysis ultra filtration.

DISCUSSION

The main findings of this study are twofold:
1. The electrocardiographic criteria for LVH are less sensitive than echocardiographic measurements and are not reliable in patients on chronic hemodialysis.
2. In patients on chronic hemodialysis, the degree of concentric left ventricular hypertrophy is not accurately predicted by the blood pressure measured prior to dialysis.

Left ventricular hypertrophy can be expected to occur frequently in patients on chronic hemodialysis, for two reasons. Adaptive increases in preload because of anemia and arteriovenous fistula may cause an increase in left ventricular mass because of dilatation. Increases in left ventricular wall thickness may also be expected to occur frequently, because of renal hypertension or fluid overload. In the latter case, the left ventricular hypertrophy results from the conversion of a non-adaptive increase in preload into afterload [13]. The latter mechanism was most likely operative in those of our patients with marked increases in left ventricular wall thickness, since the hypertension observed before dialysis decreased or disappeared altogether after dialysis in all but one patient.

In agreement with others using angiographic techniques for measuring left ventricular mass [14], we observed, using echocardiographic techniques, that the criteria used for diagnosing left ventricular hypertrophy from the ECG provided an insensitive and unreliable measure for detecting symmetrical and asymmetrical increases in left ventricular wall thickness in our patients. This unreliability is probably accounted for by two observations. The left ventricular mass measured in the echocardiogram according to the empirically obtained formula [12]:

$$LV_{MASS} = 1.04(LVID_{ED} + LVPW_{ED} + IVS_{ED})^3 - (LVID_{ED})^3 - 14\,g$$

in which LV_{MASS} = left ventricular mass
              $LVID_{ED}$ = end-diastolic left ventricular diameter
              $LVPW_{ED}$ = end-diastolic posterior wall thickness
              IVS_{ED} = end-diastolic septal thickness

This formula reflects the fact that left ventricular hypertrophy is more efficiently brought about by an increase in wall thickness than by an increase in inner diameter. This observation together with the finding [14] that, unless a sufficient degree of chamber dilatation is present, a degree of wall thickening sufficient to result in an increase in left ventricular mass usually does not result in increased voltage on the ECG.

Sasayana [2] indicates that the ECG may particularly underestimate afterload-mediated left ventricular hypertrophy. Inclusion in the electrocardiographic point score of changes with limited specificity such as left axis deviation, ST-T changes or P-wave abnormalities, all of which are used in the Romhilt and Estes point score system [8], did not enhance the sensitivity of the ECG in detecting left ventricular hypertrophy.

Although the left ventricular wall thickness and inner diameters are easily and accurately measured echocardiographically, the echocardiograms could not be used for the accurate estimation of cardiac mass because in our study, the inter-observer variation in measuring wall thickness was 3 mm and also because the left ventricular inner diameter varies with the heart rate [15]. With these restrictions, the left ventricular mass of our patients – the infarcted ventricles and those with asymmetrical hypertrophy excepted – calculated echocardiographically according to Devereux [12] was in excess of 140 grams/m², which is well above the angiographically-determined left ventricular mass for normal men and women of 120 and 80 grams/m² respectively [16, 17]. For the reasons outlined above, left ventricular wall thickness rather than calculated cardiac mass was used as measure of afterload-mediated left ventricular hypertrophy during follow-up.

Although the data obtained at entry showed the presence of an increase in left ventricular wall thickness to be invariably associated with systolic or diastolic hypertension prior to dialysis, the follow-up data indicate that a direct relationship between the degree of hypertension and the thickness of the left ventricular wall was not present in several of the patients with one or two kidneys. Firstly, a marked increase in left ventricular wall thickness developed in the presence of only very mild predialysis hypertension in one patient (§ in Figure 2) and, secondly, worsening of left ventricular hypertrophy was associated with a decrease in predialysis blood pressure in two patients. All these patients were normotensive after dialysis, suggesting that both hypertension [18] and left ventricular hypertrophy were secondary to excesses of extracellular fluid. The increased left ventricular wall thickness in these patients does not appear to be due to edema since, after abolishing the predialysis hypertension by means of oral fluid restriction and prolonged ultra filtration, it takes weeks to months before the left ventricular wall returns to a normal thickness [19].

REFERENCES

1. Dodge HT, M Frimer, DK Stewart: Functional evaluation of the hypertrophical heart in man. Circ Res supplement II 35:122–127, 1974.
2. Sasayma S, J Ross, D Franklin, CM Bloor, S Bishop, BD Dilley: Adaptations of the left ventricle to chronic pressure overload. Circ Res 38:172–178, 1976.
3. Papadimitrion JM, BE Hopkins, RR Taylor: Regression of left ventricular dilatation and hypertrophy after removal of volume overload. Circ Res 35:127–135, 1974.
4. Neff MS, KE Kim, M Persoff, G Onesti, Ch Swartz: Hemodymics of uremic anemia. Circulation 43:876–883, 1971.
5. Anderson ChB, JR Codd, RA Graff, MA Groce, HR Harter, WT Newton: Cardiac failure and upper extremity arteriovenous dialysis fistula. Arch Intern Med 136:292–297, 1976.
6. Omvik P, RC Tarazi, EL Bravo: Determination of extracellular fluid volume in uremic patients by oral administration of radiosulfate. Kidney International 15:71–79, 1979.
7. Coleman CT, JD Bower, HG Langford, AC Guyton: Resulation of arterial pressure in the anephric state. Circulation 42:509–514, 1970.
8. Romhilt DW, EH Estes: A pointscore system for the E.C.G. diagnosis of left ventricular hypertrophy. Am Heart J 75:752–758, 1968.
9. Bailey JJ, SB Itscoitz, JW Hirshfeld, LE Graner, MR Horton: A method for evaluating computer programs for electrocardiographic interpretation. Circulation 50:73–78, 1974.
10. Feigenbaum H, S Chang: Echocardiography. Lea and Febiger: 236, 311 and 464, Philadelphia, 1976.
11. Allen JW, Sun June Kim, AW Edmiston, K Venkataraman: Problems in ultrasonic estimates of septal thickness. Am J Card 42:289–296, 19 .
12. Devereux RB, N Reichek: Echocardiographic determination of left ventricular mass in man. Circulation 55:613–618, 1977.
13. Ross J jr: Afterload mismatch and preload reserve: a conceptual framework for the analysis of ventricular function. Progress Cardiov Disease 28:255–265, 1976.

14. Antman EM, LH Green, W Grossmann: Physiologic determinants of the electrocardiographic diagnosis of left ventricular hypertrophy. Circulation 60:386–396, 1979.
15. DeMaria AN, A Neuman, PJ Schubart, G Lee, DT Mason: Systematic correlation of cardiac chamber size and ventricular performance determined with echocardiography and alterations in heart rate in normal persons. Am J of Card 43:1–10, 1979.
16. Kennedy JW, WA Baxley, MM Figley, HT Dodge, JR Blackman: Quantitative angiography I the normal ventricle in man. Circulation 34:272–279, 1966.
17. Kennedy JW, DD Reichenbach, WA Baxley, HT Dodge: Left ventricular mass: a comparison of angiographic measurements with autopsy weight. Am J of Card 19:221–223, 1967.
18. Brown JJ, LR Curtis, AF Lever, JS Robertson, HE de Wardener, AJ Wing: Plasma renin concentration and the control of bloodpressure in patients on maintenance haemodialysis. Nephron 6:329–349, 1969.
19. Voogd PJ: Personal observation.

22. DETERMINATION OF QUANTITATIVE LEFT VENTRICULAR FUNCTION BY M-MODE ECHOCARDIOGRAPHY TOGETHER WITH OTHER NONINVASIVE PARAMETERS

P. Hanrath, P. Kremer, and B.A. Langenstein

M-mode echocardiography, which was first introduced in cardiology in order to identify valve disease, has since been shown to be very useful for studying left ventricular (LV) function. The advantage of this method is its noninvasive nature and therefore its suitability for sequential studies in the same patient. Due to its high repetition rate in comparison with angiography and radionuclide techniques, M-mode echocardiography allows a detailed analysis of the dynamic changes in LV dimension and wall thickness within one cardiac cycle. In order to take full advantage of the high repetition rate of this technique for LV dimension analysis, echocardiograms must be digitized. Computer analysis of the M-mode echocardiogram then enables continuous computation of a number of variables throughout one cycle and hence the possibility of following LV cavity dimension, and its rate of change, during systole and diastole. It is also possible to analyse wall thickness changes of the septum and of the left ventricular posterior wall, which is not possible using any other technique.

However, the main limitation of M-mode echocardiography is that only a relatively small part of the left ventricle can be visualized. If changes in local dimension or wall thickness are not considered in isolation but are compared with other measurements of global left ventricular function, specifically those derived from a simultaneously recorded apexcardiogram or phonocardiogram during isovolumic contraction and relaxation, the shortcomings of M-mode echocardiography can be partially overcome.

SIMULTANEOUS RECORDING OF THE APEXCARDIOGRAM AND M-MODE ECHOCARDIOGRAM

One noninvasive approach – first introduced by Venco and co-workers [1] – was the simultaneous recording of the apexcardiogram and phonocardiogram. Since the apexcardiogram is virtually synchronous with the ventricular pressure pulse, it is possible to relate regional dimension and wall thickness changes to the timing of global left ventricular function determined from the apexcardiogram. Simultaneous recordings of an apexcardiogram and echocardiogram can be used to plot uncalibrated apexcardiogram –

dimension loops in exactly the same way as the usual pressure – dimension loops [2, 3, 4].

In patients with normal left ventricular function, the apexcardiogram – dimension loop has a nearly rectangular configuration. The synchronisation of global left ventricular function and regional wall motion during the periods of isovolumic contraction and relaxation is maintained. Incoordiate wall motion of the left ventricle can be detected by this technique, due to a significant dimension change during isovolumic contraction and/or relaxation.

In patients with coronary artery disease, valvular disorders and cardiomyopathy, it has already been proven that, despite normal systolic function of the left ventricle, the timing of the wall motion of the left ventricular cavity may be disturbed. This can easily be detected using a simultaneous recording of the apexcardiogram and echocardiogram. Since this combined noninvasive method includes the time relationship between the whole left ventricular cavity and the small section of the left ventricle which is transected by the ultrasound beam, incoordinate wall motion becomes more evident and can be diagnosed easily from a premature reduction of left ventricular dimension during isovolumic contraction or from a dimension increase during isovolumic relaxation.

When a comparison study with angiographic data was carried out, approximately 85% of patients with symptomatic coronary artery disease were found to have abnormal wall movement on the M-mode during isovolumic contraction or relaxation. In these patients, digitized M-mode echocardiograms recorded simultaneously with an apexcardiogram showed an 80% specificity and sensitivity in detecting these abnormalities when compared with single plane RAO angiograms, which had been analysed by a computer in order to detect regional wall motion abnormalities [5, 6].

SIMULTANEOUS RECORDING OF THE PHONOCARDIOGRAM AND M-MODE ECHOCARDIOGRAM

A second noninvasive approach was to examine the relationship between left ventricular dimension change and valve motion, particularly during isovolumic relaxation. Mitral valve opening time can be observed directly on the echocardiogram, while the instant of aortic valve closure may be obtained from a simultaneously recorded phonocardiogram at A_2, where A_2 is defined as the onset of the first high frequency vibration of the aortic component of the second heart sound [7]. In normal subjects the instant of aortic valve closure is not synchronous with minimal LV dimension. It preceeds the instant of minimal dimension by a mean of approximately 40 msec. The time interval of left ventricular isovolumic relaxation, defined as the time from A_2 to the instant of mitral valve separation, is normally in the range of 55–70 msec [8, 9].

In patients with coronary artery disease, isovolumic relaxation may be abnormal with regard to regional left ventricular wall motion or with regard to its duration. In the majority of patients with significant coronary artery disease, the duration of left ventricular isovolumic relaxation time is normal. But both the instant of A_2 and that of mitral valve opening may be delayed with respect to minimal left ventricular dimension. The presence of such an abnormality correlates closely with a disturbed wall motion during isovolumic contraction, strongly suggesting that it is already determined at the start of the ejection, thus representing more the effect of asynchronous termination of systole than a primary abnormality of relaxation [8]. A prolongation of the isovolumic relaxation time can be observed in a smaller group of patients with coronary artery disease [8], in patients with primary as well as secondary severe left ventricular hypertrophy [8, 9, 10, 11] and various other cardiac diseases [12, 13, 14]. In these patients, the prolongation of isovolumic relaxation time is thought to be an expression of primary left ventricular relaxation disorder, which need not be associated with an abnormal left ventricular systolic function. This primary left ventricular relaxation abnormality is also thought to be responsible for the abnormal left ventricular filling pattern – reduced peak filling rate, diminished LV posterior wall

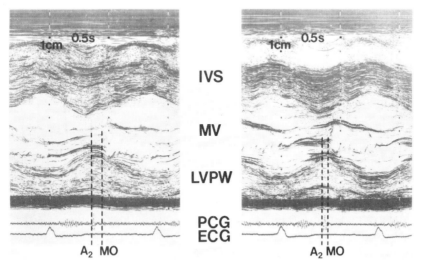

Figure 1. Simultaneous recording of the echocardiogram and phonocardiogram of a patient with secondary left ventricular hypertrophy due to severe systemic hypertension before (left panel) and after (right panel) intravenous injection of Verapamil (9.5 mg) (by permission of the American Journal of Cardiology [9]).

A_2 = aortic valve closure, MO = mitral valve opening, IVS = interventricular septum, MV = mitral valve leaflets, LVPW = posterior wall of the left ventricle.

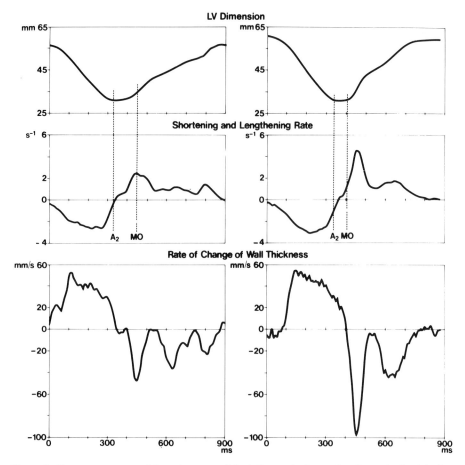

Figure 2. Computer output of the echogram of the left ventricular cavity shown in fig. 1 before (left panel) and after intravenous injection of Verapamil (right panel). After Verapamil left ventricular isovolumic relaxation time is decreased and left ventricular filling, in terms of the peak lengthening rate and the peak posterior wall thinning rate, is increased.

A$_2$ = aortic valve closure, MO = mitral valve opening.

thinning rate during early diastole and prolongation of the rapid filling phase [9, 6, 14] – often associated with a prolongation of isovolumic relaxation time.

Observations in our laboratory, which were recently confirmed by other authors [15, 16], have shown that the abnormal prolongation of left ventricular relaxation time and filling pattern in patients with primary and secondary left ventricular hypertrophy (Figures 1 and 2) can be influenced by intravenous application of calcium antagonists [9, 17] (Figure 3).

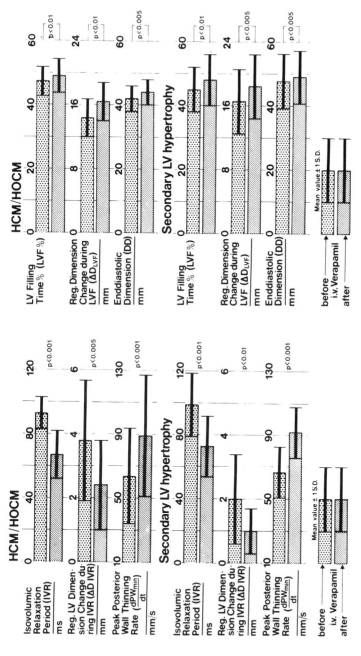

Figure 3. The effect of i.v. Verapamil upon left ventricular relaxation- and filling indices in patients with hypertrophic (obstructive) cardiomyopathy (HCM/HOCM) and secondary left ventricular hypertrophy due to hypertension.

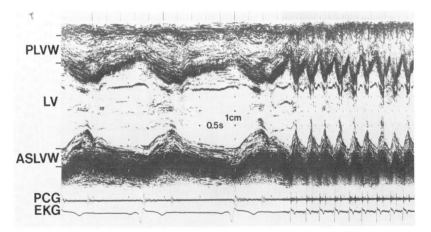

Figure 4. Recording of a trans-esophageal M-Mode-echogram of the left ventricle in a patient with aortic stenosis (with different paper speeds: 100 mm/s left hand side; 10 mm/s right hand side)

PLVW = posterior wall of the left ventricle, ASLVW = anteroseptal wall of the left ventricle, PCG = phonocardiogram, LV = left ventricle, ECG = electrocardiogram.

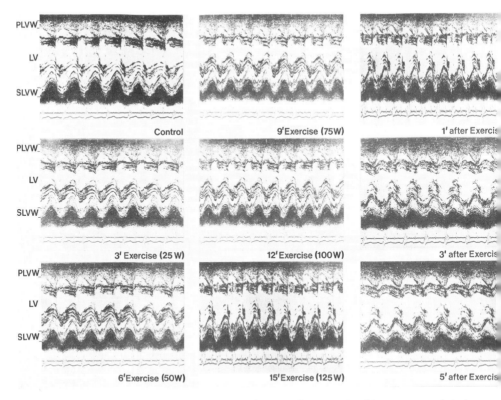

Figure 5. Trans-esophageal M-Mode echocardiogram of a normal subject at rest and during dynamic exercise at different work loads. For abbreviations see Figure 4.

SIMULTANEOUS RECORDING OF TRANS-ESOPHAGEAL ECHOCARDIOGRAM
AND PHONOCARDIOGRAM DURING DYNAMIC EXERCISE

Recently Mason [18] used M-mode echocardiography for the detection of regional left ventricular wall thickening and thinning abnormalities during exercise-induced ischemia in a selected group of patients with coronary artery disease. These authors were able to record high quality echocardiograms in only 24 out of a total of 54 patients (44%). They found an abnormally reduced thickening and thinning rate of the septum and of the left ventricular posterior wall during exercise-induced ischemia, as well as a reduced filling rate in those (echocardiographically determined) wall segments which were supplied by stenotic coronary arteries.

Since it is difficult to obtain high quality echocardiograms (undisturbed by respiration and thoracic movement) using trans-thoracic M-mode echocardiography during dynamic exercise this technique has not found wide application in clinical cardiology. In order to avoid the difficulties of trans-thoracic M-mode, we used the trans-esophageal M-mode echocardiography together with a simultaneously recorded phonocardiogram in order to evaluate left ventricular performance at rest (Figure 4) and during exercise (Figure 5). Trans-esophageal echocardiography was performed with a newly developed trans-esophageal ultrasound transducer system, which is incorporated into a gastroscope [19]. Since the ultrasound transducer can be controlled independently by the examiner as well as by moving the gastroscope up or down or by rotating it (Figure 6), high quality M-mode recordings can

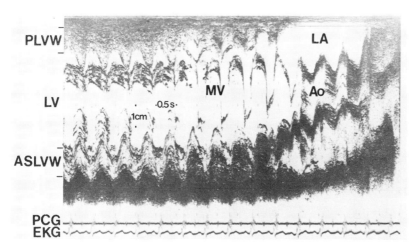

Figure 6. Trans-esophageal M-Mode scan from the aorta (right hand side) to the left ventricle at the level of the papillary muscle (left hand side).
Ao = Aorta, ASLVW = antero septal wall of the left ventricle, MV = mitral valve leaflets, LV = left ventricle, LA = left atrium, PLVW = posterior wall of the left ventricle, PCG = phonocardiogram, ECG = electrocardiogram.

196

always be guaranteed, even during supine bicycle ergometry. Trans-esophageal M-mode echocardiography thus enables the study of left ventricular systolic and diastolic performance in terms of left ventricular dimension and wall thickness changes at rest, as well as during dynamic exercise, in different physiological and pathophysiological conditions [20] (Figure 7).

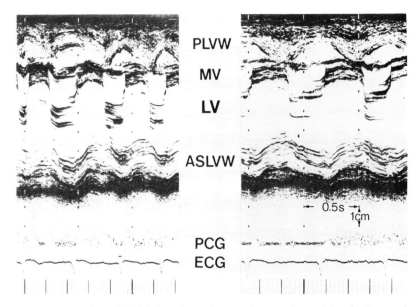

Figure 7. Trans-esophageal M-Mode echocardiogram in a patient with mitral stenosis and coronary artery disease. At rest (right hand side) mitral valve opens immediately after peak posterior wall thickening is reached.

During ergometry and exercised induced ischemia (left hand side) the coordination between regional wall motion and global LV function is disturbed. Mitral valve opens already before posterior wall thickening is terminated. For abbreviations see Figure 4.

REFERENCES

1. Venco A, DB Gibson, DJ Brown: Relation between the apexcardiogram and changes in left ventricular pressure and dimension. Brit Heart J 38:117, 1977.
2. Gibson DB, DJ Brown: Assessment of left ventricular systolic function in man from simultaneous echocardiographic and pressure measurements. Brit Heart J 38:8, 1976.
3. Roelandt J, W Walsh, PG Hugenholtz: Advantages of combined hemodynamic and ultrasonic studies in man. In: Echocardiology (Bom N, ed.), p. 95. Martinus Nijhoff, The Hague, 1977.
4. Hanrath P: Abnormal LV relaxation and filling patterns. In: Echocardiology (Lancée ChT, ed.), Martinus Nijhoff, The Hague, 1979.
5. Doran JH, TA Traill, DJ Brown: Detection of left ventricular wall movement

during isovolumic contraction and early relaxation: comparison of echo- and angiography, Br Heart J 40:367, 1978.

6. Upton MT, DG Gibson: The study of left ventricular function from digitized echocardiograms. Progress in Cardiovasc. Diseases 20:314, 1978.

7. Hirschfield S, J Lietman, G Boshat, C Borsmith: Intracardiac pressure-sound correlates of echographic aortic valve closure. Circulation 55:602, 1977.

8. Chen W, DG Gibson: Relation of isovolumic relaxation to left ventricular wall movement in man. Br Heart J 42:51, 1979.

9. Hanrath P, DG Mathey, P Kremer, F Sonntag, W Bleifeld: Effect of Verapamil on LV isovolumic relaxation time and regional left ventricular filling in hypertrophic cardiomyopathy. Am J Cardiol 45:1258, 1980.

10. Sanderson JE, TA Trail, J Sutton, DJ Brown, DG Gibson, JF Goodwin: Left ventricular relaxation and filling in hypertrophic cardiomyopathy. An echocardiographic study. Brit Heart J 40:596, 1978.

11. Gibson DG, TA Trail, RJC Hall, DJ Brown: Echocardiographic features of secondary left ventricular hypertrophy. Br Heart J 41:54, 1979.

12. Mensing H, P Kremer, P Hanrath, M Matsumoto, D Mathey, W Bleifeld, WM Meigel: Detection of cardiac involvement in patients with scleroderma by M-mode echocardiography. Transactions of the European Congress of Cardiology p 112, 1980.

13. Venco A, M Sariotti, D Besana: Noninvasive assessment of left ventricular function in myotonic muscular dystrophy. Br Heart J 40:1262, 1978.

14. Sutton John MGSt, AY Olukotun, AJ Tajik, JL Lorett, ER Giulani: Left ventricular function in Friedrich's ataxia. An echocardiographical study. Br Heart J 44:399, 1980.

15. Lorell HB, WJ Paulus, W Grossmann, J Wynne, PF Cohn, E Braunwald: Improved diastolic function and systolic performance in hypertrophic cardiomyopathy after Nifedipine. New Engl J Med 303:801, 1980.

16. Bonow RO, DR Rosing, StL Bacharach, MV Green, KM Kent, LC Lipson, JC Condt, MB Leon, StE Epstein: Left ventricular systolic function and diastolic filling in patients with hypertrophic cardiomyopathy: effect of Verapamil. (abstr.) Circulation Suppl II, 62:III-317,

17. Hanrath P, P Kremer: The effect of Verapamil on abnormal left ventricular diatolic performance in patients with secondary left ventricular hypertrophy due to hypertension. International Symposium on Calcium Antagonisms in Cardiovascular Therapy. Experiences with Verapamil. Florence, Italy October 2-4, Excerpta Medica (In Press).

18. Mason STJ, JL Weiss, ML Weisfeldt, JB Garrison, NJ Fortuin: Exercise echocardiography: detection of wall motion abnormalities during ischemia. Circulation 59:50, 1979.

19. Hanrath P, P Kremer, BA Langenstein, M Matsumoto, W Bleifeld: Transesophageale Echocardiographie – ein neues Verfahren zur dynamischen Ventrikelfunktionsanalyse. Deutsche Med Wschr 106:523, 1981.

20. Kremer P, P Hanrath, BA Langenstein, M Matsumoto, C Tams, W Bleifeld: The evaluation of left ventricular function at rest and during exercise by transesophageal echocardiography in aortic insufficiency. Am J 47–II:412, 1981.

23. MEAN VELOCITY OF FIBER SHORTENING AS LINEAR FUNCTION OF HEART RATE AND WALL STRESS: NONINVASIVE MEASUREMENTS

J. Cosyns, D. Delatte, D. Raphael, and Ch. van Eyll

Mean velocity of circumferential fiber shortening normalized for end-diastolic volume ($\overline{VCF}$) is widely accepted as a valuable index of left ventricular function [1]. This parameter can be calculated on M-mode echocardiographic tracings provided that myocardial contraction is homogeneous, without akinetic or dyskinetic segments. In these conditions, such noninvasive measurements give comparable values to those derived from angiocardiography [2]. When the contractile state is constant, $\overline{VCF}$ appears to be independent of preload but not of afterload [3]. In addition, heart rate, as a main determinant of ejection time, must affect $\overline{VCF}$ which, for this reason too, does reflect the level in sympathetic tone and contractility of the heart [4].

The aim of our study was to determine the respective role of afterload and of heart rate in the scattering of $\overline{VCF}$ values measured in normal resting subjects. We also investigated the sensitivity of $\overline{VCF}$ to acute changes in afterload, here expressed as end-systolic meridional wall stress (σ_m).

MATERIAL AND METHODS

Seventeen normal young volunteers (mean age 26.6 years) were studied. Left ventricular echoes (Irex apparatus, 2.25 MHz transducer) under the mitral level were registered on an UV recorder (100 mm/sec paper speed), simultaneously with ECG and carotid pulse tracings. Subjects were studied in a semi-recumbent position, slightly turned on the left side. Arterial brachial systolic and diastolic pressures, determined by the cuff method, permitted the calibration of the carotid pulse and the subsequent aortic pressure estimate at the time of the valve closure (dicrotic notch) [5]. Major and minor left ventricular internal diameters and maximum end-systolic posterior wall thickness in centimeters were measured to a precision of ± 1 mm. Shortening fraction (the difference between end-diastolic and end-systolic diameters, divided by end-diastolic diameter) was calculated. $\overline{VCF}$ (circ/sec) normalized for end-diastolic dimension was then obtained by dividing shortening fraction by carotid ejection time (sec). End-systolic meridional wall stress (σ_m) was calculated as follows [6]:

Rijsterborgh H, ed: Echocardiology, p 199-203. All rights reserved.

$$\sigma_m = \frac{P \cdot D \cdot 10^{-3}}{4 \cdot h \cdot (1 + h/D)} \text{ dynes/cm}^2$$

where P = end-systolic pressure (dynes/cm^2), D = end-systolic ventricular internal diameter (cm) and h = end-systolic posterior wall thickness (cm). All the data retained for this study were the means of the measurements made on five subsequent beats. After completion of the study in basal conditions, the procedure was repeated at the peak action (about 3 min) of sublingual administration of 1 mg nitroglycerin.

RESULTS

Mean values ($\pm$SD) of the different parameters in the basal state and under nitroglycerin action are presented in Figure 1. From the statistical analysis, made using the paired t-test, of the differences between the two situations, we observe that all these parameters change significantly.

Individual values of $\overline{\text{VCF}}$, RR interval (RR) and σ_m are illustrated in Figures 2 and 3, with the correlation coefficient (r) and the regression lines between $\overline{\text{VCF}}$ and σ_m and between $\overline{\text{VCF}}$ and RR.

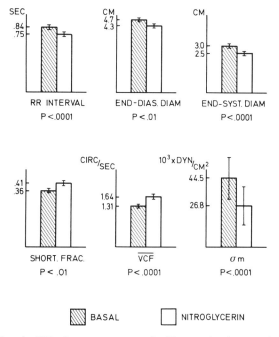

Figure 1. Mean values ($\pm$SD) of some parameters in 17 normal volunteers in basal state and at the peak action of nitroglycerin (1 mg sublingual).

In each of the two experimental situations, a regression plane between $\overline{\text{VCF}}$, RR and σ_m can be calculated by the least squares method. In this manner, $\overline{\text{VCF}}$ values can be estimated by applying the following formulas:

$$\overline{\text{VCF}}_{\text{est}} = 2.34 - 0.786 \cdot \text{RR} - 0.008 \cdot \sigma_m \qquad \text{circ/sec (SEE = 0.15)}$$

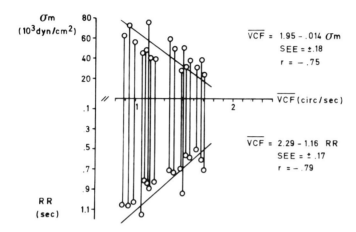

Figure 2. Correlation between $\overline{\text{VCF}}$ in the basal state with σ_m and with RR. Vertical lines join values of σ_m and RR for the same subjects. These lines intercept the horizontal axis at the corresponding values of $\overline{\text{VCF}}$.

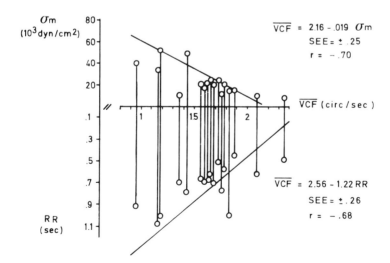

Figure 3. Correlation between $\overline{\text{VCF}}$ at the peak action of nitroglycerin with σ_m and with RR. Vertical lines join values of σ_m and RR for the same subjects. These lines intercept the horizontal axis at the corresponding values of $\overline{\text{VCF}}$.

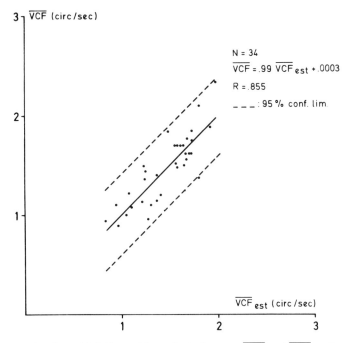

Figure 4. Regression line with 95% confidence limits between $\overline{VCF}$ and $\overline{VCF}_{est}$ after pooling the data from the control and the nitroglycerin situations.

in the basal state and

$$\overline{VCF}_{est} = 2.58 - 0.768 \cdot RR - 0.013 \cdot \sigma_m \quad \text{circ/sec (SEE = 0.23)}$$

under nitroglycerin.

The correlation coefficients between $\overline{VCF}_{est}$ and $\overline{VCF}$ in the two states are, respectively, 0.86 and 0.79. The similarity of the $\overline{VCF}_{est}$ in the two situations justifies the calculation of a common regression plane:

$$\overline{VCF}_{est} = 2.5 - 0.75 \cdot RR - 0.012 \cdot \sigma_m \quad \text{circ/sec (SEE = 0.19).}$$

Figure 4 shows the regression line with 95% confidence limits between $\overline{VCF}$ and the estimated value of $\overline{VCF}$ ($\overline{VCF}_{est}$) calculated by the last formula. This regression line is virtually a line of identity.

DISCUSSION AND CONCLUSION

This study shows that $\overline{VCF}$ is not only dependent on afterload (here expressed as end-systolic meridional wall stress) but that heart rate also plays an important role in its value. By combining these two parameters it became possible to estimate $\overline{VCF}$ in normal subjects to a good approximation. By lowering afterload, nitroglycerin, which is known to have no direct effect on myocardial function, induces a reflex tachycardia and an increase in $\overline{\text{VCF}}$. Under these conditions the relation between $\overline{\text{VCF}}$, RR and σ_m remains comparable to that found in the resting state.

Wide confidence limits are found for the relation between $\overline{\text{VCF}}_{est}$ and $\overline{\text{VCF}}$. This is not surprising when one considers that all measurements are noninvasive: dimensions of the left ventricle depend on the ultrasonic beam incidence; carotid pulse morphology and external pressure measurements only approximate the end-systolic pressure [5].

By comparing $\overline{\text{VCF}}$ with its estimated value, which is not a direct measurement of myocardial contractility, it should be possible to detect muscular dysfunction and to distinguish more accurately between myocardial and peripheral effects of drugs.

REFERENCES

1. Karliner JS, JH Gault, DL Eckberg, CB Mullins, J Jr Ross: Mean velocity of fiber shortening: a simplified measure of left ventricular myocardial contractility. Circulation 44:323, 1971.
2. Cooper RH, RA O'Rourke, JS Karliner, KL Peterson, GR Leopold: Comparison of ultrasound and cineangiographic measurements of the mean rate of circumferential fiber shortening in man. Circulation 46:914, 1972.
3. Mahler FH, J Jr Ross, RA O'Rourke, JW Covell: Effects of change in preload, afterload and inotropic state on ejection and isovolumic phase measures of contractility in the conscious dog. Am J Cardiol 35:626, 1975.
4. Hirshleifer J, M Crawford, RA O'Rourke, JS Karliner: Influence of acute alterations in heart rate and systemic arterial pressure on echocardiographic measures of left ventricular performance in normal human subjects. Circulation 52:835, 1975.
5. Marsh JD, LH Green, J Wynne, PF Cohn, W Grossman: Left ventricular end-systolic pressure-dimension and stress-length relations in normal human subjects. Amer J Cardiol 44:1311, 1979.
6. Brodie Br, LP McLaurin, W Grossman: Combined hemodynamic-ultrasonic method for studying left ventricular wall stress. Amer J Cardiol 37:864, 1976.

24. THE EVALUATION OF LEFT VENTRICULAR PERFORMANCE BY SIMULTANEOUS RECORDING OF TWO-DIMENSIONAL ECHOCARDIOGRAM AND LEFT VENTRICULAR PRESSURE

P. KREMER, M. MATSUMOTO, B. LANGENSTEIN, and P. HANRATH

Two-dimensional echocardiography [1, 2] has become a useful method for the evaluation of cardiac performance in terms of volume calculation and wall motion abnormalities. For a more detailed assessment of left ventricular (LV) performance, the simultaneous recording of two-dimensional (2D) echocardiogram and LV pressure is necessary for the calculation of special parameters, such as wall stress.

MATERIAL AND METHODS

In this study, a newly-developed analog-to-digital (AD) converter [3] was used to provide a simultaneous display of LV pressure and 2D echocardiography in order to assess LV function in 6 patients with atrial septal defect (there is a greater likelihood of being able to visualize the whole LV using 2D echo in an ASD patient).

Left ventricular pressure recordings were obtained using a high fidelity catheter-tip micromanometer. The LV pressure thus obtained was digitized by the AD-converter. Each (pressure) conversion was started at the beginning of a video frame of the imaging system and was initiated by the video frame pulse. Pressure sampling was, therefore, synchronous with the repetition rate of the two-dimensional images (50 Hz). Since the conversion time of the applied AD-converter was relatively short (35–40 μsec) compared with the duration of a video frame (20 msec), the converted value represented the pressure at the beginning of a video frame. The digitized pressure was displayed as a number, together with the two-dimensional echocardiogram, on a video monitor. The 2D echocardiograms were made with a Picker Echoview System 80 CI using a mechanical sector-scanner with a sector angle of 60° and a 3.5 MHz medium-focused 13 mm transducer. Long-axis and short-axis 2D echocardiograms of the LV were recorded successively, LV pressure was recorded simultaneously and both were recorded on a video tape recorder. Later on, the LV contour was traced with a lightpen and left ventricular diameters were digitized for computer analysis. Pressure was entered manually from the keyboard, after reading the value from the video screen.

Rijsterborgh H, ed: Echocardiology, p 205-207. All rights reserved.
Copyright © 1981 Martinus Nijhoff Publishers, The Hague/Boston/London.

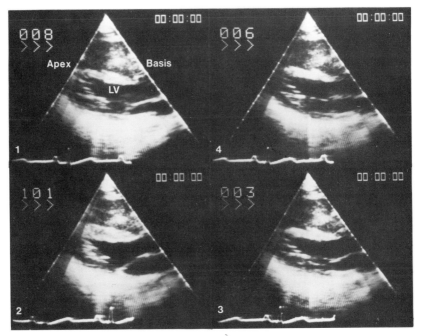

Figure 1. Four representative frames from one cardiac cycle in a case with atrial septal defect (Long-axis views).

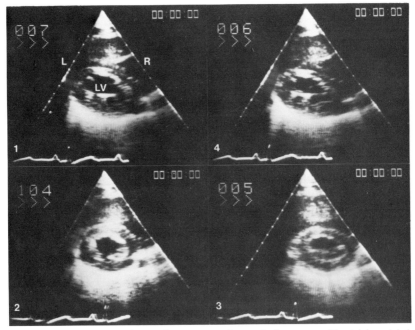

Figure 2. Four representative frames from one cardiac cycle in a case with atrial septal defect (Short-axis views).

RESULTS

Two examples are shown on the following figures: Figure 1 shows four representative frames from one cardiac cycle in one case with atrial septal defect (ASD) in long-axis view at end-diastole (frames 1 and 4) and end-systole (frame 2). Figure 2 exhibits four frames of the same patient in short-axis cross-section. Digitized LV pressure is displayed on the left upper corner of each frame.

LV circumferential and longitudinal stresses (σ_c and σ_l) at end-diastole (ED) and end-systole (ES) were calculated using the equation reported by Gould et al. [4].

The mean values of calculated stress in 6 ASD patients were as follows:

$$\sigma_c(ED) = 1.62 \pm 0.29 \text{ kPa}$$
$$\sigma_c(ES) = 15.7 \pm 5.11 \text{ kPa}$$
$$\sigma_l(ED) = 0.71 \pm 0.13 \text{ kPa}$$
$$\sigma_l(ES) = 6.15 \pm 2.16 \text{ kPa}$$

Comparison of these values with those determined by angiography showed excellent correlation ($r = 0.97$ in σ_c, $r = 0.94$ in σ_l).

DISCUSSION

This new method has the following potential advantages: the ability to calculate both longitudinal and circumferential stresses, even in a left ventricle with a non-prolate elliptic configuration, and to calculate stresses continuously, as well as to assess the response to different interventions. The major disadvantage of this method, however, is that it is only applicable to patients without dilated left ventricles and from whom high quality 2D echoes can be recorded.

REFERENCES

1. Griffith IM, WL Henry: A sector scanner for real-time two-dimensional echocardiography. Circulation 49:1147, 1974.
2. von Ramm OT, FL Thurstone: Cardiac imaging using a phased array ultrasound system. I. system design. Circulation 53:258, 1976.
3. Kamm KF: Angiographische Auswertungen mit einem Prozessrechner-System für das Herzkatheterlabor. Biomedizinische Technik 24:Suppl. 72, 1979.
4. Gould KL, K Lipscomb, GW Hamilton, JW Kennedy: Relation of left ventricular, shape, function and wall stress in man. Am J Cardiol 34:627, 1974.

I. ECHOCARDIOLOGY IN ADULTS

C. APPLICATIONS OF CONTRAST ECHOCARDIOLOGY AND DOPPLER ECHOCARDIOLOGY

25. STRUCTURE IDENTIFICATION BY CONTRAST ECHOCARDIOGRAPHY

RICHARD L. POPP and CHARLES R. TUCKER

The exciting technique of structure identification by contrast echocardiography has many developing applications and is now especially useful in defining cardiac chambers and in the recognition of congenital heart defects, as well as of complications of the abnormal flow resulting from such defects. But, if we are trying to define a given chamber, or the time sequence of flow of contrast moving from one chamber to another, the basic identity of each structure is the most important information we must begin with. Most people doing echocardiography now believe they understand cardiac anatomy very well, and in fact they do. But as the equipment has allowed us to see more and more details of the cardiac anatomy, and we are presented a more comprehensive view of the heart than has been possible in the past, the subtle details of anatomic features that were not visible or not important before become crucial to our diagnosis.

We must come to ask ourselves, "Do I understand the internal anatomy of the right atrium in enough detail to visualize it in three dimensions?", "Do I understand the attachments of the pericardium around the heart and great vessels sufficiently to know all of the potential spaces for pericardial fluid collection?" This type of detailed information is the source of diagnosis or, alternatively, the source of frustration when dealing with imaged structures that are not commonly seen. A firm basis in anatomy is the prime need of echocardiographers. Contrast echocardiography is an excellent tool for clarifying distortions of the heart due to disease superimposed on a normally formed heart, as well as for clarifying the pathophysiology of congenital defects. For example, there is a reflection of the pericardium around the right atrium in most people and, in the presence of pericardial effusion, this can give rise to some very confusing patterns. Figure 1 shows a structure which is possibly within the right atrium of a patient in whom a right atrial mass could have clinical significance. The patient also had pericardial effusion and, after injection of contrast material into the venous system, the extent of the right atrium was defined. The apparent "structure" within the right atrium was actually the posterior atrial wall, with an accumulation of pericardial effusion posterior to the atrial wall.

Further, one can inject a small amount of contrast into a needle introduced for pericardiocentesis in order to have the contrast agent circulate in the space marked by the end of the needle so one can tell if the tip of the needle is in the heart, the pericardium or the pleural space. In the usual contrast study, the contrast agent is introduced into a peripheral vein. The common defect of a persistent left superior vena cava emptying via the coronary sinus into the right atrium is well defined using injection into the left arm. The large circular space in the posterior atrioventricular groove that is present on parasternal long-axis views of the heart fills with contrast material prior to flow of the contrast agent into the right heart [1].

Structure identification by contrast echocardiography within the heart is limited by and defined by the flow patterns in a given patient. Recently several groups have primarily introduced contrast agents for echocardiogra-

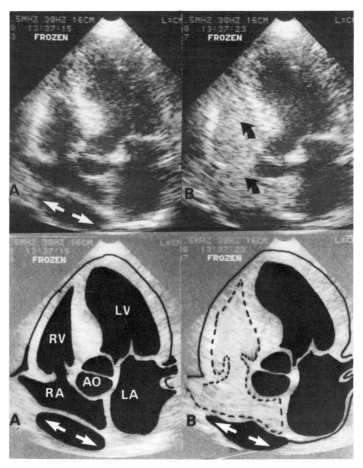

Figure 1. Apical four-chamber view prior to (panel A) and during (panel B) contrast injection. The space (white arrows), apparently part of the right atrium (RA), does not fill with contrast (black arrows) and is extracardiac. This is pericardial effusion posterior to the RA. Other abbreviations are standard.

phy by means of catheters in the left heart. However, if we do not use the newly developed technique for introducing contrast agents into the left heart via the pulmonary circulation, we should primarily concern ourselves with right heart flow. We will discuss structure identification roughly in the sequence of flow after venous injection.

The normal pattern of flow from the vena cavae to the right atrium can be well visualized in the majority of cases where adequate contrast is introduced intravenously. Reflux of contrast material into the inferior cava, after introduction of the material via the superior cava, occurs in some normal situations and several pathologic conditions. Many investigators have found M-mode records, taken through the inferior cava or hepatic veins, to be useful in precisely timing the appearance of the contrast material in the infradiaphragmatic vessels [2]. It is not at all unusual to see contrast material arrive in the inferior cava after venous injection and before ventricular systole in the presence of a relatively non-compliant right ventricle. This does not mean the patient has tricuspid regurgitation, since the contrast is refluxing into the venous system prior to ventricular systole. With a comprehensive view of the atrial-caval junction, such as is seen with subcostal views, one can get a good idea of the sequence of flow and of the timing of this flow. Nevertheless, the average observer cannot keep track of the electrocardiogram and the two-dimensional image at one time and so it is necessary to use M-mode recording or an audible signal, such as a signal joined to the QRS complex, if one wishes to adequately assess the timing of flow using contrast agents. Flow within the right atrium is generally viewed as a reference for flow targets passing into the left atrium or some other structure. When trying to track this flow, or when looking for negative contrast effects of flow from the left atrium to the right, we must be aware of the right atrial anatomy. The ostium of the coronary sinus, the valve of the inferior cava, the Chiari network, and the potential flow from the thebesian veins may lead to confusion in interpreting right atrial flow. When analyzing the echocardiogram for possible defects in the interatrial septum, one should be very clear on the anatomy of the septum primum and septum secundum. Figure 2 is a diagrammatic representation of the anatomy of the interatrial septum pertinent to the views used with most two-dimensional systems. This figure shows some of the anatomic features of the atrium and indicates the usual sites of ostium secundum, ostium primum, and sinus venous atrial septal defects.

Right atrial anatomy is generally termed "complex" or "variable" and can be properly described by both of these terms. However, the amount of trabeculation within the right ventricle, the general form of the right ventricle, and the anatomic definition of the tricuspid valve and the pulmonic valve within the normal right ventricle are rather uniform. The anatomy of the great vessels is extremely consistent in most adults, but may

214

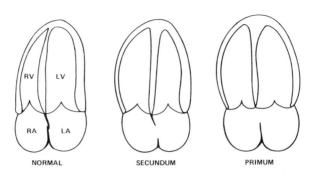

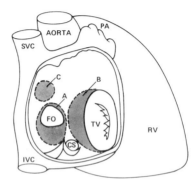

Figure 2. Diagrams of atrial septal defects as viewed by echocardiography (above) and right atrial anatomy (below). The locations of (A) ostium secundum, (B) ostium primum and (C) sinus venosus defects are indicated.

CS = coronary sinus, FO = fossa ovalis, IVC = inferior vena cava, SVC = superior vena cava, TV = tricuspid valve, RV = right ventricle.

be arranged along a full spectrum of interrelationships in patients with congenital malformations. Because the current limitations of display give us only black, white and gray pictures of the structures, it is not possible to consistently record a given chamber in a contrasting color for consistent identification. If we could do this it would not be necessary to standardize our examination techniques. Actually this is just the reason that forces us to use standardized examination techniques for transducer placement and manipulation [3]. Once the anatomy is firmly visualized and the examiner has a clear idea of the three-dimensional anatomy involved, innovative examination techniques can be used. Methods to visualize the right ventricular inflow tract, the junction of the right ventricular outflow and the pulmonary artery, and the extent of the pulmonary artery and its bifurcation, are available (Figure 3).

Transducer positions at the cardiac apex are most consistently useful for evaluation of intracardiac flow when the question of shunt is being explored. From this apical position, the four-chamber view can be used to interrogate

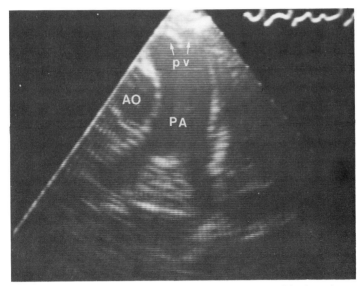

Figure 3. Echo image of the main pulmonary artery and its branches.
AO = aorta, PA = pulmonary artery, pv = pulmonary valve.

the volume which includes virtually all of the heart. Choosing the appropriate level for imaging, one can then observe the timing of the contrast echocardiographic target's appearance in the various chambers and structures. In the presence of a post-infarction ventricular septal defect, for example, one may choose parasternal or other views to further localize and define the nature of the defect once the four-chamber views have clarified the general level of the defect. As in most shunt lesions, there is some bidirectional flow across such ventricular septal defects as shown in Figure 4.

We have commented little on the identification of left heart structures since generally one needs to have a catheter introduced into the left heart in order to visualize these structures. In the presence of a large volume right-to-left shunt the identification of left heart structures has more pertinence. When injecting contrast agents into the left heart by catheter, the velocity of flow in the left heart often presents a problem for structure identification since there is very rapid washout of contrast material from the left heart. Also there may be considerable streaming of blood within the left heart.

Some very exciting studies have recently been performed with catheters placed in the coronary vessels and special contrast agents introduced selectively into the coronary arteries in animals [4]. In these studies there is considerable enhancement of reflectance of the myocardium after contrast injection. Sub-selective coronary artery injections show the distribution of coronary flow by segmental myocardial contrast enhancement and, with

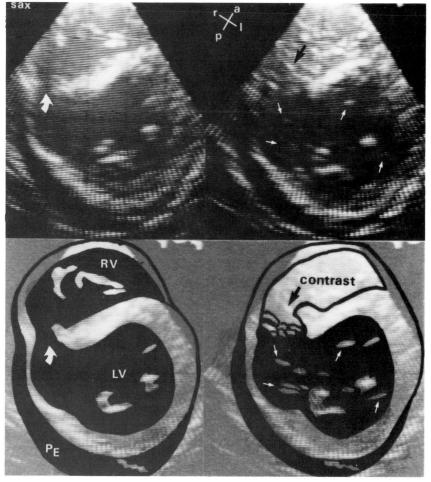

Figure 4. Short-axis (sax) parasternal views of a heart with post-infarction ventricular septal defect (large arrow). After peripheral contrast injection (right panel) contrast echoes are seen in the left ventricle (LV) (small arrows).

PE = pericardial effusion, a = anterior, p = posterior, r = right, l = left, RV = right ventricle.

some agents, slow egress of contrast agent appears to occur, indicating the level of flow present. This is an exciting area for the future.

LIMITATIONS

Structure identification by contrast echocardiography is limited by several factors. First among these is the introduction of contrast material into the venous system and its adequate transmission into the right heart. We will not go into this in detail here but, when very slow venous flow is occurring, there will obviously be an effect on transmission of the contrast agent to the right heart. Also, if the patient is in the left lateral decubitus position and the left arm is used for injection, there is sometimes an apparent compression of the left venous vessels with ineffectual contrast introduction. In general, the more proximal the injection site, the more reproducible and adequate will be the contrast visualization. Of course if one uses artificial targets or commercially produced contrast material, the reproducibility of contrast delivery is improved. Any contrast agent may be introduced into the heart and be virtually invisible if the imaging system is so noisy that a great amount of random signal is occurring and obscuring the transit of contrast through the heart. Conversely, if the system is either so insensitive or the gains are reduced to such an extent that the contrast signals are not made visible by the instrument, no structure identification can take place. It is important to note that the signal distal to a chamber highly filled with gaseous contrast material may not be well visualized. This is because a great deal of the sound transmitted into the chamber containing contrast is scattered or absorbed, with little remaining sound to be transmitted to the subsequent potential sound reflectors [5].

A different type of physical limitation relates to the volume of resolution of ultrasonic imaging systems. While we commonly speak of the axial resolution of an ultrasound system, this measurement seldom comes into consideration with contrast echocardiography. We are not trying to resolve two sides of the contrast target but we are only asking the instrument to present a single interface (the leading edge of the target) defining the location of the contrast agent. The lateral spread of such highly reflective structures may lead to apparent spread of the signal into a chamber where the contrast is not truly present. This is not usually a problem when dealing with lateral resolution in the plane of scan. In this case one can tell if the signals are being spread in both lateral directions from a location representing the true reflector site. If there is spread of the signal into a neighboring chamber, the observer can generally perceive this. There is more of a problem when we consider resolution out of the plane of scan. Resolution in this third dimension is usually worse than in either of the other two directions because of transducer construction. At least this has been true in studies done at Stanford by our group. If a signal appears in the chamber because of highly reflective targets being "behind" or "in front of" the visualized scan-plane, the observer has virtually no way of knowing that these echoes are spuriously presented. The recognition of this phenomenon goes some way toward avoiding improper diagnoses resulting from this error. As instrument sensitivity improves, this problem could become more prevalent, but as the equipment is improved with regard to transducer design, the volumetric resolution should be better and the problem just described should be reduced. It is important for each person working with contrast echocardiography to understand the physical limitations of the equipment in order to avoid problems now while the equipment is being improved beyond our current levels.

REFERENCES

1. Snider RA, TA Ports, NH Silverman: Venous anomalies of the coronary sinus: Detection by M-mode, two-dimensional and contrast echocardiography. Circulation 60:721–727, 1979.
2. Wise NK, S Myers, JA Stewart, R Waugh, T Fraker, J Kisslo: Echo inferior venacavography: A technique for the study of right sided heart disease. Circulation (Suppl II) 59 and 60:II–202, 1979.
3. Henry WL, A DeMaria, R Gramiak, DL King, JA Kisslo, RL Popp, DJ Sahn, NB Schiller, A Tajik, LE Teichholz, AE Weyman: Report of the American Society of Echocardiography Committee on Nomenclature and Standards in Two-dimensional Echocardiography. Circulation 62:212–217, 1980.
4. DeMaria AN, WJ Bommer, K Riggs, A Dajee, M Keown, OL Kwan, DT Mason: Echocardiographic visualization of myocardial perfusion by left heart and intracoronary injections of echo contrast agents. Circulation (Suppl III) 62:III–143, 1980.

26. CONTRAST ECHOCARDIOGRAPHY OF THE LEFT VENTRICLE

J. ROELANDT, R.S. MELTZER, and P.W. SERRUYS

1. INTRODUCTION

Rapid injection of biologically compatible solutions produces a "cloud of echoes" in the blood which is otherwise echo free. The source of this echocardiographic contrast is microbubbles of air introduced during injection [1, 2].

Left ventricular catheter injections have been employed to identify left side structures from M-mode echocardiograms [3, 4] and to validate cardiac views imaged by two-dimensional echocardiography [5, 6]. The method has also been found to be accurate and sensitive for the demonstration of small, intracardiac, left-to-right shunts and of minimal degrees of aortic and mitral valve regurgitation [7, 8, 9].

Injection of echo contrast material into the left ventricle, however, requires cardiac catheterization, making it an invasive procedure. This probably explains why left ventricular contrast echocardiography has not gained widespread clinical application.

Recently the possibility of transmitting echo contrast material across the capillary bed of the lungs to the left heart with pulmonary wedge injections [10, 11, 12] or with peripheral venous injections using experimental contrast agents [13, 16] has been demonstrated. These possibilities show great promise and may stimulate an increasing interest in ultrasonic left heart opacification. This chapter aims to review some methodological and clinical aspects of left ventricular contrast echocardiography. Most of this area is still investigational.

2. METHODOLOGIC ASPECTS OF LEFT VENTRICULAR CONTRAST ECHOCARDIOGRAPHY

At present, echocardiographic contrast studies of the left ventricle are performed in the catheterization laboratory. M-mode or two-dimensional techniques can be employed, each having its specific advantages and limitations for clinical problem-solving and research.

2.1. Two-dimensional echocardiographic views employed

Our experience with left ventricular echo contrast has been mainly with two-dimensional echocardiography, using a dynamically focussed linear-array instrument (Fociscan, Organon Teknika) or a phased-array sector-scanner (Toshiba SSH-10A). The long-axis and short-axis views from the parasternal transducer position as well as the four-chamber and long-axis views from apical transducer position are routinely recorded [6, 14]. The apical views are especially useful for quantitative left ventricular studies, since the entire left ventricle from apex to base can often be recorded.

2.2. Left ventricular injection of echocardiographic contrast material

The rapid injection through a catheter of any biologically compatible fluid into the left ventricle causes echocardiographic contrast. We routinely use a manual flush of 5 to 10 ml of 5% dextrose in water.

Indocyanine green dye may yield a better contrast effect because of its surfactant properties, which keep the microbubbles of air, resulting from the vigorous shaking during preparation, stabilized in the solution [2]. One milliliter of indocyanine green solution (5 mg/ml for adults) is injected into the catheter and manually flushed with 5 to 10 ml of physiologic saline or 5% dextrose [7]. We have never observed any adverse patient reaction to direct left ventricular injections during echocardiographic contrast studies [15].

2.3. Pulmonary wedge injection of echocardiographic contrast material

Bommer et al. [10] reported in 1979 that catheter injections in the pulmonary wedge position in dogs cause echocardiographic contrast on the left side of the heart. Reale et al. [11] studied 43 patients with acquired or congenital heart disease and injected different echo-producing substances (indocyanine green dye, saline and carbon dioxide) via a balloon-tipped catheter in the pulmonary wedge position. Echocardiographic contrast was seen in the left ventricle in all patients studied. No complications or side effects were observed. We have studied 41 patients, using a Cournand 7F catheter alone in 27, a Swan-Ganz 7F catheter alone in 3 and both catheters in 11, for pulmonary wedge injections. Left ventricular echocardiographic contrast was seen in 3 out of 14 patients with the Swan-Ganz catheter and in 30 out of 38 patients when the Cournand catheter was used (Figure 1). We found that injection pressure proximal to the catheter had to be more than 40 kPa (300 mmHg) in order to obtain left side echocardiographic contrast.

Angiocardiographic studies with injections of Amipaque® further demon-

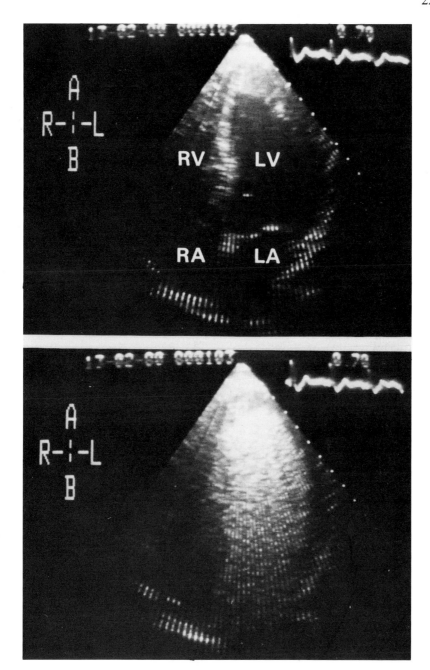

Figure 1. Stop-frame, apical four-chamber views obtained from a patient with a normal left ventricle immediately before (upper panel) and after pulmonary wedge injection of echocardiographic contrast (lower panel). The echo contrast fills both the left atrium (LA) and left ventricle (LV), of which the cavity contour becomes clearly delineated.

A = apical; B = basal; L = left; R = right; RA = right atrium and RV = right ventricle.

strated that a complete occlusive wedge position of the catheter must be achieved. The latter finding probably explains the higher success rate with a Cournand catheter: its higher stiffness allows more complete occlusion. It is conceivable that the pressure applied during occlusive injections may allow deformation of the air bubbles into a "dumbbell" shape resulting in their intact passage, rather than being retained by the "sieve" action of the capillary bed [16]. Apart from coughing, none of our patients had symptoms or worsening of their cardiopulmonary status related to the pulmonary wedge injections. Nonetheless, the method must still be considered as an experimental procedure until its safety has been finally established [12, 16].

2.4. Transmission of peripherally injected contrast through the lungs

Microbubbles of gas larger than the capillary diameter (approximately 8 microns) are stopped by the "sieve" action of the pulmonary capillary bed. On the other hand, microbubbles small enough to pass the pulmonary capillaries have an internal pressure which is significantly higher than the ambient blood pressure. Gas inside the microbubble therefore dissolves down its concentration gradient into the surrounding blood. The duration of this process is shorter than the pulmonary transit time and explains why the commonly employed contrast materials for peripheral venous injection are removed from the circulation before they reach the left side cavities [17].

We have created left side echocardiographic contrast in pigs by the injection of diethyl ether and hydrogen peroxide in the right heart or proximal pulmonary artery. Our studies demonstrated, however, that these agents are potentially dangerous [16]. Recently, transmission of echocardiographic contrast through the pulmonary capillary bed following peripheral venous injection has been demonstrated in dogs by Bommer et al. [10] using 2 to 10 micron diameter microbubbles. Human application must await toxicity studies.

Opacification of the left ventricle following peripheral venous injection is thus a valid research goal. A better understanding of physical characteristics and physiological behaviour of microbubbles will probably permit successful attainment of this goal in the not too distant future.

3. CLINICAL APPLICATIONS OF LEFT VENTRICULAR CONTRAST ECHOCARDIOGRAPHY

3.1. Demonstration of valvular insufficiency

Systolic regurgitation of echo contrast material to the left atrium after left ventricular injection is indicative of mitral regurgitation. The method is sensitive and minimal amounts of regurgitation are readily detected [9, 18]. In moderate to severe degrees of mitral incompetence, the clearance time of the echo contrast from both the left atrium and left ventricle is considerably prolonged. Normally, echo contrast material remains from 4 to 10 cycles in the left ventricle and from 4 to 6 cycles in the left atrium. Uchiyama et al. [19] were able to determine the site of regurgitation in two patients with mitral valve prolapse syndrome using the echo contrast technique. Aortic regurgitation is demonstrated with a high degree of sensitivity by injecting echo contrast material in the aortic root and detecting its appearance in the left ventricle during diastole. The clearance time of the echo contrast from the left ventricle is much prolonged (15 to 50 cycles). In some instances, the regurgitant pattern of echo contrast may be observed as a "shower of echoes" hitting the anterior mitral valve or interventricular septum. Clearance time cannot be used to quantify mitral or aortic regurgitation reliably. It may serve, however, to confirm or exclude its presence in patients in whom roentgenographic contrast studies are contraindicated due to pregnancy [20] or angiographic dye allergy.

3.2. Demonstration of left-to-right shunts

Echo contrast flow patterns after left ventricular injection are helpful in identifying ventricular septal defects with left-to-right shunting and are at least as sensitive as indicator-dilution studies. Appearance of the echo contrast in the right ventricle or right ventricular outflow tract may be simultaneous with injection or be delayed by one cycle. The appearance time is dependent upon the timing of injection during the cardiac cycle and the position of the catheter in the left ventricle. A left-to-right shunt as small as 5 % of the pulmonary flow may be detected [8]. We have experience with two patients in whom a ventricular septal defect was missed by oximetry and diagnosed by left ventricular contrast echocardiography (Figure 2). The method is useful for the demonstration of a left ventricular to right atrial shunt and the localization of small defects in the trabecular septum using the apical four-chamber view. Recently, Reale et al. [11] have demonstrated the possibility of using pulmonary wedge injections (see paragraph 2.3) for direct visualization of a left-to-right shunt at atrial or ventricular level, thus obviating left heart catheterization. They rightly concluded that the method could be used as a simple screening procedure during right heart catheterization to avoid invasion of the left heart in some patients. The toxicity of pulmonary wedge injections and the sensitivity of this approach as compared to oximetry and indicator dilution techniques need further evaluation.

224

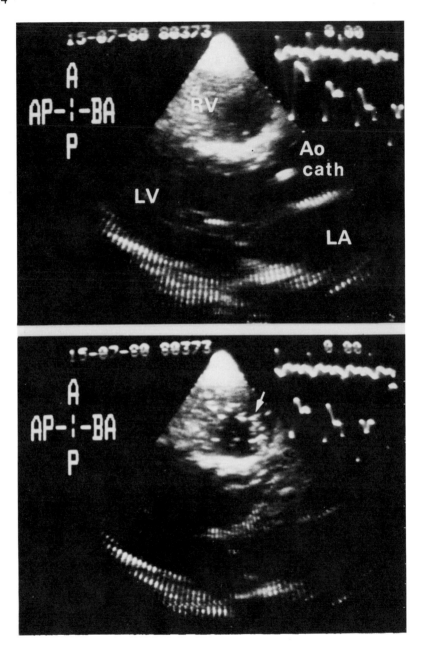

Figure 2. Parasternal long-axis views of a patient with a small ventricular septal defect before (upper panel) and after (lower panel) catheter injection of echo contrast in the left ventricular outflow tract. Echoes appear in the right ventricular outflow tract (arrow) proving the existence of a small left-to-right shunt.

A = anterior; AP = apical; BA = basal; P = posterior; Ao = aorta; cath = catheter; LA = left atrium; LV = left ventricle; RV = right ventricle.

225

3.3. Delineation of the left ventricular cavity

Feigenbaum et al. [4] utilized left ventricular injections of indocyanine green dye to identify the endocardium from other echoes within its cavity. Even when using newer equipment, non-structural echoes often obscure the endocardial boundaries and make proper delineation of the left ventricular cavity difficult or even impossible [21]. It is conceivable that opacification of the left ventricular cavity with echocardiographic contrast would improve border recognition. An illustrative case of a patient with clinical features of restrictive (obliterative) cardiomyopathy is shown in Figure 3. The size and shape of the left ventricle could not be appreciated from the routine echocardiographic study because the apical area was obliterated by non-structural echoes (Figure 3, upper panel). After opacification with echocardiographic contrast via a pulmonary wedge injection, a bilocular deformity of its shape was demonstrated (Figure 3, lower panel).

It would seem likely that improved cavity delineation by echocardiographic contrast would increase the accuracy of left ventricular volume determination from two-dimensional images. We therefore made recordings of the left ventricle in four views (parasternal long-axis view and short-axis view, at mitral level; apical four-chamber view and long-axis view) before and during left ventricular injections of 5% dextrose in water in 13 patients (Figures 1 and 4). Long axis length and surface area within the endocardial contours were measured from stop-frame images, independently, from recordings with and without contrast, using a lightpen system and a digital computer. The measurements were repeated by the same investigator one month later. Long axis length was 71.5 ± 14.0 mm without and 70.8 ± 12.0 mm with contrast (mean ± 1 SD). This difference was not statistically significant. For the surface area, the measurement with contrast was 1.5 cm^2 larger than without contrast and this was significant ($P > 0.001$). Thus, the use of echo contrast did not affect measurement of the long axis length but did increase the value for surface area. To our surprise, measurements on contrast images showed a higher intra-observer variability. In another series of 18 patients we compared left ventricular volumes determined by angiocardiography with these measured from two-dimensional echocardiographic views (apical four-chamber view and apical long-axis view) before and after injections of echocardiographic contrast. The use of contrast did not improve the correlation between echocardiographic and angiocardiographic volumes. Our studies, although preliminary, indicate that contrast echocardiography does not improve the accuracy of quantitation of the left ventricle from echocardiographic stop-frame images.

226

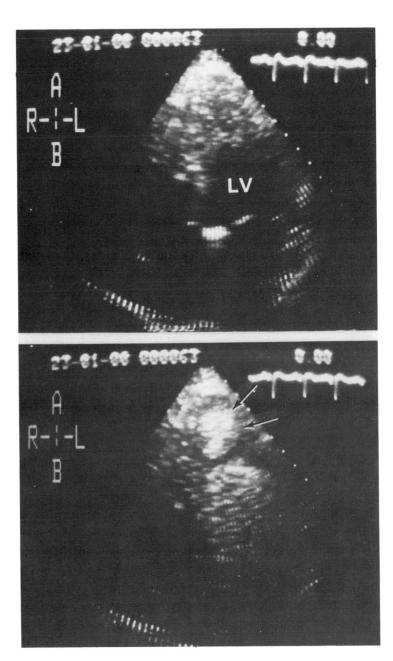

Figure 3. Apical four-chamber views of a patient with Loefflers eosinophilia. Before opacification, the contour of the left ventricle cannot be appreciated because of non-structural echoes filling its cavity, mainly in the apical area (upper panel). After a pulmonary wedge injection of echo contrast, a bilocular shape of the left ventricular cavity is demonstrated (lower panel).

A = apical; B = basal; R = right; L = left; LV = left ventricle.

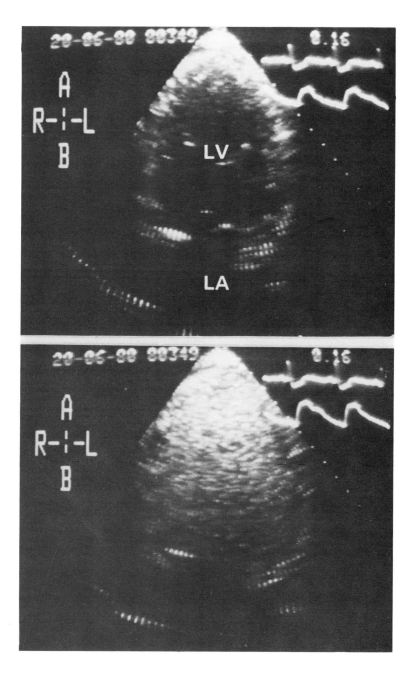

Figure 4. Stop-frame images of apical four-chamber views obtained from a patient with a dilated left ventricle before (upper panel) and after (lower panel) catheter injection of echo contrast in the left ventricle (LV). The left atrium remains echo free, which excludes mitral insufficiency. Border recognition is not facilitated after its opacification.

A = apical; B = basal; L = left; R = right; LA = left atrium.

3.4. Study of blood flow patterns

The non-contrast blood flowing from the left atrium into the left ventricle after its opacification with echo contrast allows us to observe transmitral blood flow. The negative contrast shadow delineates the functional mitral valve orifice. This is demonstrated in Figure 5, obtained from a patient with mitral valve stenosis. The anatomical dimension of the valve is visualized during the baseline study in the parasternal long-axis view (Figure 5, upper panel). The functional dimension is visualized by the echo-free blood entering the left ventricle after its opacification and appears smaller in the same cross-section (Figure 5, middle panel). Intracavitary flow patterns produced by a mitral valve prosthesis can be followed after pulmonary wedge injections. Occasionally one may observe a vortex of echo contrast circulating within an ischaemic aneurysm in patients with coronary artery disease (Figure 6). Left ventricular contrast echocardiography thus allows a new type of study on local flow, turbulence and stasis, which promises to become more useful in the future if transpulmonary echo contrast transmission becomes available.

3.5. Densitometric dilution curves of echocardiographic contrast

Bommer et al. [22] described in 1978 a method of obtaining dilution curves of echocardiographic contrast by videodensitometry. They focused an analog photometer upon the screen of the videomonitor over the middle of the right ventricular cavity during two-dimensional echocardiographic contrast studies. The dilution curves were reproducible on multiple echocardiographic contrast injections to an accuracy of 15%. The time course of decay made it possible to separate patients with normal from those with low cardiac output and/or tricuspid regurgitation. Echo-contrast indicator dilution curves of the left ventricle were subsequently performed in dogs using injections of 10 ml of a 1:100,000 concentration by volume of 30 micron diameter microballoons. Good correlations with cardiac output measurements were found [23]. We have used an image-processing computer to analyze video recordings of contrast injections in order to follow the decay of density after left ventricular and pulmonary wedge injections in 17 patients. A meaningful calculation of the area under the curve could not be made because of limitations due to video "overload" immediately after injection. In consequence, contrary to the studies by DeMaria et al. [23], it seems that cardiac output measurements cannot be estimated reliably using routine contrast dilution techniques. The decay phase was found to be exponential and has characteristics of indicator-dilution curves, as predicted theoretically. Preliminary data indicate that R-wave gating may allow estimation of ejection fraction [24].

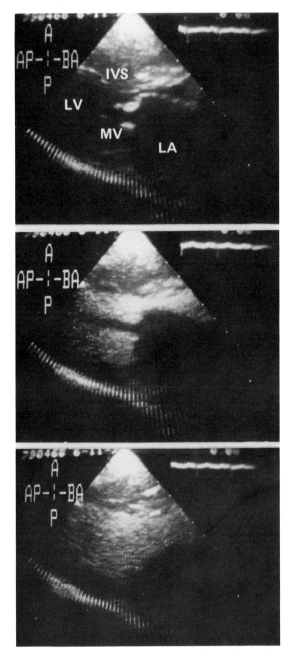

Figure 5. Stop-frame photographs of parasternal long-axis views of a patient with mitral valve stenosis before (upper panel) and after injection of echo contrast via a catheter in the left ventricle. The middle panel shows a frame recorded during diastole. The negative shadow caused by the non contrast blood flowing from the left atrium into the ventricle visualizes the transmitral blood flow pattern. During systole (lower panel), the echo contrast does not pass into the left atrium, excluding mitral incompetence.

A = anterior; AP = apical; BA = basal; P = posterior; IVS = interventricular septum; LA = left atrium; LV = left ventricle; MV = mitral valve.

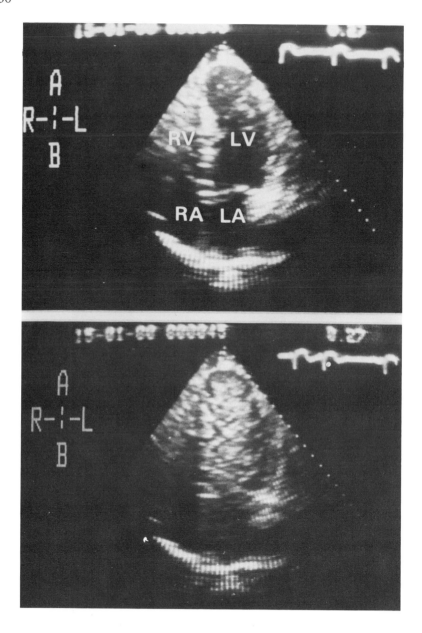

Figure 6. Apical four-chamber views before (upper panel) and after (lower panel) left ventricular opacification by echo contrast via a pulmonary wedge injection in a patient with an apical aneurysm. Wash-out of echo contrast from within the aneurysm was delayed.

A = apical; B = basal; L = left; R = right; LA = left atrium; LV = left ventricle; RA = right atrium; RV = right ventricle.

Hagler et al. [25] used computer-based videodensitometric techniques to analyze video recordings of left ventricular contrast echocardiograms to quantitate left-to-right shunts. Time-density histograms were generated from the right and left ventricular cavities after injection of echo contrast in the left ventricle in 7 patients with a ventricular septal defect. Their results indicate the possibility of quantitating shunts with these techniques.

ACKNOWLEDGEMENT

The authors wish to thank Willem Gorissen, Jackie McGhie and Wim Vletter for technical assistance and Machtelt Brussé for help in manuscript preparation.

REFERENCES

1. Gramiak R, PM Shah: Echocardiography of the aortic root. Invest Radiol 3:356, 1968.
2. Meltzer RS, EG Tickner, TP Sahines, RL Popp: The source of ultrasonic contrast effect. J Clin Ultrasound 8:121, 1980.
3. Gramiak R, PM Shah, DH Kramer: Ultrasound cardiography: contrast studies in anatomy and function. Radiology 92:939, 1969.
4. Feigenbaum H, JM Stone, DA Lee, WK Nasser, S Chang: Identification of ultrasound echoes from the left ventricle by use of intracardiac injections of Indocyanine green. Circulation 41:614, 1970.
5. Sahn DJ, DE Williams, S Shackelton, WF Friedman: The validity of structure identification for cross-sectional echocardiography. J Clin Ultrasound 2:201, 1975.
6. Tajik AJ, JB Seward, DJ Hagler, DD Mair, JT Lie: Two-dimensional real-time ultrasonic imaging of the heart and great vessels: technique, image orientation, structure identification and validation. Mayo Clin Proc 53:281, 1978.
7. Seward JB, AJ Tajik, JG Spangler, DE Ritter: Echocardiographic contrast studies. Mayo Clin Proc 50:163, 1975.
8. Pieroni DR, J Varghese, RM Freedom, RD Rowe: The sensitivity of contrast echocardiography in detecting intracardiac shunts. Cathet Cardiovasc Diagn 5:19, 1979.
9. Kerber RE, JM Kioschos, RM Lauer: Use of ultrasonic contrast method in the diagnosis of valvular regurgitation and intracardiac shunts. Am J Cardiol 34:722, 1974.
10. Bommer WJ, DT Mason, AN DeMaria: Studies in contrast echocardiography: development of new agents with superior reproducibility and transmission through lungs. Circulation 59 and 60 (Suppl II):II-17, 1979 (abstract).
11. Reale A, F Pizzuto, PA Giaffré, A Nigri, F Romeo, E Martuscelli, E Mangier, G Scibilia: Contrast echocardiography: transmission of echoes to the left heart across the pulmonary vascular bed. Europ Heart J 1:101, 1980.
12. Meltzer RS, PW Serruys, J McGhie, N Verbaan, J Roelandt: Pulmonary wedge injections yielding left-sided echocardiographic contrast. Brit Heart J 44:390, 1980.

232

13. Bommer WJ, EG Tickner, J Rasor, T Grehl, DT Mason, AN DeMaria: Development of a new echocardiographic contrast agent capable of pulmonary transmission and left heart opacification following peripheral venous injection. Circulation 62 (Suppl III):III–34, 1980 (abstract).
14. Meltzer RS, C Meltzer, J Roelandt: Sector Scanning views in echocardiography: a systematic approach. Europ Heart J 1:379, 1980.
15. Serruys PW, F Hagemeijer, J Roelandt: Echocardiological contrast studies with dynamically focussed multiscan. Acta Cardiol 34:283, 1979.
16. Meltzer RS, OEH Sartorius, CT Lancée, PW Serruys, PD Verdouw, CE Essed, J Roelandt: Transmission of ultrasonic contrast through the lungs. Ultrasound in Med & Biol (In press).
17. Meltzer RS, EG Tickner, RL Popp: Why do the lungs clear ultrasonic contrast. Ultrasound in Med & Biol 6:263, 1980.
18. Amano K, T Sakamoto, Y Hada, T Yamaguchi, T Ishimitsu, H Adachi: Contrast echocardiography: application for valvular incompetence. J Cardiography 9:697–716, 1979.
19. Uchiyama I, T Isshiki, K Koizumi, Y Ohuchi, K Kuwako, T Umeda, K Machii, S Furuta: Detection of the site and severity of mitral valve prolapse by real-time cross-sectional echocardiography with contrast technique. J Cardiography 9:689–696, 1979.
20. Meltzer RS, PW Serruys, J McGhie, PG Hugenholtz, J Roelandt: Cardiac catheterization under echocardiographic control in a pregnant woman. Amer J Med (In press).
21. Roelandt J, WG van Dorp, N Bom, PG Hugenholtz: Resolution problems in echocardiology, a source of interpretation errors. Amer J Cardiol 37:256, 1976.
22. Bommer W, J Neef, A Neumann, L Weinert, G Lee, DT Mason, AN DeMaria: Indicator-dilution curves obtained by photometric analysis of two-dimension echo-contrast studies. Amer J Cardiol 41:370, 1978 (abstract).
23. DeMaria AN, W Bommer, K Riggs, A Dajee, L Miller, DT Mason: In vivo correlation of cardiac output and densitometric dilution curves obtained by contrast two-dimensional echocardiography. Circulation (III–101) 1980 (abstract).
24. Bastiaans OL, J Roelandt, L Piérard, RS Meltzer: Ejection fraction from contrast echocardiographic videodensity curves. Clin Res (In press).
25. Hagler DJ, AJ Tajik, JB Seward, DD Mair, DG Ritter, EL Ritman: Videodensitometric quantitation of left-to-right shunts with contrast sector echocardiography. Circulation 57 and 58 (Suppl II), II–70, 1978 (abstract).

27. CONTRAST ECHOCARDIOGRAPHY IN VALVULAR REGURGITATION

R.S. Meltzer, P.W. Serruys, and J. Roelandt

1. INTRODUCTION

1.1. Contrast echocardiography in aortic, mitral or pulmonic valvular regurgitation

For the first few years after the introduction of contrast echocardiography by Gramiak, its use was limited to structure identification and shunt detection. In 1974, Kerber reported the use of an ultrasonic contrast method in the diagnosis of valvular regurgitation and intracardiac shunts [1]. He noticed contrast appearing in the left atrium after left ventricular injection in 14 out of 16 patients with mitral regurgitation, and in the left ventricle after aortic root injections in 13 out of 16 patients with aortic regurgitation. Valvular regurgitation as low as 10%, according to angiographic calculations, was detected by this method. One false positive study due to catheter-induced mitral regurgitation was noted. The authors concluded that M-mode ultrasonic monitoring of catheter injections distal to a regurgitant valve is a sensitive and specific – though qualitative – technique for detecting valvular regurgitation. Other laboratories, including our own, have confirmed that intracardiac injections during catheterization can be monitored by echocardiography and that this is a sensitive method for the detection of valvular regurgitation. Little further work has been reported in this area, and this invasive technique probably has only limited applications in the occasional patient where there is a strong contraindication to the use of ionizing radiation, for example in early pregnancy [2].

This chapter will deal largely with a newer application of contrast echocardiography in the diagnosis of valvular regurgitation:

1.2. Contrast echocardiography for the diagnosis of tricuspid valvular regurgitation

In 1978, the group from Duke University reported on a contrast echocardiographic method for the diagnosis of tricuspid regurgitation [3]. Their subsequent experiences were detailed at the symposium in Rotterdam in 1979 [4],

Rijsterborgh H, ed: Echocardiology, p 233-243. All rights reserved.
Copyright © 1981 Martinus Nijhoff Publishers, The Hague/Boston/London.

and at the American Heart Association meeting in late 1979 [5]. Their technique involved upper extremity injections of ultrasonic contrast material during two-dimensional echocardiographic imaging of the inferior vena cava, trying to detect retrograde flow of contrast agents into the inferior vena cava. They reported that the appearance of contrast during systole in the inferior vena cava was a sensitive and specific diagnostic sign for the presence of tricuspid regurgitation. We noticed the presence of systolic contrast in several patients without tricuspid regurgitation, and undertook the following study in order to: 1) examine sensitivity and specificity of peripheral contrast echocardiography in the diagnosis of tricuspid regurgitation, 2) attempt to ascertain the reason for false positive and false negative studies and 3) examine the utility of M-mode echocardiography in the diagnosis of tricuspid regurgitation [6].

2. METHODS

2.1. Patient population

We studied 62 patients with both M-mode and two-dimensional echocardiography of the inferior vena cava during upper extremity injections of 5% dextrose in water. Ten patients had a definite clinical diagnosis of tricuspid regurgitation, based on the jugular venous pulse, the holosystolic murmur increasing with respiration and, frequently, a pulsating liver.

Forty patients were studied because they had cardiac disorders frequently associated with tricuspid regurgitation, such as mitral stenosis, pulmonary hypertension, or former tricuspid valve surgery. Twelve further patients were included in the study because they were normal, as judged by history, physical examination and echocardiography.

Patients were divided into three groups on the basis of clinical and/or invasive evaluation of the tricuspid valve. Group A included 21 patients: 10 with clinically definite tricuspid regurgitation (5 also had the diagnosis confirmed by invasive studies) and 11 with clinically uncertain tricuspid regurgitation but positive invasive studies. Group B also comprised 21 patients: 12 normal subjects and 9 patients from the group with uncertain tricuspid regurgitation who had no tricuspid regurgitation at invasive studies. The remaining 20 patients with clinically uncertain tricuspid regurgitation and no invasive studies constituted group C.

2.2. Echocardiographic methods

All patients were studied in the supine position with the knees and hips slightly flexed to achieve maximal abdominal relaxation. The M-mode or two-dimensional echocardiographic transducer was placed in the subcostal position, just to the right of the midline, and the inferior vena cava was imaged in a sagittal plane by two-dimensional echocardiography [7]. A number 16 or 18 gauge intravenous cannula was introduced into an antecubital vein and a three-way stopcock was attached. Repeated, rapid, hand injections of 5-8 cc of 5% dextrose solution were made, using a 10 cc syringe. In some patients 1 cc to 3 cc of carbon dioxide were added to the 5% dextrose solution to insure adequate echocardiographic contrast [8]. M-mode echocardiograms were obtained with an EchocardioVisor SE (Organon Teknika) interfaced to a Honeywell LS6 stripchart recorder. Two-dimensional echocardiograms were recorded using a Toshiba SSH-10A phased-array sector-scanner or an Organon Teknika EchocardioVisor 03 multielement linear-array instrument. They were stored on videotape for subsequent analysis.

2.3. Diagnosis of tricuspid regurgitation

On right ventricular angiograms, tricuspid regurgitation was diagnosed if contrast appeared in the right atrium in the absence of premature beats. Intraoperative diagnosis of tricuspid regurgitation involved palpation of a thrill on the right atrium prior to cannulation for cardio-pulmonary bypass, making sure that there was no traction on the heart that might cause false tricuspid regurgitation [9].

3. RESULTS

3.1. Patterns of inferior vena cava contrast appearance

Using M-mode tracings of the inferior vena cava, we identified four different patterns of contrast appearance after upper extremity intravenous injections. The first is the pattern of tricuspid regurgitation, which we call the v-wave synchronous pattern. This is illustrated in Figure 1. The second pattern, the a-wave synchronous pattern, is characterized by the appearance of contrast in the inferior vena cava during the a-wave of the right atrial pressure tracing or jugular venous pulsation or even inferior vena cava "a" pulsation. The contrast reverses direction and, in the early part of systole, is seen returning to the right atrium, as illustrated in Figure 2. Both of these patterns give one pulsation per beat on the two-dimensional echocardiogram, and are very difficult to separate in real-time. Slow motion and stop frame analysis is necessary to analyze timing of inferior vena cava contrast appearance

236

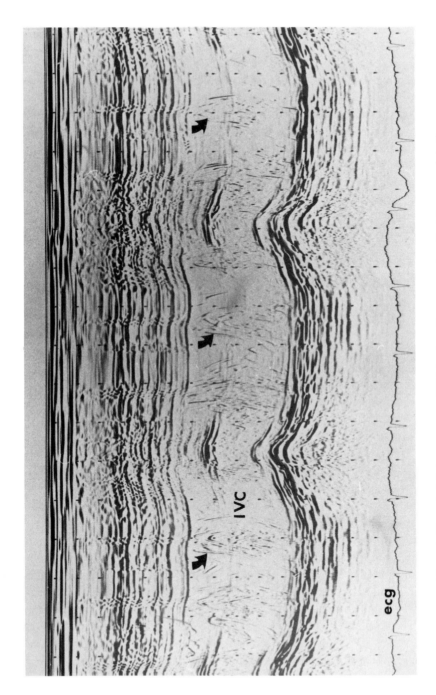

Figure 1. M-mode inferior vena cava (IVC) tracing after upper extremity intravenous injection of 5% dextrose solution in a patient with tricuspid regurgitation. Note appearance of *v*-wave synchronous contrast (arrows) in the IVC – a pattern diagnostic for tricuspid regurgitation.

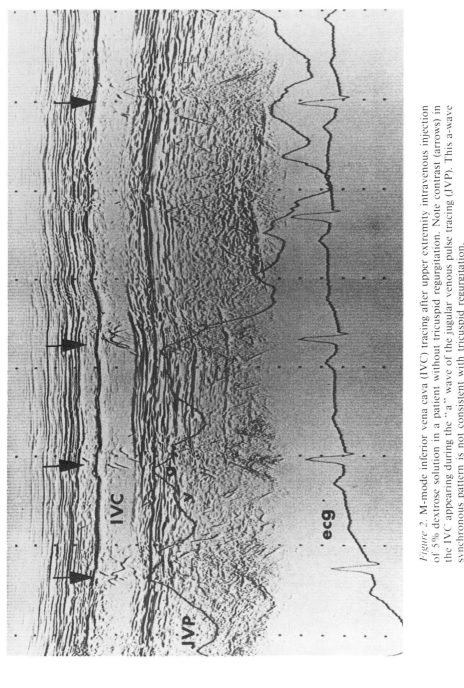

Figure 2. M-mode inferior vena cava (IVC) tracing after upper extremity intravenous injection of 5% dextrose solution in a patient without tricuspid regurgitation. Note contrast (arrows) in the IVC appearing during the "a" wave of the jugular venous pulse tracing (JVP). This a-wave synchronous pattern is not consistent with tricuspid regurgitation.

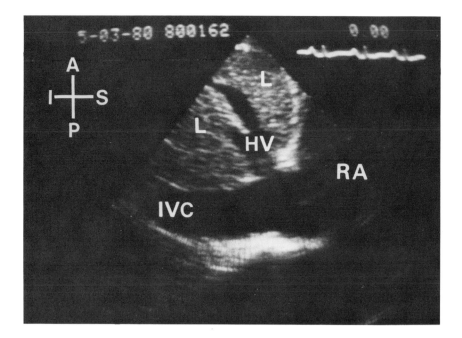

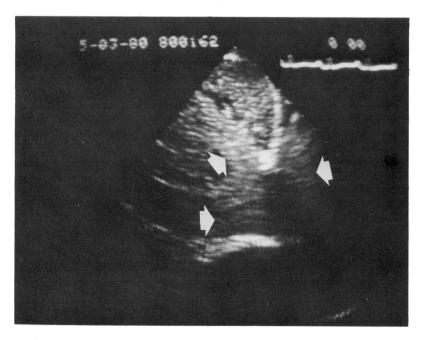

Figure 3. Upper panel: right parasagittal two-dimensional echocardiogram in a patient with tricuspid regurgitation, before upper extremity intravenous injection of 5% dextrose solution. Lower panel: 15 seconds later, with contrast now filling the right atrium (RA), inferior vena cava (IVC) and hepatic vein (HV). Further abbreviations: L = liver; A = anterior; P = posterior; I = inferior; S = superior.

properly from two-dimensional echocardiograms (Figure 3). The initial appearance during normal respiration is the most important indication for diagnosis. Timing analysis is considerably simplified using M-mode echocardiography. We have called the third pattern of contrast appearance in the inferior vena cava the "random" pattern. In this pattern, contrast is seen in the inferior vena cava with no definite relation to the cardiac cycle and mainly appears during deep inspiration. The "random" pattern is the false positive most frequently associated with atrial fibrillation, where an a-wave synchronous pattern is not possible. The last pattern identified was designated "no contrast appearance". That is, despite echocardiographic imaging of the inferior vena cava during and immediately after a peripheral contrast injection, no contrast is seen moving retrograde into the inferior vena cava at any time.

3.2. Relation of echocardiographic pattern to presence or absence of tricuspid regurgitation

The distribution of the four echocardiographic patterns among patient groups A, B and C is displayed in Table 1. It is clear from this table that the

Table 1. Distribution of patterns among patients groups (TR = tricuspid regurgitation).

Group	v-wave synch.	a-wave synch.	random	no contrast
A (n = 21) TR	19	0	0	2
B (n = 21) no TR	0	6	5	10
C (n = 20) ? TR	11	6	3	0

Table 2. Sensitivity and specificity of contrast echo in the diagnosis of tricuspid regurgitation.

		Presence of TR	
		+	−
Contrast	+	19	0
Echo	−	2	21

Sensitivity   19/21 = 90%
Specificity   21/21 = 100%

240

v-wave synchronous pattern is the diagnostic pattern of tricuspid regurgitation, with a sensitivity of 90% and specificity of 100% in our patient population (Table 2). However, group B patients frequently have contrast in the inferior vena cava during systole, particularly in relation to deep inspiration or at the end of a Valsalva maneuver, but its initial appearance is always either an a-wave synchronous or a random pattern.

3.3. M-mode versus two-dimensional echocardiography in the diagnosis of tricuspid regurgitation

The title of this section is misleading, since M-mode and two-dimensional echocardiography are complementary and not inimical techniques. However, we wished to examine the utility of M-mode echocardiography in the diagnosis of tricuspid regurgitation, since the original report from Duke was only concerned with two-dimensional echocardiography [3]. We had the impression that M-mode echocardiography might be at least as good, and perhaps preferable.

The 62 study subjects had both M-mode and two-dimensional contrast echocardiograms. Each study was categorized as one of the four patterns mentioned above (v-wave synchronous, a-wave synchronous, "random", or no contrast appearance). Fifty-one patients had the same M-mode and two-dimensional echocardiographic patterns of contrast appearance in the inferior vena cava, divided as follows: 27 v-wave synchronous, 13 no contrast, 8 a-wave synchronous, and 3 random. Within this group, timing analysis was always easier by M-mode than by two-dimensional studies. Eleven patients had contrast seen in the inferior vena cava on the M-mode study but not during two-dimensional imaging after upper extremity contrast injection. All 11 had verification of adequate right heart contrast during the two-dimensional study. The distribution of M-mode patterns was as follows: 4 a-wave synchronous, 4 random, 3 v-wave synchronous. Only two of these eleven patients had invasive diagnostic tests for tricuspid regurgitation. Both of these were patients with no regurgitation; one had an M-mode a-wave synchronous pattern. Two further clinically normal subjects had small amounts of a-wave synchronous contrast in the inferior vena cava on the M-mode study but not on the two-dimensional study.

Some signs of tricuspid regurgitation have been proposed that are unique either to M-mode or to two-dimensional echocardiography. The "back-and-forth motion" of contrast echo across the tricuspid valve during the cardiac cycle on two-dimensional echocardiography has been proposed as a sign of tricuspid regurgitation. It has also been proposed as a sign of regurgitation of other cardiac valves. We found this to be an extremely subjective sign, lacking either sensitivity or specificity. There is a normal retrograde motion of contrast in both the right ventricle and right atrium as the tricuspid valve closes, and it was nearly impossible to differentiate reliably between where this normal retrograde movement ended and where abnormal "back-and-forth motion" began. A possibly more useful sign, but one which needs further study, is an M-mode sign: a large number of highly negatively-sloping contrast lines, seen in the right atrium just below the tricuspid valve during systole. We have noticed this sign in several patients, but have not systematically studied its sensitivity or specificity.

3.4. Studies after tricuspid valve surgery

Ten patients were studied more than one month after a De Vega tricuspid valvuloplasty for tricuspid regurgitation. Nine of these were in atrial fibrillation, and all nine had a "v-wave synchronous" pattern on echocardiography suggesting continued tricuspid regurgitation. Only 4 of these had tricuspid regurgitation clinically. Two patients were studied pre and postoperatively, and little change in their "v-wave synchronous" pattern could be detected. The patient in normal sinus rhythm had the "random" pattern suggesting the absence of significant tricuspid regurgitation.

Four patients were studied after tricuspid valve replacement with a porcine bioprosthesis. Three were in atrial fibrillation and demonstrated a "v-wave synchronous" pattern, with small amounts of inferior vena cava contrast, as assessed subjectively (one was positive only during end-inspiration, another had a positive M-mode but a negative two-dimensional study). The fourth, in normal sinus rhythm, had an "a-wave synchronous" pattern.

4. DISCUSSION

As indicated on Table 2, peripheral contrast echocardiography is a sensitive and specific test for the diagnosis of tricuspid insufficiency. However, this is the case only if the following precautions have been taken: studies must not be considered negative unless the echocardiographer is sure that adequate right heart opacification has been achieved on multiple injections, timing analysis has excluded v-wave synchronous inferior vena cava contrast appearance, and the operator is aware of the causes of false positive and false negative studies listed in Table 3.

Since timing analysis is improved when using M-mode, and we have encountered two-dimensional studies where contrast was not imaged in the inferior vena cava when it was seen by M-mode (but not vice versa), we feel that M-mode inferior vena cava imaging should always be used – either alone or in combination with two-dimensional studies.

Table 3. Contrast inferior vena cava echo for tricuspid regurgitation diagnosis.

False positive	False negative
— a-wave synchronous pattern	— Failure to achieve adequate central contrast
— Randon pattern	— Failure to use M-mode
— Deep inspiration	— M-mode beam too inferior
— M-mode beam too superior	

Our experience that tricuspid regurgitation in general does not completely resolve after tricuspid surgery is in line with other recently reported angiographic data [10]. We wish to emphasize, though, that contrast inferior vena cava echocardiography, as we report it, is not a quantitative technique. Perhaps Doppler echocardiography, either alone or possibly in combination with contrast, may help to further refine the noninvasive diagnosis and quantification of tricuspid regurgitation [11].

The role of contrast echocardiographic techniques in diagnosing non-tricuspid valvular regurgitation is at present minor, though it is conceivable that a large number of upward-sloping contrast trajectories during diastole may be an important M-mode diagnostic sign for pulmonary regurgitation [12]. Since, clinically, creation of left-sided contrast now requires cardiac catheterization, the use of contrast echocardiography to diagnose aortic or mitral regurgitation is rarely necessary. Even with transpulmonary transmission of contrast, the "back-and-forth" sign is unlikely to have sufficient sensitivity or specificity to aid considerably in the diagnosis of left-sided valvular regurgitation. It is conceivable that combined Doppler/contrast techniques may be useful in this setting in the future, if noninvasive trans-pulmonary transmission of echocardiographic contrast becomes available [13].

REFERENCES

1. Kerber RE, JM Kioschos, RM Lauer: Use of an ultrasonic contrast method in the diagnosis of valvular regurgitation and intracardiac shunts. Am J Cardiol 34:722, 1974.
2. Meltzer RS, PW Serruys, J McGhie, PG Hugenholtz, J Roelandt: Cardiac catheterization under echocardiographic control in a pregnant woman. Am J Med (In press).
3. Lieppe W, VS Behar, R Scallion, JA Kisslo: Detection of tricuspid regurgitation with two-dimensional echocardiography and peripheral vein injections. Circulation 57:128, 1978.
4. Kisslo JA: Usefulness of M-mode and cross-sectional echocardiography for analysis of right-sided heart disease. In: Echocardiology (Lancée, CT, ed.), pp 37–47, Martinus Nijhoff, The Hague, 1979.

5. Wise NK, S Myers, JA Stewart, R Waugh, T Fraker, J Kisslo: Echo inferior venacavography: a technique for study of right sided heart disease. Circulation 59–60 (suppl II): II–202, 1979.
6. Meltzer RS, DCA van Hoogenhuyze, PW Serruys, MMP Haalebos, J Roelandt: The diagnosis of tricuspid regurgitation by contrast echocardiography. Circulation (In press).
7. Meltzer RS, C Meltzer, J Roelandt: Sector scanning views in echocardiography: a systematic approach. Europ Heart J 1:379, 1980.
8. Meltzer RS, PW Serruys, J Roelandt: Intravenous carbon dioxide as an echocardiographic contrast agent. J Clin Ultrasound 9:127, 1981.
9. Pepine CJ, WW Nichols, JH Selby: Diagnostic tests for tricuspid insufficiency: How good? Cath & Cardiovasc Diagnosis 5:1, 1979.
10. Simon R, H Oelert, HG Borst, PR Lichtlen: Influence of mitral valve surgery on tricuspid incompetence concomitant with mitral valve disease. Circulation 62 (suppl I):I–152, 1980.
11. Fantini F, A Magherini: Detection of tricuspid regurgitation with pulsed Doppler echocardiography. In: Echocardiology (Lancée CT, ed.), pp 233–235, Martinus Nijhoff, 1979.
12. Gullace G, M Savoia, V Locatelli, F Schubert, C Ranzi: Evaluation of linear contrast echo on pulmonary valve echogram. International Meeting on Bidimensional Echocardiography, Milan, 1980, pp 72–73 (abstract).
13. Meltzer RS, OEH Sartorius, CT Lancée, PW Serruys, PD Verdouw, C Essed, J Roelandt: Transmission of echocardiographic contrast through the lungs. (Submitted for publication to Ultrasound in Medicine and biology).

28. DETERMINATION OF CARDIAC OUTPUT BY TWO-DIMENSIONAL CONTRAST ECHOCARDIOGRAPHY

Anthony N. DeMaria, William Bommer, Julia Razor, Glenn Tickner, and Dean T. Mason

Contrast echocardiography refers to the process of opacifying cardiac chambers and major vessels with dense "clouds" of reflected echoes by means of the intravascular injection of a variety of fluids [1]. Although the exact source of the contrast effect is not known, available evidence overwhelmingly points to the role of microscopic air bubbles in the genesis of the contrast effect [2]. Although indocyanine green, saline, and dextrose in water have been the solutions most routinely used to produce contrast echocardiograms, even intravascular injection of the patient's own blood can elicit similar phenomena. Recently a variety of gas containing substances have been utilized in the experimental laboratory to standardize the contrast recordings obtained [3].

Contrast echocardiography has found a variety of applications in clinical cardiology. Initially, contrast injections within the central circulation were utilized during echocardiography to verify ultrasonically determined cardiac anatomy [4]. Subsequently, contrast echocardiography has been utilized to evaluate blood flow patterns, especially in regard to intracardiac communications [5]: Since the contrast effect is removed by the transit of blood through the lungs, contrast is not normally seen in the left side cardiac chambers following intravenous injection, and the technique may therefore be of particular value in the recognition of right-to-left intracardiac shunting by either atrial or ventricular septal defects. In addition, a contrast free jet (negative contrast) may be observed during opacification of the right side chambers in patients with left-to-right shunting [6], and reflux of contrast into the inferior vena cava has proven to be of value in the detection of tricuspid regurgitation [7]. Unfortunately, none of these applications or approaches have yielded any quantitative data from contrast echocardiograms.

In the course of analysis of a number of two-dimensional contrast echocardiograms performed in our laboratory for clinical purposes, the qualitative observation was made that the time-course of appearance and disappearance of the contrast effect in an individual patient seemed to be related to the status of overall cardiac function at the time of the study. These initial qualitative observations were confirmed by the simple procedure of timing with a stopwatch the duration of the ultrasonic contrast effect in patients with varying levels of cardiac function. Stimulated by these findings, a series of projects were undertaken by which to obtain quantitative information from the appearance and disappearance characteristics of two-dimensional contrast echocardiograms.

PHOTOMETRIC AQUISITION OF INDICATOR DILUTION CURVES

The contrast effect obtained by two-dimensional echocardiography is presented as luminescence upon a video monitor or cathode ray oscilloscope. Further, the luminance may be readily recorded by means of a photometer (lightmeter) which is focused upon the screen of the monitor (Figure 1).

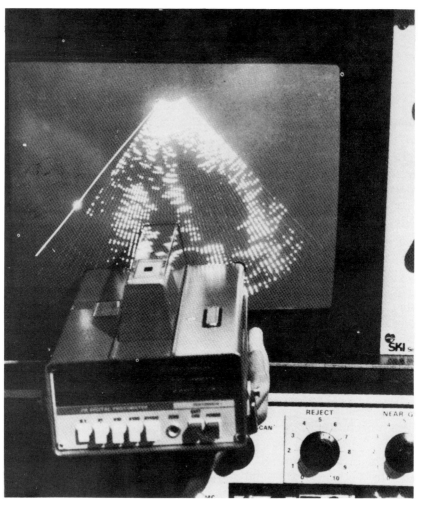

Figure 1

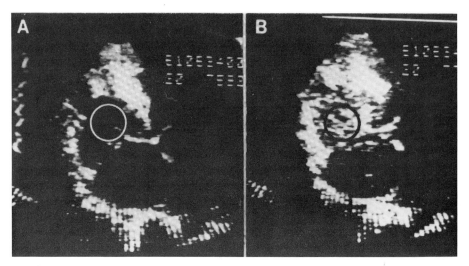

Figure 2

Accordingly, a system was developed whereby the luminescence emitted by a video monitor during a two-dimensional contrast echocardiogram was continuously recorded by a photometer focused upon the screen, and the analog signal was transferred to a stripchart recorder for a paper printout [8]. The photometer utilized was a Tektronics model J6503 with a light-sensitive area one centimeter in diameter which yielded readings expressed in foot-lamberts. The signal from the photometer was recorded by means of a standard fiberoptic Honeywell model 1856 stripchart recorder.

Indicator dilution curves were obtained from two-dimensional echocardiograms performed from the cardiac apex in the four-chamber view, with the transducer manipulated to maximize the size of the right ventricular and right atrial chambers. The contrast agent utilized for the initial studies was 10 cc of normal saline, which was delivered into an indwelling 19 gauge plastic cannula inserted in the brachial vein. Contrast visualization was recorded onto video tape for subsequent playback, during which the photometer was focused upon an area of interest centered in the right ventricular cavity (Figure 2) and the analog signal was continuously recorded on paper.

The result of photometric analysis of two-dimensional contrast echocardiograms was to yield an indicator dilution type curve whose upstroke was related to luminescence created by the appearance of contrast on the video screen and whose downslope was created by the disappearance or washout of the contrast agent (Figure 3). Although contrast indicator dilution curves appeared similar to those produced by indocyanine green or thermodilution, the ultrasonic opacification was removed in the lungs and therefore a break in the downslope was not observed in patients with left-to-right cardiac

248

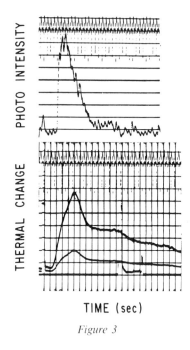

TIME (sec)

Figure 3

shunts. A series of studies was performed to assess the reproducibility of photometric indicator dilution curves in patients. Utilizing the methodology described, a variability of approximately plus or minus fifteen percent was found in consecutive curves. Further central circulatory injections yielded data which was only slightly superior to those from injections in peripheral veins. Accordingly, a method was developed which was capable of yielding reasonably reproducible indicator dilution curves from two-dimensional contrast echocardiograms.

The initial quantitative analysis of the photometric indicator dilution curves was confined to the disappearance phase of the tracing. Two parameters were defined for each contrast curve, the time from peak contrast effect (peak of the curve) to the point of 50% decrease in amplitude (DT/50) and the time from the peak of the curve to 90% reduction in amplitude (DT/90). Application of the measurement of either DT/50 or DT/90 immediately revealed a striking separation between groups of normal subjects or patients with atrial septal defect and patients with either markedly reduced cardiac indices or tricuspid regurgitation [9] (Figure 4). In addition, when either DT/50 or DT/90 were subjected to linear regression analysis in comparison with thermodilution measurements of cardiac output, good correlations were obtained with the correlation coefficient ranging from r = 0.70 to 0.92. Importantly, when patients were divided into two groups, one with reduced cardiac index (below 2.5 liters/minute/m^2) and one having normal cardiac index, striking differences existed for both DT/50 and DT/90 (1.3 versus 8.9

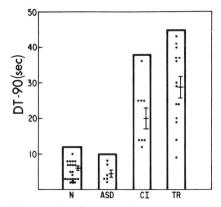

Figure 4. Measurements of DT/90 in different study groups.
N = normal, ASD = atrial septal defect, CI = reduced cardiac index, TR = tricuspid regurgitation.

seconds and 3.6 versus 23.0 seconds respectively, $p < 0.01$). Thus, even simple measurements obtained from the disappearance phase of echocardiographic contrast curves showed good correlation with cardiac output measurements.

ADVANCES IN THE QUANTITATION OF ECHOCARDIOGRAPHIC INDICATOR DILUTION CURVES

Although the early experiments demonstrated that the disappearance characteristics of the indicator dilution curves from contrast echocardiography yielded information regarding cardiac output, a direct calculation of cardiac output was not possible from such recordings. The calculation of cardiac output (CO) from any indicator dilution curve is usually computed by means of the Hamilton equation as $CO = i/(\bar{c} \cdot t)$, where i is the mass of the indicator, $\bar{c}$ is the mean concentration of the indicator during its initial pass through the sampling area, and t is the total duration of the curve obtained. Accordingly, it was necessary to determine the mass of the contrast agent injected as well as to develop a method for the computation of the mean concentration of the agent during transit through the heart in order to calculate actual cardiac output from two-dimensional contrast echocardiograms.

In order to determine the mass of the injectate, it was necessary to utilize an agent which yielded a constant and predictable contrast effect. Since the contrast effect was predominately referrable to microscopic air bubbles within the injected solution, an effort was undertaken to develop microbubbles of uniform size. Two agents were acquired: plastic microballoons whose size varied in a bell-shaped distribution about a mean of 30 microns in diameter and, secondly, gelatin-encapsulated microbubbles of precise size (each measuring exactly 10 microns), developed by Razor Associates of Sunnyvale, California [10]. Initial studies indeed confirmed that the newer substances yielded contrast intensities which were both more reproducible and of consistantly higher amplitude when compared to commonly utilized contrast agents. Accordingly, utilizing these new contrast agents the mass of the contrast injected could be predicted.

In order to determine the mean concentration of contrast during a recording it was necessary to develop a system in which the analog signal obtained from the luminance of opacification was linear with respect to the concentration of the contrast present. To accomplish this, a videodensitometer was constructed which sensed the voltage peaks from a video signal over a triangular sample volume and expressed its output as the sum of the products of voltage and time. The ultrasound/videodensitometer system was tested by examining a series of plastic bags containing 30 micron microballoons suspended at various concentrations by volume, ranging from 1.7 to 6.3×10^{-5} in a viscous medium. The system was found to yield a linear signal throughout the concentrations evaluated. The final requirement was, of course, a calibration factor representing the analog signal which would be obtained by a known amount of contrast diluted in a known amount of blood from within the patient. Unfortunately, at present a calibration factor from which to determine absolute concentration of the contrast agent has not been developed.

IN VITRO EVALUATION OF VIDEODENSITOMETRIC CONTRAST INDICATOR DILUTION CURVES

The availability of an injectate of uniform and predictable mass, and ultrasonic videodensitometer system capable of yielding linear analog signals with regard to contrast amplitude enabled the evaluation of contrast curves to indicate directional changes in cardiac output. Therefore, a series of studies were undertaken to determine whether indicator dilution curves obtained by this method of contrast echocardiography could be correlated with measurements of flow and cardiac output.

Initially, in vitro studies were performed in a mechanical simulated heart and lung system in which pump flow could be adjusted to any rate. Gelatin encapsulated precision 10 micron microbubbles were utilized as the contrast agent for these studies.

A fixed concentration of gelatin microballoons dissolved in a vehicle was injected into the right atrial port of the heart-lung simulator while echocardiograms were performed from a water bath surrounding the pulmonary artery segment of the model. Multiple contrast injections were performed at simulated cardiac output flow rates varying from 4 to 12 liters per minute, and indicator dilution curves were obtained by videodensitometry of these ultrasonic recordings. The area under these curves was then determined by simple planimetry. Analysis of this data yielded a correlation coefficient of $r = 0.99$ between the inverse planed area under the curve and model flow rate [11]. Accordingly, it was documented that indicator dilution curves obtained by contrast echocardiography in vitro were capable of yielding estimates of cardiac output which correlated extremely closely with actual measurements.

IN VIVO EVALUATION OF VIDEODENSITOMETRIC INDICATOR DILUTION CURVES

Subsequently, a series of studies were performed to determine if indicator dilution curves obtained by two-dimensional contrast echocardiography were capable of yielding estimates of cardiac output in vivo [12]. Studies were carried out in a group of open-chested mongrel dogs in whom cardiac output was measured by thermodilution techniques with the thermister positioned in the pulmonary artery and in whom alterations of cardiac output were induced by the administration of either isoproterenol, propranolol, or blood withdrawal. Contrast was produced by the left atrial injection of 10 cc of 1:100,000 concentration by volume of 30 micron plastic microballoons. Echocardiograms were performed in the long-axis plane of the left ventricle by means of the direct epicardial positioning of a wide-angle, rotatory, mechanical sector-scanner. The two-dimensional contrast echocardiograms were recorded on videotape, and subsequently analyzed by ultrasonic videodensitometry with the sample volume in the left ventricle to yield indicator dilution curves (Figure 5). Five injections were carried out at each cardiac output in every animal, and a total of 60 cardiac outputs were

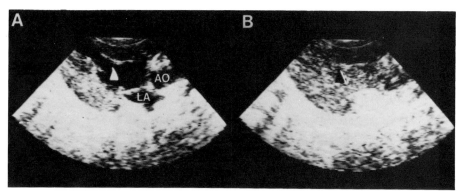

Figure 5

obtained in the group of animals studied. The indicator dilution curves obtained were quantified by means of planimetry to obtain the total area under the curve, as well as the extrapolated area under the curve using the forward triangle method.

When the area measurements of the indicator dilution curves were compared to actual measurements of cardiac output by thermodilution, an extremely close correlation was obtained in each of the individual animals studied. However, the number of cardiac output levels in individual animals were limited, and ranged from 4 to 7, with the mean of 5.2 per·experiment. Nevertheless, it was clear that the indicator dilution curves obtained by two-dimensional contrast echocardiograms in vivo correlated extremely closely with thermodilution cardiac output in individual animals. Further, when the data for all cardiac outputs in all animals was evaluated, a general correlation was observed between the area under the curve, expressed as either total area or extrapolated by the forward triangle method, and thermodilution cardiac output, with correlation coefficients being $r = 0.65$ and 0.61, respectively.

Although these data indicating good correlation between the contrast indicator dilution curves and thermodilution cardiac output are most encouraging, several important limitations to this technique must be kept in mind. Firstly, no method of obtaining a calibration factor has yet been devised for this procedure. Accordingly, at the present time this method is capable of yielding estimates of cardiac output which are of value only in terms of directional changes within an individual subject. Secondly, despite utilizing a closed system in all studies, it was never possible to totally eliminate the extraneous introduction of micro quantities of air into the animal, thereby resulting in the inclusion of a contrast effect unrelated to the injectate itself. However, the intensity of such extraneous contrast was small in comparison to that introduced by the actual agent, and was constant after the initial 1 to 2 injections. Finally, in utilizing this methodology it is necessary to avoid producing a quantity of contrast which is so great that it saturates the ultrasonic videodensitometry system. Although studies in our laboratory determined a suitable concentration for this animal model, similar data will have to be accumulated in a clinical setting, and may vary from patient to patient.

CONCLUSION

Contrast echocardiography offers exciting new potentials for the application of ultrasonic methods in the diagnosis and management of patients with heart disease. However, in order to realize the full potential of contrast echocardiography it will be necessary to apply quantitative methods to the analysis of these recordings. Studies in our laboratory in association with Razor Associates have demonstrated that biodegradeable contrast agents of uniform size can be utilized to yield indicator dilution curves from the videodensitometric analysis of two-dimensional echocardiograms. Further, such indicator dilution curves have been demonstrated to correlate well with cardiac flow and cardiac output measurements both in vitro and in vivo. It is fully anticipated that further developments in this area will enable the determination of cardiac output in man by means of two-dimensional contrast echocardiography.

REFERENCES

1. Seward JB, AJ Tajik, DJ Hagler, DG Ritter: Peripheral venous contrast echocardiography. Am J Cardiol 39:202–209, 1977.
2. Meltzer RS, EG Tickner, RL Popp: The source of ultrasound contrast effect. J Clin Ultrasound 8:121, 1980.
3. Bommer WJ, DT Mason, AN DeMaria: Studies in contrast echocardiography: Development of new agents with superior reproducibility and transmission through lungs. Circulation 60 (Suppl II):II–17, 1979.
4. Gramiak R, PM Shaw, DH Kramer: Ultrasound cardiology: Contrast studies in anatomy and function. Radiology 92:939–946, 1969.
5. Kerber RE, JM Kioschos, RM Lauer: Use of an ultrasonic contrast method in the diagnosis of valvular regurgitation and intracardiac shunts. Am J Cardiol 34:722–730, 1974.
6. Weyman AE, LS Wann, RA Hurwitz, et al.: Negative contrast echocardiography: A new technique for detecting left-to-right shunts. Circulation 56 (Suppl III):III–26, 1977.
7. Lieppe W, VS Behar, R Scallion, JA Kisslo: Detection of tricuspid regurgitation with two-dimensional echocardiography and peripheral vein injections. Circulation 57:128–32, 1978.
8. Bommer WJ, J Neef, A Neumann, L Weinert G Lee, DT Mason, AN DeMaria: Indicator-dilution curves obtained by photometric analysis of two-dimensional echo-contrast studies. Am J Cardiol 41:370, 1978 (abstract).
9. DeMaria AN, W Bommer, L George, Neumann, L Weinert, DT Mason: Combined peripheral venous injection and cross-sectional echocardiography in the evaluation of cardiac disease. Am J Cardiol 41:370, 1978 (abstract).
10. Bommer WJ, G Tickner, J Rasor, T Grehl, DT Mason, AN DeMaria: Development of a new echocardiographic contrast agent capable of pulmonary transmission and left heart opacification following peripheral venous injection. Circulation 62 (Supp III):III, 1980 (abstract).
11. Bommer W, Lantz Bo, Miller, Larry, Naifeh, Jerome, Riggs, Kay, Kwan, Oi Ling, DT Mason, AN DeMaria: Advances in Quantitative contrast echocardiography: Recording and calibration of linear time-concentration curves by videodensitometry. Circulation 60 (Part II-18), 1979 (abstract).
12. DeMaria AN, W Bommer, K Riggs, A Dajje, L Miller, DT Mason: In vivo correlation of cardiac output and densitometric dilution curves obtained by contrast two-dimensional echocardiography Circulation (Supp III):III–101, 1980 (abstract).

29. ANALYSIS OF RIGHT HEART BLOOD FLOW FROM CONTRAST PATTERNS ON THE ECHOCARDIOGRAM

TASSILO BONZEL, DIETER FASSBENDER, NIKOLAI BOGUNOVIC, GUNTHER TRIEB, and ULRICH GLEICHMANN

Flow velocity measurements are common diagnostic procedures during invasive hemodynamic studies [1, 2]. In noninvasive cardiovascular investigation, however, flow velocity analysis is still a major problem, though highly sophisticated Doppler systems have been applied for flow measurements with increasing success [2, 3, 4]. Contrast echocardiography has been used for the detection of shunts and of tricuspid regurgitation. The advantage of one-dimensional (1D) echocardiography is the excellent time resolution, routinely used for the calculation of the mitral valve EF-slope and the slopes of other moving structures. Blood flow lines can be visualised on M-mode echocardiograms by injection of ultrasound-reflecting substances or microspheres. The slope and direction of these flow lines can be analysed in order to obtain the component of flow direction and velocity along the main transducer axis [6, 7]. As far as we know, no other groups have published experiences with the technique described in this study.

MATERIAL AND METHODS

M-mode echocardiograms were recorded from the left sternal border with a commercially available M-mode echocardiograph (Organon Teknika). After location of the tricuspid valve, a bolus of 8 cc of a mixture of saline and indocyanine solution was injected into the left or right antecubital vein. M-modes were recorded at 100 mm/sec paper speed, when typical "bubble" flow lines appeared in the right atrium, tricuspid orifice and adjacent right ventricle (Figures 1 and 2).

Normal and abnormal flow directions and peak early diastolic (EFV) and peak late diastolic flow velocities (AFV) were analysed in 40 subjects, including 13 normals and 27 patients with various primary or secondary right heart myocardial or valvular disorders, but excluding patients with intracardiac shunts. In normals cardiac disorders were ruled out by history, ECG and clinical investigation. In abnormals end-diastolic right ventricular pressure was more than 0.8 kPa (6 mmHg), mean 1.2 kPa (9 mmHg), systolic right ventricular pressure was more than 4.0 kPa (30 mmHg), mean 6.1 kPa (46 mmHg), by right heart catheterisation. 14 patients had tricuspid regurgi-

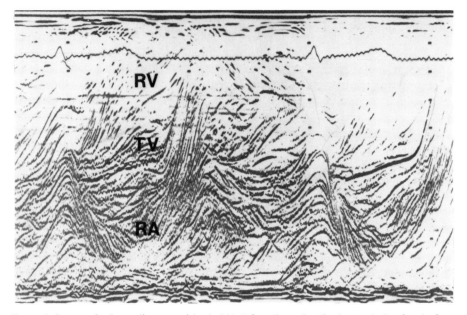

Figure 1. A normal echocardiogram with "bubble" flow lines. Qualitative analysis of main flow patterns see Figure 3.
RV = right ventricle, TV = tricuspid valve, RA = right atrium.

tation by angiography and/or clinical investigation; 12 patients were in atrial fibrillation; 12 patients had the auscultatory finding of pulmonic regurgitation, in these patients aortic regurgitation was excluded by aortic root angiography.

RESULTS

The following typical flow patterns were found (Figure 3).
Normal flow:
1) early diastolic flow lines across the tricuspid valve (for calculation of EFV).
2) reduced mesodiastolic flow.
3) late diastolic flow lines across the tricuspid valve (for calculation of AFV).
4) retrograde flow with tricuspid valve closure.
5) systolic flow acceleration within the right ventricle.
6) turbulent flow against the tricuspid valve during right ventricular systole.

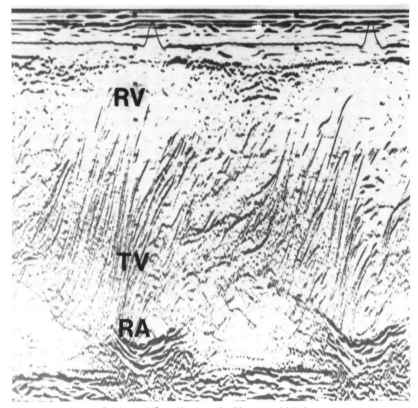

Figure 2. Normal flow lines, as in Figure 1; high heart rate.

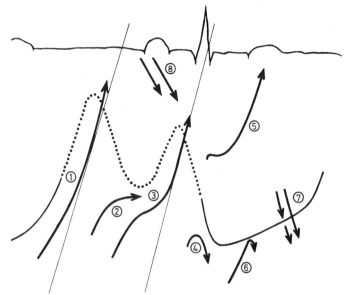

Figure 3. Main flow patterns. For explanations see results.

258

Abnormal flow:
7) in all 14 patients with tricuspid regurgitation straight systolic flow lines across the tricuspid valve (Figure 4).
8) in 6 of the 7 patients with pulmonic regurgitation retrograde diastolic flow lines from the right ventricular outflow tract against the anterior tricuspid leaflet, resulting in tricuspid valve preclosure in 2 patients (Figure 5). 7) and 8) were not observed in normals.

Velocity of bloodflow in the direction of the transducer could be determined by measuring the slopes of the recorded flow lines. The difference between this measurement and the true velocity will depend on the angle between the ultrasound beam and the true direction of the flow. For the estimation of the right ventricular (diastolic) dysfunction, this handicap can be overcome by introducing a diastolic flow index (RVI). RVI was defined as the ratio of the peak diastolic flow velocities in early and late diastole (RVI = EFV/AFV). The diastolic flow index is independent of the angle between the ultrasound beam and the true direction of flow, provided that the difference between the true directions of flow in early and late diastole is small.

The measurements of EFV, AFV and RVI are listed in Table 1.

AFV was significantly higher (p<0.001) in patients with right ventricular dysfunction than in normals. RVI was less than 1.3 in 11 and less than 1.1 in 9 patients with right ventricular dysfunction, while in normals it was greater

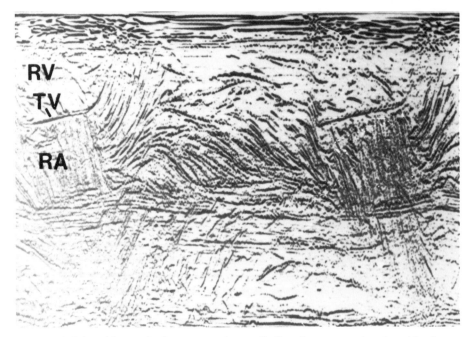

Figure 4. Tricuspid regurgitation: retrograde systolic flow lines across the tricuspid valve.

Table 1. Diastolic flow velocities (± 1 SD), early diastolic peak flow velocity (EFV), late diastolic peak flow velocity (AFV), diastolic flow index (RVI = EFV/AFV).

	n	EFV mm/sec	AFV mm/sec	RVI
Normals	13	455 ± 135	284 ± 72	1.7 ± 0.4
RV-dysfunction	14	397 ± 61	385 ± 101	1.0 ± 0.3
Atrial fibrillation	11	479 ± 123	(0)	:

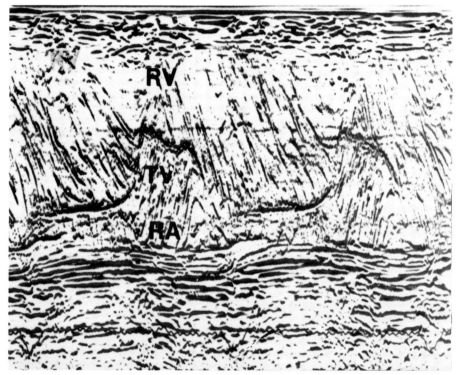

Figure 5. Pulmonic regurgitation: retrograde diastolic flow lines from the right ventricular outflow tract against the anterior tricuspid leaflet.

than 1.3 for 10 normals and greater than 1.1 in all cases (Figure 6). EFV was highest in patients with atrial fibrillation without atrial contribution to ventricular filling, where flow was decreasing to zero during diastole with occasional retrograde flow lines (Figures 6, 7).

DISCUSSION

We proved that right heart flow lines can be visualised by contrast M-mode echocardiography. These flow lines can yield important information on

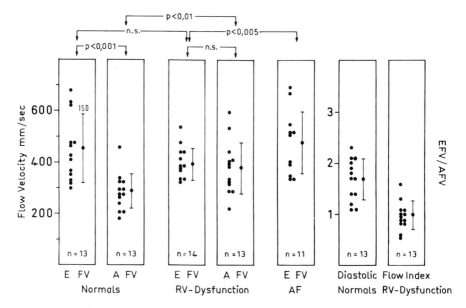

Figure 6. Flow velocities, diastolic flow index and significant flow velocity differences (Student's t-test) in 40 patients and normals. For details see text.

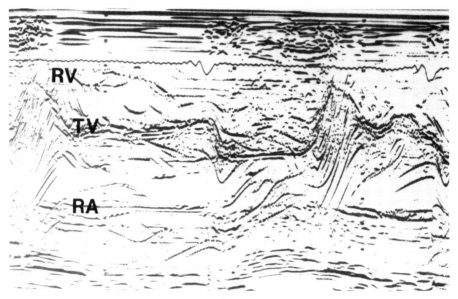

Figure 7. Diastolic flow lines in atrial fibrillation, decreasing flow to zero after high early diastolic flow. Occasional retrograde diastolic flow lines in the tricuspid orifice during late diastole.

1) flow direction in relation to the position of the transducer and 2) diastolic flow velocities across the tricuspid valve. Since only the component of flow along the transducer axis can be estimated, the difference between measured and true flow velocity will depend on the angle between the ultrasound beam and the true direction of flow. For the estimation of right ventricular (diastolic) dysfunction this handicap can be overcome by introducing a diastolic flow index RVI. Right ventricular dysfunction was diagnosed with high probability when RVI was less than 1.3 and was always present when RVI was less than 1.1. These findings go together with previously published results regarding the atrial contribution to ventricular filling in ventricular dysfunction [8, 9, 10]. Atrial contraction not only increases end-diastolic pressure (booster pump, [8]), but also provides adequate ventricular filling.

In our experience, tricuspid and pulmonic regurgitation can be detected with high specificity and sensitivity from the observation of flow direction. The method described is probably as valuable in predicting these disorders as are two-dimensional (2D) echocardiography or Doppler echocardiography, and might be superior for the detection of tricuspid regurgitation to the technique of visualising contrast bubbles in the inferior vena cava.

When comparing with 2D echocardiography and Doppler techniques, the advantages of our method are the nearly unlimited time resolution, the simultaneous visualisation of flow and of structures within one image and the ability to dispense with highly sophisticated techniques.

The most important disadvantage, so far, is the limitation to the right heart. The method can be performed essentially without risk and – in the absence of right to left shunts – can be repeated for additional interventional studies.

SUMMARY

Contrast M-mode echocardiography enables noninvasive quantitative and qualitative flow analysis, helps in the detection of tricuspid and pulmonic regurgitation and in the diagnosis of right ventricular dysfunction. The method can be easily performed with conventional M-mode systems and can be repeated, in the absence of right to left shunts, without the risk e.g. for interventional studies.

REFERENCES

1. Mason et al.: Application of the catheter-tip electromagnetic velocity probe in the study of the central circulation in man. Amer J Med 49:465, 1970.
2. Redel et al.: Vergleichende Flußanalysen am Herzen mit invasiver und nichtinvasiver Ultraschallmethode. Z Kardiol 69:222, 1980 (Abstr.).

3. Brubakk et al.: Diagnosis of valvular heart disease using transcutaneous Doppler ultrasound. Cardiovasc Res 11:461, 1977.
4. Kalmanson et al.: Noninvasive recording of mitral flow velocity patterns using pulsed-Doppler echocardiography. Brit Heart J 39:517, 1977.
5. Bom et al.: Current instrumentation. In: Echocardiology (Lancée, ChT, ed.), pp 373–383. Martinus Nijhoff, The Hague, 1979.
6. Bonzel et al.: Diagnose myokardialer und klappenbedingter Funktionsstörungen des rechten Ventrikels durch qualitative und quantitative Flußmessungen mittels Kontrastmittel M-Mode Echokardiographie. V. Münchner Echosymposium, 17–18 November 1980 (In press).
7. Bonzel et al.: Quantitation of right ventricular flow by contrast M-mode echocardiography for detection of right ventricular dysfunction. International meeting on bidimensional echocardiography, Milan, 29–31 October, 1980.
8. Mitchell et al.: The transport function of the atrium: factors influencing the relation between mean left atrial pressure and left ventricular end-diastolic pressure. Am J Cardiol 9:237, 1962.
9. Bonzel et al.: Pulmonalarteriendrücke und linksventrikulärer enddiastolischer Druck in Ruhe und unter dynamischer Belastung. Vergleichende Untersuchungen zur Druckübertragung im Kleinen Kreislauf bei simultaner Messung. Z Kardiol 65:1088, 1976.
10. Giambartholomei et al.: Behaviour of echocardiographic parameters following acute hemodynamic interventions. Circulation 58:II–52, 1978 (Abstr.).

30. COMPARISON OF MICROBUBBLE DETECTION BY M-MODE ECHOCARDIOGRAPHY AND TWO-DIMENSIONAL ECHO/DOPPLER TECHNIQUES

STANLEY J. GOLDBERG, LILLIAM M. VALDES-CRUZ,
YVONNE CARNAHAN, HEINZ HOENECKE, HUGH D. ALLEN,
and DAVID J. SAHN

1. INTRODUCTION

Blood flow tracking by M-mode echocardiography has proven to have considerable clinical utility [1, 2, 3]. Tracking is accomplished by imaging microbubbles during their passage from chamber to chamber. Timing of initial appearance usually allows determination of flow direction. Debate continues as to the best manner for injecting and generating microbubbles, but it is clear that once injected, these microbubbles act as ultrasonic reflectors. Microbubbles are created by injection of solutions, or of the patient's own blood, via catheters or needles. However, use of microbubbles as tracers has several problems. First, generation of sufficient microbubbles for tracking is not always possible. Secondly, microbubbles generally produce weak echoes, and these echoes can be eliminated by echo processing adjustments. Finally, microbubbles do not pass through the lung. The former two problems might be approached by use of a detection system which is designed to process low level echoes, and echo/Doppler is such a system.

The objective of our investigation was to determine the efficacy of blood flow tracking by echo/Doppler techniques.

2. METHODOLOGY

Microbubble detection by Doppler was studied during routine cardiac catheterization. Microbubbles were created by injection of saline in volumes of 5 ml for patients more than 10 kg and 2 ml for those under 10 kg body weight. We utilized injection sites from peripheral vessels, as well as from catheters in specific chambers. Two Doppler instruments were used to image passage of contrast material. The first was an ATL 500, equipped with a second generation time interval histographic frequency output and a trace which indicates strength of the Doppler signal. The ATL 500 also had an M-mode output which allowed simultaneous comparison of M-mode contrast and Doppler output. This M-mode output was shown to be substantially similar to the M-mode tracings for contrast produced by a Smith Kline 20A. The second Doppler instrument was a prototype two-dimensional

Rijsterborgh H, ed: Echocardiology, p 263-267. All rights reserved.
Copyright © 1981 Martinus Nijhoff Publishers, The Hague/Boston/London.

echo/Doppler (Honeywell). The latter instrument is operative in two modes, 1) a two-dimensional image with a movable cursor for range-gating and 2) a Doppler output with only an ECG reference signal. Frequency analysis for the latter instrument was accomplished with a fast Fourier transform. With our Honeywell instrument, simultaneous M-mode and frequency analysis was not possible.

M-mode contrast was identified according to earlier descriptions [1, 2, 3]. Doppler detection of microbubbles was judged positive if 1) a frequency dispersion greater than 1 vertical cm occurred after microbubble injection [4], and 2) a rise occurred in the Doppler signal strength indicator. Records recorded with the Honeywell instrument were evaluated for obvious

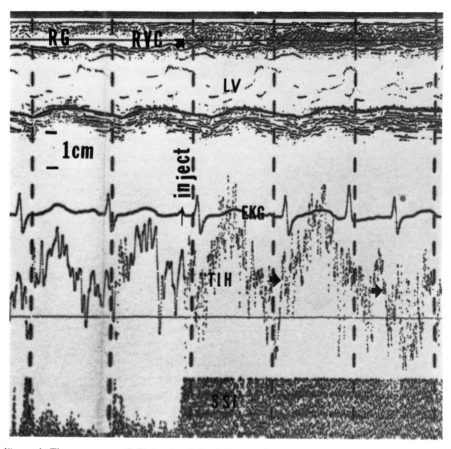

Figure 1. The range-gate (RG) is placed in right ventricular cavity (RVC). An injection was performed in the right atrium. Contrast is visualized in the RVC of the M-mode after the arrow. The time interval histogram (TIH) shows a frequency dispersion post-injection which exceeds 1 cm of vertical distance. Arrows point to areas of significant dispersion. The signal strength indicator (SSI) shows a marked rise after injection. Other abbreviations: LV = left ventricular cavity.

addition of a spectral dispersion imprinted on top of the standard velocity pattern.

3. RESULTS

Eighty-eight studies were performed in 16 children, 78 with the M-mode system and 10 with the prototype two-dimensional system. No complications were encountered. Three of the seventy-eight M-mode studies were unsatisfactory because of equipment failure, leaving 75 for analysis.

For studies with the ATL 500 instrument [5], the Doppler signal reflected from the microbubbles caused a frequency dispersion and a marked rise in the Doppler signal strength indicator (Figure 1). The contrast result of the simultaneous M-mode was almost always less diagnostic than the Doppler result, and in 36 instances the contrast effect was detected only with difficulty on M-mode, while the Doppler registered a very strong signal. In all instances (n = 20), in which microbubbles were not expected on the basis of flow patterns, none were detected by Doppler, and one error occurred for M-mode. In the error instance, microbubbles were detected in the right ventricular outflow tract immediately after injection into the left ventricle of a patient with no left-to-right shunt demonstrated by angiography. The range-gate of the Doppler had been placed into the aorta and, therefore, it did not test the right ventricular outflow tract in that instance. We could not duplicate this result. In instances in which microbubbles were expected (n = 55), five failures occurred for Doppler and 15 for M-mode. Three of the five failures occurred with injection and range-gating in the same chamber, and this may be due to streaming. The reason for M-mode failure was not apparent.

The two-dimensional echo/Doppler system depicted microbubbles as a background haze overlying the original wave form. Appropriate detection occurred in 8 out of 10 instances (Figure 2). Positive identification was missed in two instances in which injection and range-gating was placed in the same chamber. Fast Fourier transform displayed the contrast effect differently than the time interval histogram. The fast Fourier transform allowed visualization of the velocity pattern while registering the microbubbles as a background signal. The time interval histogram totally obscured the velocity wave form when microbubbles were present.

4. DISCUSSION

This investigation demonstrates that echo/Doppler is an effective method for tracing blood flow, and the reflected signals from microbubbles are more

266

readily detected by Doppler than by M-mode techniques. Both time interval histographic and fast Fourier transform spectral analysis techniques may be used to record the Doppler signal. Each of the two spectral analysis techniques has advantages and disadvantages. The fast Fourier transform allows simultaneous visualization of the velocity signal and the microbubble reflection, but is less sensitive to passage of microbubbles. The time interval

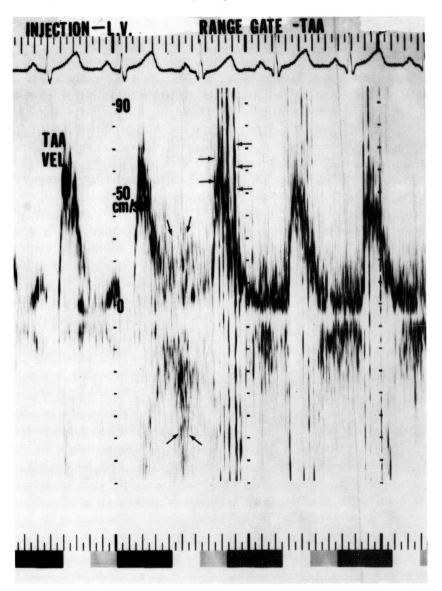

Figure 2. Velocities are inscribed positively and negatively from the zero (0) baseline. Injection is in left ventricle (LV) and the range-gate in the transverse aortic arch (TAA). Arrows point to the frequency dispersion due to microbubbles.

histogram is very sensitive to detection of microbubbles but the velocity signal is masked. Doppler appears to have significant clinical utility for microbubble tracing.

REFERENCES

1. Gramiak R, PM Shah, DH Kramer: Ultrasound cardiography: Contrast studies in anatomy and function. Radiology 92:939, 1969.
2. Valdes-Cruz LM, DR Pieroni, J Roland, PJ Varghese: Echocardiographic detection of intracardiac right-to-left shunts following peripheral vein injections. Circulation 54:558, 1976.
3. Sahn DJ, HD Allen, W George, M Mason, SJ Goldberg: The utility of contrast echocardiographic techniques in the care of critically ill infants with cardiac and pulmonary disease. Circulation 56:959, 1977.
4. Areias JC, SJ Goldberg, SEC Spitaels, VH de Villeneuve: An evaluation of range gated pulsed Doppler echocardiography for detecting pulmonary outflow tract obstruction in d-transposition of the great vessels. Am Heart J 96:467, 1978.
5. Goldberg SJ, LM Valdes-Cruz, L Felderman, DJ Sahn, HD Allen: Range dated Doppler ultrasound detection of contrast echographic microbubbles for cardiac and great vessels blood flow patterns. Am Heart J (in press.).

31. PULSED-DOPPLER SYSTEMS AND CARDIOVASCULAR DISEASE *

R.S. RENEMAN, A. HOEKS, C. RUISSEN, and F. SMEETS

1. INTRODUCTION

A variety of Doppler methods is in use to evaluate the functional state of the peripheral arterial circulation [20, 22]. Among these methods the detection of disturbances in the flow pattern is drawing attention because of the increasing evidence that these disturbances occur at relatively slight degrees of stenosis [3, 10, 24] and hence can be considered as an important parameter in the diagnosis of arterial lesions at an early stage of the disease.

In the clinic rather detailed information about the disturbances in the flow pattern along stenosed arteries can be obtained by using a continuous wave (CW) Doppler device with imaging system and audio spectrum analysis [23]. Velocity imaging is used to localize properly the site of recording of the audio spectrum in relation to the position of the stenosis. Another approach is to combine audio spectrum analysis with a single-channel pulsed-Doppler device and to localize the site of sampling by using a B-mode image of the vessel wall [4]. Although with audio spectrum analysis valuable information can be obtained about the flow disturbances in stenosed arteries, this method certainly has its limitations. Firstly, spectral broadening is used to diagnose disturbances in the flow pattern. Spectral broadening, however, does not only occur in turbulent flow, but also when plug flow changes into parabolic flow, the dimensions of the sample volume in the velocity direction increase in relation to the artery dimensions or the sound beam is non-homogeneous. Therefore, spectral broadening does not necessarily represent pathology. Secondly, no information can be derived from the audio spectra about the velocity profile – that is the velocity distribution over the cross-sectional area of the blood vessel – at discrete time intervals during the cardiac cycle. This limits the applicability of this approach in diagnosing peripheral arterial disease because in the vicinity of a stenosis the velocity profile was found to change locally during one cardiac cycle [28]. Velocity profiles at discrete time intervals during one cardiac cycle can be recorded on-line with multi-channel

* In part supported by the Dutch Heart Foundation and the Foundation for Medical Research FUNGO which is subsidized by the Netherlands Organization for the Advancement of Pure Research (ZWO).

pulsed-Doppler systems [1, 5, 12, 18]. Besides, these systems allow the on-line recording of the relative diameter changes of an artery during the cardiac cycle [14].

In clinical cardiology pulsed-Doppler systems have mainly been used in combination with echocardiography to diagnose valvular disease [8, 11, 16, 27]. In this technique single-channel pulsed-Doppler systems are used and flow disturbances are detected with audio spectrum analysis. So far, in adults multi-channel pulsed-Doppler devices have hardly been used to diagnose flow disturbances in and near the heart, mainly because of the problems encountered in recording accurately velocity profiles at a certain depth.

In the present survey the advantages and limitations of pulsed-Doppler devices as well as their possible usefulness in diagnosing cardiovascular disease are discussed.

2. PERIPHERAL VASCULAR APPLICATIONS

In pulsed-Doppler instruments usually one single crystal, operating alternately as transmitter and receiver, is used. The crystal receives the back-scattered signals from the red blood cells (RBC's) and the vessel wall during the interval between pulses. An electronic gate allows selection of scatterings either from the vessel or the RBC at a given distance from the transducer. This makes it possible to determine the mean velocity as an instantaneous function of time in a small sample volume at various sites in an artery thus avoiding contamination of the desired signal by unwanted signals.

In single-channel pulsed-Doppler systems, during one cardiac cycle the velocity as an instantaneous function of time can only be determined at one site in the vessel. Therefore, synthesis of the velocity profile during a cardiac cycle requires that the instantaneous velocity signals at various sites in an artery are assessed during consecutive heart beats. This limits the applicability of these systems in the diagnosis of peripheral artery diseases because in the vicinity of stenotic lesions the velocity profile was found to change locally during one cardiac cycle [28]. Besides, the positioning and maintenance of the sample volume at the site of interest requires some skill. Combining pulsed-echo (M-mode or two-dimensional) and pulsed-Doppler systems [2, 19] will facilitate this task, but introduces other limitations [12].

Recently multi-channel pulsed-Doppler systems have been developed that have the ability to detect simultaneously and instantaneously velocities over the full range of interest [1, 5, 12]. With these systems the velocity profile can be recorded on-line at discrete time intervals during one cardiac cycle. To obtain reliable velocity profiles, the sample resolution has to be high and the sample distance along the ultrasonic beam must be small. A limited number of independent samples along the cross-section of the vessel provides more parabolic velocity profiles and significantly overestimates vessel diameter [1]. Small sample volumes can only be obtained if the effective duration of the measurement is small and the beam width is narrow. The effective duration is set by the duration of emission combined with the bandwidth of the receiver section and the gate-width [18]. Increasing the bandwidth and shortening the duration of emission (high emission frequency) and the gate-width will reduce the sample volume, but will decrease the signal-to-noise ratio. In the present generation of the system developed in Maastricht, velocity samples can be taken along the vessel diameter at distances of 0.5 mm (sample volume about 1 mm^3) and as close to the vessel wall as 0.5 mm. Besides, the relative changes in artery diameter during the cardiac cycle can be obtained on-line by means of this system. An additional

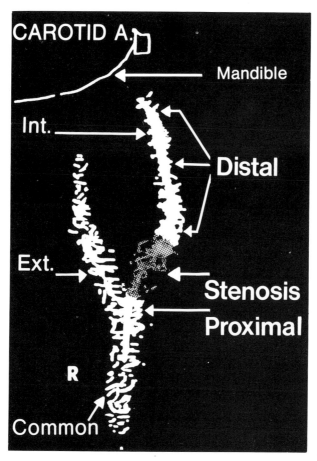

Figure 1. Cervical carotid image with sites of recording in a patient with an internal carotid artery stenosis [20].

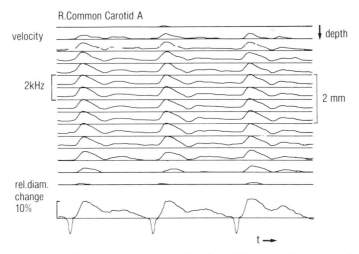

velocity

2kHz

2 mm

depth

rel.diam.
change
10%

t →

Figure 2. The mean velocity as an instanteneous function of time at various sites in the common carotid artery as recorded in a healthy volunteer of 20 years. The relative diameter changes of the artery during the cardiac cycle are shown as well. The negative deflection coincides with the R-wave of the ECG [22].

advantage of pulsed devices is that small volume samples are taken along the vessel diameter so that a narrow frequency spectrum is fed into the zero-crossing meter. Hence the error made in determining the mean frequency of the Doppler spectrum with this meter is small.

For proper localization of the disturbances in the velocity profile, the multi-channel pulsed-Doppler system is combined either with velocity imaging or B-mode imaging of the vessel wall. In velocity imaging a focussed transducer of a directional CW [25] or pulsed-Doppler [9, 17] flow system is connected to a mechanical scanning arm. The position of the transducer and beam is electronically sensed by position sensing circuitry which causes the beam of an image storage oscilloscope to move in correspondence with the position of the transducer. If for a given direction of flow the velocity exceeds a present threshold, the Z-axis of this oscilloscope is activated. By passing repeatedly the transducer over the artery and following the artery along its course a two-dimensional picture of arteries can be made (Figure 1).

The mean velocity as an instantaneous function of time at various sites in the common carotid artery as recorded in a young, healthy adult is presented in Figure 2. The data in this figure show that the phase shift between the velocity signal and the relative diameter change of the artery during the cardiac cycle, the latter being largely determined by the pressure pulse, is minimal. This observation indicates that arterial wall compliance can be estimated from the relative diameter changes and the instantaneous velocity tracings during systole.

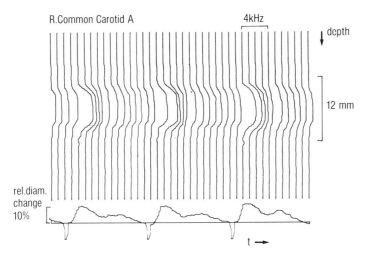

Figure 3. The velocity profile in the common carotid artery at discrete time intervals during the cardiac cycle as synthetized from the analog velocity tracings shown in Figure 2. The relative diameter changes of the artery during the cardiac cycle are shown as well. The negative deflection coincides with the R-wave of the ECG [22].

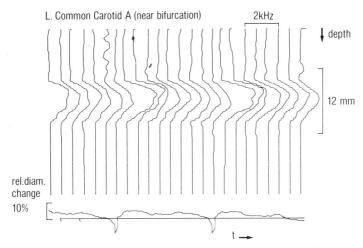

Figure 4. The velocity profile in the common carotid artery at discrete time intervals during the cardiac cycle as recorded near the bifurcation in a healthy volunteer of 45 years. Note the asymmetry of the velocity profile during systole. The relative diameter changes of the artery during the cardiac cycle are shown as well. The negative deflection coincides with the R-wave of the ECG [22].

The velocity profile in the common carotid artery at discrete time intervals during the cardiac cycle as synthetized from the analog velocity tracings in Figure 2 is shown in Figure 3. The velocity profile in this artery is flat, representing plug flow. Near the carotid bifurcation the velocity profiles become asymmetric, especially at peak velocity during systole (Figure 4).

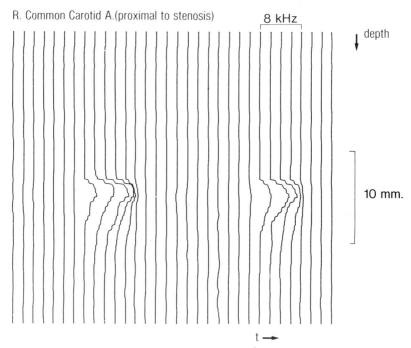

R. Common Carotid A.(proximal to stenosis) 8 kHz

depth

10 mm.

t →

Figure 5. The velocity profile at discrete time intervals during the cardiac cycle as recorded proximal to a slight stenosis in the common carotid artery. Note the asymmetric velocity profile [22].

Reflections from a small stenotic lesion cause asymmetry of the velocity profile, recorded proximal to the lesion (Figure 5).

Distorsion of the velocity waveforms and oscillations on these tracings are indicative for the existence of turbulence. These disturbances can easily be detected distal to a stenosis with multi-channel pulsed-Doppler systems [20]. In young adults the relative diameter changes of the carotid artery during systole are in the order of 10%, while in older healthy volunteers relative diameter changes of about 6% are recorded (cf. Figures 3 and 4).

Although the advantages of pulsed-Doppler systems are obvious, it should be noticed that in these devices problems are encountered which are not met in CW systems. The circuitry of pulsed devices is complex and the maximum Doppler frequency that can be detected unambiguously is limited and depends on the distance between transducer and vessel and the transmitter frequency [13, 21]. The distance sets an upper bound to the pulse repetition frequency, which should exceed the maximum Doppler frequency at least twice.

3. CARDIAC APPLICATIONS

In peripheral arterial applications a high emission frequency can be used, while maintaining a good signal-to-noise ratio, because of the shallow site of investigation. In pulsed-Doppler systems a high emission frequency (5 to 10 MHz) offers the advantage of a high spatial resolution.

Application of pulsed-Doppler systems in cardiology, especially in adults, requires a modification of the system. Because the site of investigation is more profound a sufficient signal-to-noise ratio in the Doppler signals can only be attained with a considerably lower emission frequency (2 to 5 MHz). Decreasing the emission frequency, however, enhances the amplitude of the unwanted low-frequency signals reflected by tissue interfaces with respect to the amplitude of the Doppler signals originating from blood particles. This problem is even more severe when the tissue interfaces are perpendicular to the ultrasound beam. Therefore, the cut-off frequency of the high-pass filter for the Doppler signals is set at a relatively high frequency which is at the expense of discarding low velocity information. The maximum velocity that can be detected unambiguously with pulsed-Doppler systems in the cavities of the heart is in the same order of magnitude as in peripheral vascular applications (approximately 1 m/sec) because the reduced pulse repetition frequency due to the increased depth of investigation is compensated by the reduced emission frequency. This maximum velocity, however, is hardly acceptable because velocities in the order of 1 m/sec can easily be present in heart valves even under physiological circumstances.

In clinical cardiology the experience with pulsed-Doppler devices is practically limited to single-channel systems, generally combined with pulsed-echo techniques. Although valvular disease can be diagnosed with these systems [7, 11, 26, 27], the use of single-channel pulsed-Doppler instruments has its limitation. As mentioned before, the spatial resolution, both axial and lateral, has to be high to be able to obtain detailed information. But maintaining a small sample volume in a stable position in relation to a moving structure is impossible. Moreover, small variations in position of the probe will largely affect the position of the sample volume because of the distance between probe and site of measurement. To overcome these problems, in single-channel pulsed-Doppler systems generally large sample volumes are used at the cost of spatial resolution. In this respect multi-channel pulsed-Doppler systems yield some advantages because detailed velocity information can be obtained with these systems in moving structures. The sample volume can be kept small because the velocity will be detected automatically in the adjacent channel in case of moving structures. Moreover, the displacement of this structure can be determined.

Beside in the estimation of aortic regurgitation [15], multichannel pulsed-Doppler systems have hardly been used in clinical cardiology. Theoretically

276

these systems offer the possibility to detect disturbances in the velocity profile within and distal to diseased valves and to assess simultaneously forward and backward flow, for instance, in aortic insufficiency and in case of bidirectional shunting. It is likely that velocities can be determined relatively easily in aorta-to-coronary bypass grafts with multi-channel systems. After all, velocity measurements in bypass grafts could be made [6] with single-channel pulsed-Doppler systems although localization of the vessel is more problematic in these systems.

Real-time assessment of volume flow in the ascending aorta with pulsed-Doppler devices remains problematic, mainly because the simultaneous determination of the average velocity over the cross-sectional area of the vessel and the absolute vessel diameter, both as an instantaneous function of time, cannot be performed accurately. First of all, the angle between the ultrasonic beam and the flow direction, necessary to correct the measured velocities for the angle of insonation, is not precisely known. Secondly, determination of the average velocity over the cross-sectional area requires that the sample volume envelops the vessel which is generally not the case. Thirdly, the accuracy with which the position of the vessel wall can be determined is, even for high resolution echo systems, beyond 0.5 mm which means an error of 5% in assessing the diameter and of 10% in assessing the cross-sectional area of a vessel of 20 mm in diameter. Fourthly, real-time assessment of volume flow requires that the angle of insonation for Doppler and the vessel diameter are detected simultaneously. Although a pulsed-echo system combined with a pulsed-Doppler system may provide this information, both systems are competitive, i.e. the use of the echo device reduces the maximum velocity that can be assessed with the Doppler device.

4. CONCLUSION

Multi-channel pulsed-Doppler systems combined with an imaging technique are likely to be an asset in the diagnosis of peripheral arterial disease because they can detect disturbances in the velocity profile induced by vascular lesions with slight narrowing of the artery. These lesions can generally not be detected with CW Doppler instruments. However, it should be noticed that quantification of these flow disturbances will be difficult. The use of multi-channel pulsed-Doppler systems in clinical cardiology may have some advantage, but further evaluation is required.

ACKNOWLEDGEMENTS

The authors are indebted to Mariet de Groot and Joke Hoozemans-Koreman for their help in preparing the manuscript.

REFERENCES

1. Anliker M: Diagnostic analysis of arterial flow pulses in man. In: Cardiovascular system dynamics. (Baan J, A Noordergraaf, J Raines eds.), p 113. MIT Press Cambridge, 1978.
2. Barber FE, DW Baker, DE Strandness, GD Mahler: Duplex Scanner II. Ultsym Proc IEEE, Cat = 74 CHO 8961 SU, 1974.
3. Barnes RW, Ge Bone, J Reinertson, EE Slaymaker, DE Hokanson, DE Strandness: Noninvasive ultrasonic carotid angiography: Prospective validation by contrast arteriography. Surgery 80:328, 1976.
4. Blackshear WM, DJ Phillips, DE Strandness: Pulsed-Doppler assessment of normal human femoral artery velocity patterns J Surg Res 27:73, 1979.
5. Brandestini M: Topoflow – A digital full range Doppler velocity meter. IEEE-SU-25:187, 1978.
6. Diebold B, PA Peronneau: Noninvasive assessment of aortocoronary bypass graft patency, using pulsed-Doppler echocardiography. Am J Cardiol 43:10, 1979.
7. Diebold B, P Theroux, MG Bourassa, C Thuillez, P Peronneau, JL Guermonprez, M Xhaard, DD Waters: Noninvasive pulsed-Doppler study of mitral stenosis and mitral regurgitation: Preliminary study. Br Heart J 42:168, 1979.
8. Fantini F, A Magherini: Detection of tricuspid regurgitation with pulsed-Doppler Echocardiography. In: Echocardiology (Lancée CT, ed.) p 233. Martinus Nijhoff, The Hague, 1979.
9. Fish PJ: Multichannel, direction-resolving Doppler angiography. Excerpta Medica International Congress Series no. 363, p 153. Excerpta Medica, Amsterdam, 1975.
10. Giddens DP, RF Mabon, RA Cassanova: Measurements of disordered flows distal to subtotal vascular stenoses in the thoracic aortas of dogs. Circ Res 39:112, 1976.
11. Hatle L, B Angelsen, A Tromsdal: Noninvasive assessment of atrioventricular pressure half-time by Doppler ultrasound. Circulation 60:1096. 1979.
12. Hoeks APG, RS Reneman, PA Peronneau: A multigate pulsed-Doppler system with serial data-processing. IEEE-SU (In press).
13. Hoeks APG, RS Reneman, CJ Ruissen, FAM Smeets: Possibilities and limitations of pulsed-Doppler systems. In: Echocardiology (Lancée CT, ed.), p 413. Martinus Nijhoff, The Hague, 1979.
14. Hoeks APG, CJ Ruissen, RS Reneman: A multi-gate multi-purpose pulsed-Doppler system. Fed Proc 39:1177, 1980.
15. Jenni R, W Hübscher, M Casty, M Anliker, HP Krayenbuehl: Quantitation of aortic regurgitation by a percutaneous 128-channel digital ultrasound Doppler instrument. In: Echocardiology. (Lancée, CT, ed), p 241. Martinus Nijhoff, The Hague, 1979.
16. Johnson SL, DW Baker, RA Lute, HT Dodge: Doppler echocardiography – The localization of cardiac murmers. Circulation 48:810, 1973.
17. Mozersky DJ, DE Hokanson, DS Sumner, DE Strandness: Ultrasonic visualization of the arterial lumen. Surgery 72:253, 1972.
18. Peronneau PA, JP Bournat, A Bugnon, A Barbet, M Xhaard: Theoretical and practical aspects of pulsed-Doppler flowmetry: Real-time application to the measure of instantaneous velocity profiles in vitro and in vivo. In: Cardiovascular applications of ultrasound. (Reneman RS, ed.), p 66. North-Holland/American Elsevier Publishing Company, Amsterdam, London, New York, 1974.
19. Pourcelot L: Echo-Doppler systems – Applications for the detection of cardiovas-

cular disorders. In: Echocardiology with Doppler applications and real time imaging. (Bom N, ed.), p 245. Martinus Nijhoff, The Hague, 1977.

20. Reneman RS: What measurements are necessary for adequate evaluation of the peripheral arterial circulation. Cardiovasc Dis (In press).

21. Reneman RS, A Hoeks: Continuous wave and pulsed-Doppler Flowmeters – a general introduction. In: Echocardiology with Doppler applications and real time imaging. (Bom N, ed.), p 189. Martinus Nijhoff, The Hague, 1977.

22. Reneman RS, A Hoeks, MP Spencer: Doppler ultrasound in the evaluation of the peripheral arterial circulation. Angiology 30:526, 1979.

23. Reneman RS, MP Spencer: Local Doppler audio spectra in normal and stenosed carotid arteries in man. Ultrasound Med Biol 5:1, 1979.

24. Sandmann W, P Peronneau, G Schweins, J Bournat, J Hinglais: Turbulenzmessung mit dem Doppler-Ultraschallverfahren: Eine neue Methode der Qualitätskontrolle in der Arterienchirurgie. In: Ultraschall-Doppler-Diagnostik in der Angiologie. (Kriesmann A, A Bollinger, eds.), p 77. Thieme Verlag, Stuttgart, 1978.

25. Spencer MP, JM Reid, DL Davis, PS Paulson: Cervical carotid imaging with a continuous wave Doppler flowmeter. Stroke 5:145, 1974.

26. Thuillez C, P Théroux, MG Bourassa, D Blanchard, P Peronneau, JL Guermonprez, B Diebold, DD Waters, P Maurice: Pulsed-Doppler echocardiographic study of mitral stenosis. Circulation 61:381, 1980.

27. Veyrat C, N Cholot, G Abitbol, D Kalmanson: Validity of echopulsed-Doppler velocimetry for assessing the diagnosis and severity of aortic valve disease and prosthetic valve function. In: Echocardiology. (Lancée CT, ed.), p 261. Martinus Nijhoff, The Hague, 1979.

28. Wille SØ: Numerical models of arterial blood flow. Thesis. Institute of Informatics, University of Oslo, 1979.

32. DOPPLER ECHOCARDIOGRAPHY AND VALVULAR REGURGITATION, WITH SPECIAL EMPHASIS ON MITRAL INSUFFICIENCY: ADVANTAGES OF TWO-DIMENSIONAL ECHOCARDIOGRAPHY WITH REAL-TIME SPECTRAL ANALYSIS

D. Kalmanson, C. Veyrat, G. Abitbol, and M. Farjon

1. INTRODUCTION

Since one-dimensional (1D) and two-dimensional (2D) echocardiography in combination with pulsed-Doppler (DE) allow the detection of localized turbulence and of reversal flow velocities, they provide a unique tool for diagnosing and evaluating regurgitation of all heart valves [1, 2, 3, 4, 5, 6, 7, 9, 10]. Since these diagnostic capabilities have been already substantiated by previous publications, we shall focus our attention on recent developments in the exploration of mitral valve regurgitation by two-dimensional Doppler echocardiography (2D DE).

2. MITRAL VALVE REGURGITATION

2.1.. Materials

We studied a control group of 20 normal subjects and a group of 28 patients with confirmed mitral valve regurgitation. These patients included 9 males and 19 females, from 20 to 69 years old. 13 of these patients (group I) had pure mitral regurgitation, with mitral valve prolapse (12) or a dilated annulus (1); 5 had a Barlow syndrome, associated in one case with atrial septal defect; 5 had one or more ruptured or elongated chordae tendinae, of rheumatic (3 cases) or Oslerian (2 cases) origin. There was one case of endocardial fibroelastosis and one case associated with mitral valve papillary dysfunction; 8 were in sinus rhythm, 5 in atrial fibrillation. The anterior leaflet was involved in 5 cases, the posterior one in 6 cases, both leaflets in 2 cases. The remaining 15 patients (group II) had combined mitral regurgitation and stenosis, of rheumatic origin. 13 were in atrial fibrillation, 2 in sinus rhythm. In all cases, the diagnosis was confirmed by cardiac catheterization and left ventriculography in right anterior oblique view, and a frame-by-frame study of the film was performed in order to substantiate the existence of the regurgitant jet, its origin, width, direction and depth. The severity of the regurgitation was established according to Sellers' criteria [8] on a 3 grade scale: mild, moderate and severe. In 19 patients who underwent surgery, the surgical findings were compared to the Doppler data.

Rijsterborgh H, ed: Echocardiology, p 279-290. All rights reserved.
Copyright © 1981 Martinus Nijhoff Publishers, The Hague/Boston/London.

2.2. Apparatus

We used the 851 ATL 3 MHz Cardiac Duplex, whose description, use and performance have been previously published [3, 4], together with two video monitors, one for cross-sectional imaging and the other for Doppler display, a videotape recorder and an Irex I fiberoptic stripchart recorder for simultaneous recording of M-mode echocardiogram including Doppler gate localization, ECG (lead 2) and frequency-selected phonocardiogram. Hard copies were obtained on a 4633 TEKTRONIX. In one series of patients, a Fast Fourier Transform device (Angioscan/Uniscan*) was connected to the 851 ATL in order to obtain a real-time spectral analysis. Analysis speed was 6.5 msec for one 128-point frequency spectrum (Figures 10, 11).

2.3. Recording technique

(Figure 1) Summarizing briefly, the technique requires two sequential procedures: first, the mitral valve is explored using the standard cross-sectional echocardiographic technique with various approaches (long-axis, short-axis, four-chamber view). Once the proper image has been obtained, the Doppler beam, displayed on the monitor as a continuous bright line, is swept across the plane and positioned in such a way that it always transsects the mitral area or the left atrium at the chosen angle, while the Doppler gate is adjusted in depth and made to coincide with the desired point in the area. The image is then frozen, while the apparatus is automatically switched to the Doppler mode. If a satisfactory "Doppler" sound is heard, a valid flow velocity recording can be made, either as an (analog) velocity curve or as a (digital) spectral frequency display. If not, the procedure has to be performed again with the Doppler gate slightly displaced until a satisfactory sound is heard. Thus the whole mitral valve area and the left atrium are systematically scanned and screened in order to obtain the maximum information. A set of flow velocity curves can be recorded and points of turbulent flow detected at the mitral annulus and within the left atrium, which can thus be "mapped".

The following approaches were studied sequentially:

2.3.1. Long-axis view (Figure 1)

The atrial side of the mitral annulus, as well as the whole left atrium, were screened. However, particular attention was paid to three directions. Starting from the centre of the annulus these were: 1) downwards and posteriorly,

---

* Unigon, Mount Vernon, New York, U.S.A.

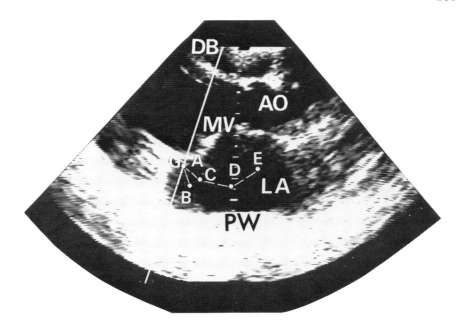

Figure 1. 2D scan/Doppler image of the mitral valve and of the left atrium. Long-axis view.
DB = Doppler beam, AO = aorta, MV = mitral valve, LA = left atrium, G = Doppler gate, A to E = points in the left atrium where a negative wave was recorded.

towards the inferior and posterior wall of the left atrium including the orifices of the pulmonary veins whenever possible; 2) axially, horizontally and posteriorly; 3) upwards and posteriorly, toward the posterior wall of the aortic root. Both types of recording were essential, an analog flow velocity trace in order to detect the presence of negative systolic waves, and a spectral display in order to detect turbulent flow (from of the spectrum). Finally the left atrium could be "mapped" into zones of turbulence, zones of negative systolic waves, and "zones of silence" as well as any zones of normal atrial flow velocity.

2.3.2. Short-axis view (Figure 5)
a. *Vertically:* a search was made within the orifice and below the posterior leaflet for zones of turbulent flow.

b. *Horizontally:* the postero-internal commissure, the centre and the antero-external commissure and the adjoining regions were explored carefully.

2.3.3. Transverse aortic view
This approach completed the preceding one.

282

2.3.4. Four-chamber view

The centre of the annulus, the juxta-septal zone, as well as the region close to the free wall of the left atrium and the atrial cavity were explored.

2.4. Results

In normal subjects, the flow velocity patterns of the mitral valve, and of the left atrial cavity, were consistent with those previously described [2, 3]. Neither systolic turbulence nor systolic negative waves could be detected at the mitral valve or within the left atrium.

2.5. Mitral insufficiency

a) *Detection of the regurgitation*

A systolic anomaly could be detected in 26 out of the 28 patients studied. In 11 out of the 13 patients in group I and 14 out of 15 patients in group II, systolic turbulence was detected during all or part of systole. In 26 patients out of 28 a negative wave was recorded during part or all of systole.

b) *Determination of the regurgitant jet*

1. *Pure insufficiency:* In 11 of the 13 patients with mitral prolapse, a linear sequence of turbulent zones could be determined, starting at the middle of

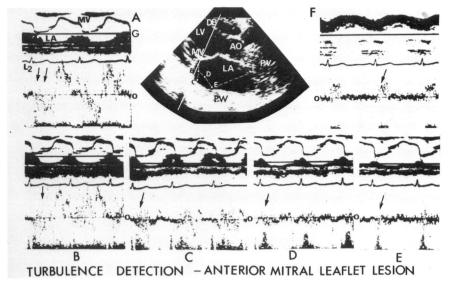

TURBULENCE DETECTION – ANTERIOR MITRAL LEAFLET LESION

Figure 2. Detection of turbulence in mitral regurgitation due to anterior valve prolapse. Doppler scan of the mitral valve and left atrium. Display of turbulent flow (arrows) recorded at points A to F.

the valve in the long-axis view (Figures 2 and 3), oriented posteriorly and either inferiorly (anterior leaflet prolapse) or superiorly (posterior leaflet prolapse, Figure 4) or horizontally (both leaflets prolapsed). The broadening of the spectrum decreased from the mitral valve to the end of this linear sequence, which in severe cases extended into the pulmonary veins. Other points showing a lesser degree of turbulence and/or showing a negative systolic wave on the analog velocity curve, could be detected at a small distance from the line of maximum turbulence (Figure 3), thus providing an estimate of the width of the jet along the long axis of the heart. In one case with a dilated annulus jets with different orientations (superior, inferior, and horizontal) were seen. In the short-axis view (Figure 5), turbulent flow was detected at the centre of the annulus and sometimes at one or both commissures, between the mitral valve leaflets and/or below the posterior leaflet. Such findings gave a first approximation of the width of the jet along the short axis.

In the four-chamber view, turbulent zones were detected at the centre and, sometimes, at the septal or the free wall part of the valve (Figure 6).

2. *Associated lesions.* In 14 of the 15 patients studied, turbulent zones and negative waves could be detected at the centre of the valve, extending laterally to either one or both commissures, and horizontally more or less deeply into the left atrium.

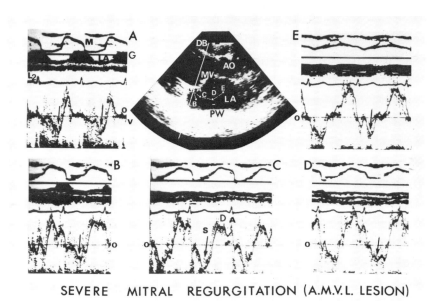

SEVERE MITRAL REGURGITATION (A.M.V.L. LESION)

Figure 3. Detection of negative waves in mitral regurgitation due to anterior valve prolapse. Same patient as in Figure 2. Compare with the angiogram in Figure 7.

284

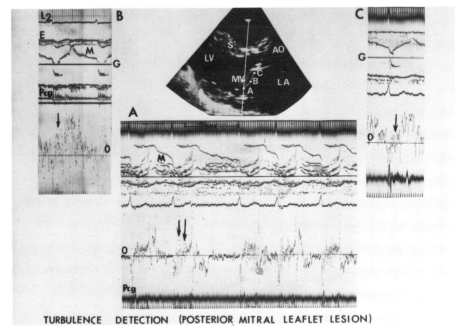

TURBULENCE DETECTION (POSTERIOR MITRAL LEAFLET LESION)

Figure 4. Detection of turbulence in mitral regurgitation due to posterior valve prolapse. Note the ascending direction of the jet and compare with the jet of the angiogram in Figure 8.

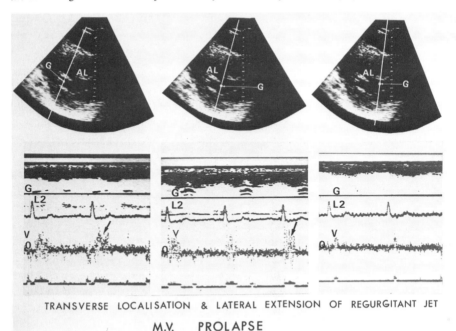

TRANSVERSE LOCALISATION & LATERAL EXTENSION OF REGURGITANT JET

M.V. PROLAPSE

Figure 5. Doppler scan of the mitral valve. Short-axis view.

G = Doppler gate, AL = anterior leaflet of the mitral valve. Left: posterior commissure; middle: center of the valve; right: anterior commissure. Turbulence is indicated by the spectral broadening.

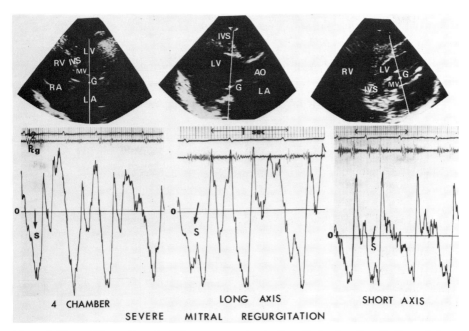

Figure 6. Three different Doppler 2D scan approaches to the mitral valve. Despite the variations in the angle between the beam and direction of flow, a negative wave, demonstrating mitral regurgitation, can be recorded in all 3 approaches.

2.6. Correlation with the angiographic findings

In all cases where the jet could be detected using DE, its origin, direction, length and width correlated fairly well with the features of the angiographic jet, providing a rough estimate of its shape and importance (Figures 7 and 8).

3. DISCUSSION

Thus 2D Doppler echocardiography appears to be an extremely useful and reliable method for the noninvasive detection of mitral regurgitation and assessment of the general shape, location and extent of the mitral regurgitant jet and providing a good idea of the severity of the mitral insufficiency. In the case of mitral valve prolapse, it can furthermore help to indicate the prolapsed leaflet, and even single out the scallop involved. However, some restrictions should be mentioned: 1) the possibility of overlooking a very small jet; 2) detection of a central jet does not always enable one to identify the prolapsed leaflet; 3) discrepancies in assessing the severity of the insufficiency may stem from the size of the left atrium: considerable

286

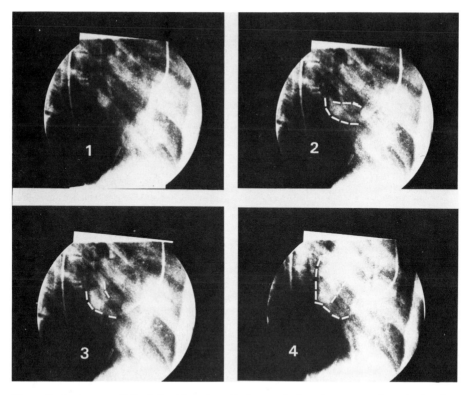

Figure 7. Angiogram of the left atrium in mitral regurgitation due to anterior mitral valve prolapse (same patient as in Figures 2 and 3). Note the right anterior oblique view, which gives a symmetrical image of the jet in contrast to the views in Figures 2 and 3.

enlargement of the atrium may mislead one into underestimating the importance of the mitral regurgitation.

The additional technical problems associated with the physics of ultrasound and Doppler technique have been published previously [2, 3]. However, the inconvenience of using the inadequate zero-crossing detector was overcome by adding an online spectrum analyzer. The spectra so recorded confirmed the clinical validity of the previously obtained velocity patterns in all cases. The usefulness of the additional information provided is currently under investigation.

4. AORTIC VALVE REGURGITATION (AR)

The results of investigations using the suprasternal notch approach supplemented by the parasternal one, together with 1D and 2D DE, have been previously published [4, 9]. In 31 patients with confirmed AR (19 pure, 12

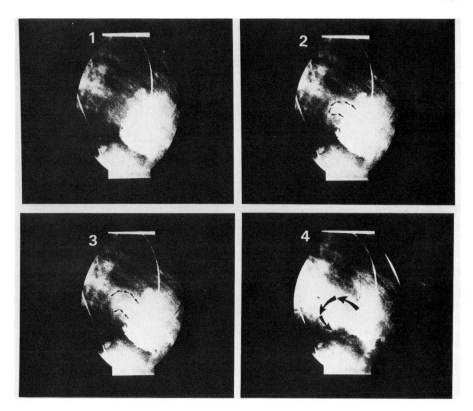

Figure 8. Left atrial angiogram. Mitral regurgitation due to posterior valve prolapse. Same patient as in Figure 4. Note the counter-clockwise direction of the jet, which is symmetrical, unlike the jet in Figure 4, due to the right anterior oblique view.

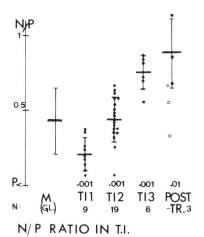

N/P RATIO IN T.I.

Figure 9. Assessment of severity of tricuspid regurgitation using N/P ratio index.
M = mean of all 37 patients; TI 1 = mild cases; TI 2 = moderate, TI 3 = severe cases; Post-Tr. = values in patients having had a tricuspidectomy. The open circles indicate the value in the same patients before tricuspidectomy.

288

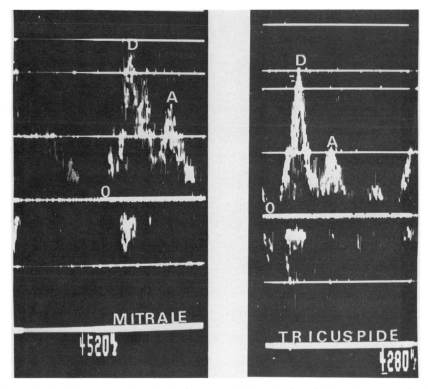

Figure 10. Real-time spectral analysis of normal mitral and tricuspid Doppler output signal. D = initial filling wave, A = end-diastolic filling wave, 0 = zero line (2 kHz).

associated) both sensitivity and specificity reached 90% for pure AR, and 85% for AR combined with stenosis. Correct grading of severity was respectively 81% and 83%, based on a three-grade scale.

5. TRICUSPID VALVE REGURGITATION (TR)

Technique and results have been published previously [3, 4, 10]. In 37 patients with confirmed TR, sensitivity was 83%, specificity 86% and correct grading 80% (Figure 9), using a negative over positive wave amplitude ratio as index.

6. PULMONARY VALVE REGURGITATION

Previously published results [2b, 4] using 1D and 2D DE, on a small series of patients (3) showed that in all cases the positive diagnosis and correct grading of severity could be established.

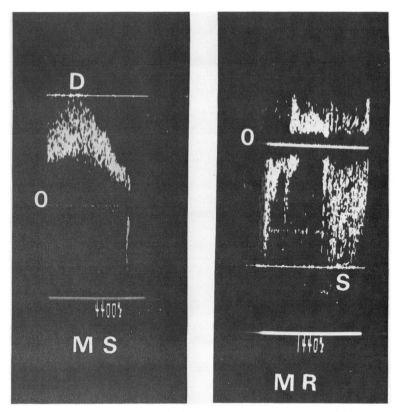

Figure 11. Real-time spectral analysis of mitral valve Doppler output signal in case of mitral regurgitation. S = systolic negative wave. The diastolic components of the spectrum were cutoff due to the format of the oscilloscope.

CONCLUSION

In summary, 1D and 2D Doppler echocardiography turns out to provide the most reliable noninvasive method, to date, for diagnosing and evaluating valvular regurgitation. In spite of some shortcomings, particularly the fact that the technique is not quantitative, it nevertheless provides qualitative and semiquantitative information, enhanced by the combined use of the Fast Fourier Transform spectral analyzer, which is largely sufficient for clinical purposes. The technique therefore desires to be more widely and more routinely used in clinical cardiology.

REFERENCES

1. Johnson S, D Baker, R Lute, H Dodge: Doppler echocardiography localization of cardiac murmurs. Circulation 48:810, 1973.

2a. Kalmanson D, C Veyrat, F Bouchareine, A Degroote: Non invasive recording of mitral flow velocity patterns using Doppler echocardiography. Br Heart J 39:517, 1977.

2b. Kalmanson D, C Veyrat: Echo-Doppler velocimetry in cardiology. In: Quantitative Cardiovascular Studies. Clinical and Research Applications of Engineering Principles. (Hwang NH, R Gross, D Patel, eds), pp 689–714, University Park Press, Baltimore, 1979

3. Kalmanson D, C Veyrat, G Abitbol: Two-dimensional echo-Doppler velocimetry in mitral and tricuspid valve disease. In: Recent advance in Ultrasound Diagnosis. (Kurjak A, ed.), pp 335–348. Excerpta Medica, Amsterdam, 1980.

4. Kalmanson D, C Veyrat, G Abitbol: L'exploration valvulaire non invasive par vélocimétrie Scanner-Doppler pulsé. Cœur et Médecine Interne 19:237–246, 1980.

5. Kinoshita N, K Miyatake, H Sakakibara, Y Nimura: Studies of regurgitant flow in mitral regurgitation with the combined use of the pulsed-Doppler and cross-sectional echocardiography. Abstr. 3rd Symposium of Echocardiology. Rotterdam, June 1979.

6. Matsuo H, A Kitabatake, M Asso, M Mishima, H Abe: Detection of the regurgitant flow direction in mitral valve prolapse syndrome using a combined ultrasound system. Proceedings of the 2nd Meeting of the WFUMB, Miyazaki, Japan, Excerpta Medica, Amsterdam, 1980.

7. Pearlman A, R Gentile, S Rubenstein, T Dooley, D Franklin: Echocardiographic detection of mitral regurgitation in mitral valve prolapse. In: Echocardiology (Lancée, CT, ed.), pp 255–260. Martinus Nijhoff, The Hague, 1979.

8. Sellers R, M Levy, K Amplatz, C Lillehei: Left retrograde cardioangiography in acquired cardiac diseases. Technique, indications and interpretation. Am J Cardiol 14:437, 1964.

9. Veyrat C, N Cholot, G Abitbol, D Kalmanson: Noninvasive diagnosis of aortic valve disease and evaluation of aortic prosthesis function using echo pulsed-Doppler velocimetry. Brit H J 43:393–413, 1980.

10. Veyrat C, G Abitbol, M Berkmann, MC Malergue, D Kalmanson: Diagnostic et évaluation par Echo-Doppler pulsé des insuffisances tricuspidiennes, des communications interauriculaires et interventriculaires. Archives des maladies du cœur et des vaisseaux 73:1037–1051, 1980.

33. COMBINED PULSED-DOPPLER ECHOCARDIOGRAPHY FOR THE INVESTIGATION OF VALVULAR HEART DISEASES: ONE-DIMENSIONAL VERSUS TWO-DIMENSIONAL APPROACH

C. Veyrat, D. Kalmanson, M. Farjon, J.P. Guichard, D. Sainte-Beuve, and G. Abitbol

In the last few years, the combined pulsed-Doppler echocardiographic technique, by providing a means of recording blood flow velocity patterns at various points in the heart cavities and great vessels, has led to a new noninvasive method for diagnosing and assessing cardiac valvular disorders and shunts [3, 4, 5, 6, 11, 12, 13]. The original combined one-dimensional (1D) apparatus has been replaced recently by a two-dimensional (2D) unit in order to improve performance. Instead of using two separate transducers, as in the first 2D units [2, 10], the one we use in our laboratory employs a single transducer for both techniques [7, 8]. This paper reports the results of a comparative study using 1D and 2D pulsed-Doppler echocardiographic velocimetry (PDEV) sequentially on a group of patients with valvular heart disorders.

1. MATERIAL

We examined a control group of 25 normal subjects, 9 females and 16 males, ranging in age from 8 to 61 years (mean = 32), and a group of 107 patients, with 150 valvular lesions, 62 females and 45 males, ranging in age from 8 to 77 years (mean = 48). The lesions comprised:

1) 71 mitral lesions (38 stenoses MS, 18 regurgitations MR, 15 associated lesions MS + MR);

2) 19 tricuspid lesions (14 regurgitations TR, 5 associated lesions TS + TR);

3) 25 aortic lesions (8 stenoses AS, 11 regurgitations AR, 6 associated lesions AS + AR);

4) 9 pulmonary lesions (7 stenoses PS, 2 regurgitations PR). The diagnosis was confirmed in 86% of the cases using the usual invasive procedures, including surgery when appropriate. For 14 patients, with minimal valvular lesions, the diagnosis was confirmed by the usual noninvasive procedures (ECG, echo, phonocardiogram with vasoactive drugs, auscultation). The severity of the lesions was established on a 3 grade scale for each type of lesion (1 = mild, 2 = moderate, 3 = severe), taking into account the Gorlin

Rijsterborgh H, ed: Echocardiology, p 291-298. All rights reserved.
Copyright © 1981 Martinus Nijhoff Publishers, The Hague/Boston/London.

formula and/or surgical data for stenosis, angiographic and/or pressure and/or surgical data for regurgitation.

2. TECHNIQUES AND APPARATUS

We used an ATL pulsed-Doppler 500 A velocimeter operating at 3 MHz, whose characteristics have already been described [1, 11], combined with either a 1D echocardiograph, or an ATL 851 90° wide-angle mechanical scanner (Cardiac Duplex). In the latter case, the scanhead included the Doppler probe in the same transducer. A lever built in the scanhead could be tilted (in one plane only) in order to move the Doppler beam (schematically represented as a white line) in the plane of the sector scan. The position of the gate (schematically represented as a bright point) was adjusted along the Doppler beam to any given point between 3 and 17 cm from the chest wall. In addition, we used two video monitors, one for the real-time scanning, and the other for the Doppler display. All the data were recorded on video tape, using a Sony video tape recorder. Hard copies were obtained on a Tektronix 4633 recorder. Doppler (analog) flow velocity curves, (digital) spectral frequency displays, M-mode echocardiographic tracings, ECG (lead 2) and frequency-selected phonocardiograms were recorded simultaneously on an IREX I fiberoptic stripchart recorder.

2.1. Recording method

Since the technique has already been described [6, 7, 8] it is only necessary to summarize the respective advantages of each approach for 2D PDEV:

a) *Mitral flow velocity patterns*. The long-axis view provided accurate location of the sample with regard to the annulus and, by translating or rotating the transducer laterally, to its internal or external regions. The short-axis view provided accurate location of the gate with regard to the center and the commissural areas. These two approaches are recommended for turbulence detection. The apical view is particularly suitable since the Doppler beam can be threaded through the mitral valve, parallel to the flow axis.

b) *Tricuspid flow velocity patterns*. We alternated the short-axis transsecting the aorta and left ventricle), four-chamber and subcostal views.

c) *Aortic valve and flow velocity patterns*. Parasternal approaches (long-axis and short-axis) are indicated for turbulence detection at the orifice. Suprasternal or right supraclavicular approaches were regularly used for recording the aortic flow.

d) *Pulmonary artery flow velocity patterns*. We used the short-axis view (aortic base) for the valvular area; the pulmonary trunk and branches were visualized from one intercostal space higher (supravalvular aortic area); the right branch was also obtained from the suprasternal notch.

Table 1. Correlation between 1D and 2D PDEV and invasive procedures.

n Pts: 107	Diagnosis				Correct assessment of severity		
Invasive procedures	1D PDEV		2D PDEV		1D	2D	Identification of anatomic lesions (2D)
	sensi-tivity %	speci-ficity %	sensi-tivity %	speci-ficity %	%	%	
Mitral lesions (71)							
MS (38)	97	97	97	98	89	92	Commissure 92%
MR (18)	77	96	88	98	72	83	Valve 80%
MS+MR (15) S.	86	95	93	100	73	86	Central regurgitation
R.	80	95	93	96	73	80	9 out of 9
Tricuspid lesions (19)							
TR (14)	80	95	86	98	73	80	
TR+TS (5) S.	80	98	80	99	80	80	
R.	80	90	80	95	66	80	
Aortic lesions (25)							
AS (8)	87	100	87	100	87	75	
AR (11)	90	90	81	98	81	81	
AS+AR (6) S.	83	92	83	99	83	83	
R.	85	86	85	98	66	83	
Pulmonary lesions (9)							
PS (7)	85	89	85	94	71	83	
PR (2)		No Discrepancy				No Discrepancy	

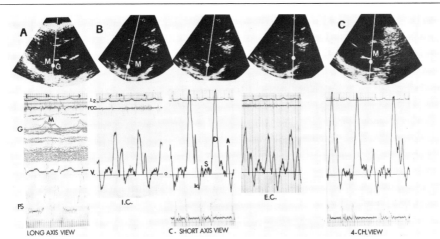

Figure 1. Cardiac Duplex recording: normal mitral flow velocity pattern: A) long-axis, B) short-axis (IC = internal commissure, EC = external commissure), C) four-chamber view (G = Doppler gate, M = mitral valve, ic = isometric contraction, S = systolic segment, D and A = early diastolic and presystolic filling waves, V = velocity curve).

RESULTS AND CORRELATIONS WITH INVASIVE DATA (Table 1)

The patterns are shown in Figures 1 to 4. They were found to be similar to those previously reported using 1D PDEV, for normals as well as for patients [5, 6, 11, 13], (Figures 5 to 6). The latter group showed the previously noted characteristic anomalies with both 1D and 2D PDEV, consisting of spectral broadening with indentations on the corresponding part of the analog curve for stenosis, and of a reversal wave with or without spectral disturbance for regurgitation. The assessment of severity relied on the spatial

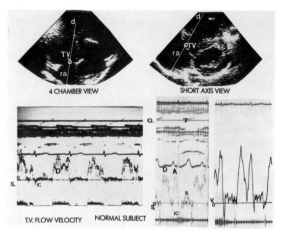

Figure 2. Cardiac Duplex recording: normal tricuspid flow velocity pattern: same abbreviations as in Figure 1.
  TV = tricuspid valve, ra = right atrium, d = Doppler beam.

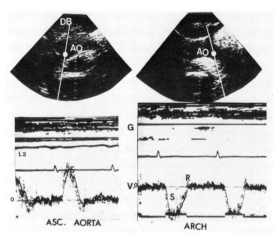

Figure 3. Cardiac Duplex recording: normal aortic flow velocity patterns.
  AO = aorta, ASC. = ascending, DB = Doppler beam, S = systolic wave, R = R wave.

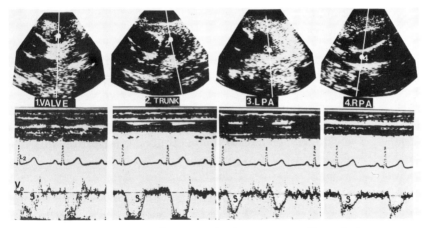

Figure 4. Cardiac Duplex recording: normal pulmonary artery flow velocity patterns.
LPA = left pulmonary artery, RPA = right pulmonary artery suprasternal approach.

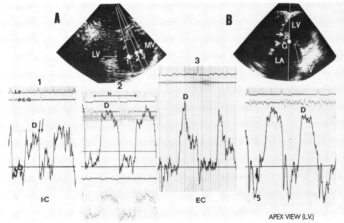

Figure 5. Contribution of Cardiac Duplex in the investigation of an associated mitral lesion: predominant stenosis is disclosed at the internal commissure, whereas central regurgitation is elicited using the four-chamber approach.

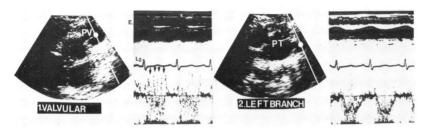

Figure 6. Moderate pulmonary stenosis: the anomalies do not spread far from the valvular area in this case.
PV = pulmonary valve, PT = pulmonary trunk

extension to the annulus for atrioventricular valve, and along the vessel for arterial valvular lesions.

DISCUSSION

Focussing the investigation on the presence and severity of a lesion, Table I shows that, for pure stenoses, comparable results are obtained for the two techniques. The cumbersomeness of the 2D probe even led to poorer results for aortic lesions, because it was impossible to record two cases.

On the other hand, 2D has a clear advantage over 1D for associated lesions, with particular emphasis on the assessment of the regurgitant factor and for pure mitral regurgitation. These advantages of 2D for diagnosing atrioventricular regurgitation stem from the multiple approaches used, specially recommended in cases of non-axial jets. Moreover, by allowing sampling all over the spatially visualized atria and afferent veins, 2D provides a better assessment of the importance of the regurgitant flow than does 1D. It is also more sensitive in cases of associated lesions, such as shunts for instance. But, above all, even when the results have equal percentages, the basic improvement of 2D PDEV is to provide a new insight of the valvular lesions than that suggested by 1D PDEV; because of the far more accurate location of the sample with regard to valvular structures, a functional and anatomic evaluation of the diseased valve enables one to detect *where* the predominant flow disturbances are with respect to the orifice. These refined qualitative data introduce new items in the correlative study, such as for instance, for mitral lesions, the assessment of each commissure and of the site of regurgitation (central and/or lateral), and the identification of the regurgitant valves [9]. For great vessel valvular lesions, despite the sometimes difficult suprasternal location of the probe for the aorta, 2D PDEV provides a better assessment by avoiding confusion between a branch vessel and the aortic arch, and enables one to combine the finding of a more or less far downstream extension of the anomalies with the presence or absence of a dilated aorta. For the pulmonary artery, although this limited group prompts us to make only preliminary statements, 2D PDEV appears most promising, since it is easier to perform and since it visualizes not only the valvular area but also the trunk and the branches, thus allowing a better assessment of the lesions on the basis of the spatial extension of the anomalies.

LIMITATIONS OF THE METHOD

The same general and technological limitations already mentioned [1, 7, 8, 11] apply to the two devices. Primarily, this technique is still not quantitative, it still uses a zero-crossing detector, with its well known deficiencies; in particular, for 2D devices, we must recall the lesser flexibility of the probe and the less satisfactory signal-to-noise ratio than in 1D devices. Further improvements must be made to the technique in this respect.

CONCLUSION

The above mentioned considerations should not overshadow the fact that, even if 1D PDEV is still a nearly comparable technique and even in the present state of the Duplex technique, 2D PDEV represents a conspicuous breakthrough among the available noninvasive methods. It provides much more refined qualitative information on the functional anatomy of the normal and diseased valves and, therefore, turns out to play a prominent role in the routine discussions about management of valvular heart diseases.

REFERENCES

1. Baker DW, S Rubenstein, G Lorch: Pulsed-Doppler echocardiography. Principles and applications. Am J Med 63:69, 1977.
2. Henry W, G Griffith: Combined Doppler cross-sectional echocardiographic system for measuring cardiac bloodflow velocities in man, Ultrasound in Medicine, vol. 3b (White D, R.E. Brown, eds), p 1375. Plenum Press, NY, 1977.
3. Johnson J, D Baker, R Lute, H Dodge: Doppler echocardiography. localization of cardiac murmurs. Circulation 48:810, 1973.
4. Kalmanson D, C Veyrat, A Degroote et al.: Enregistrement par voie transcutanée des courbes de vélocité sanguine mitrale normales et pathologiques par la technique Doppler. Rapport préliminaire. CR Acad Sci (Paris) D, 282:937, 1976.
5. Kalmanson D, C Veyrat, F Bouchareine et al.: Noninvasive recording of mitral flow velocity patterns using Doppler echocardiography. Brit H J 39:517, 1977.
6. Kalmanson D, C Veyrat: Echo-Doppler Velocimetry in cardiology. In: Quantitative Cardiovascular Studies. Clinical and Research Applications of Engineering Principles. (Hwang HN, R Gross, D Patel, eds) pp 689–714. University Park Press, Baltimore, 1979.
7. Kalmanson D, C Veyrat, G Abitbol: Two-dimensional echo-Doppler velocimetry in mitral and tricuspid valve disease. In: Recent Advances in Ultrasound Diagnosis (Kurjak A, ed.), pp 335–348. Excerpta Medica, Amsterdam, 1980.
8. Kalmanson D, C Veyrat, G Abitbol: L'exploration valvulaire non invasive par vélocimétrie Scanner-Doppler pulsé. Cœur et Médecine Interne 19:237–246, 1980.
9. Kalmanson D, C Veyrat, G Abitbol et al.: Doppler echocardiography and valvular regurgitation, with special emphasis on mitral insufficiency; advantages of two-dimensional echocardiography with real-time Fourier transform. In: this volume, pp 279-290.
10. Matsuo H, A Kitabatake, T Hayashi et al.: Intracardiac flow dynamics with

bidirectional ultrasonic pulsed-Doppler Technique. Japan Circulation J 41:515, 1977.

11. Veyrat C, N Cholot, G Abitbol et al.: Noninvasive diagnosis of aortic valve disease and evaluation of aortic prosthesis function using echo pulsed-Doppler velocimetry. Brit Heart J 43:393–413, 1980.

12. Veyrat C, N Cholot, M Berkmann et al.: Diagnostic non-traumatique des communications interventriculaires par la vélocimétrie Doppler-pulsé. Acta Cardiol (Bruxelles) 34:401, 1979.

13. Veyrat C, G Abitbol, M Berkmann et al.: Diagnostic et évaluation par Echo-Doppler pulsé des insuffisances tricuspidiennes, des communications interauriculaires et interventriculaires. Archives des maladies du cœur et des vaisseaux 73:1037–1051, 1980.

34. DIAGNOSIS AND ASSESSMENT OF TRICUSPID REGURGITATION WITH DOPPLER ULTRASOUND

T. Skjærpe and L. Hatle

Velocity of blood flow through the tricuspid valve was recorded noninvasively by Doppler ultrasound with a combined pulsed and continuous wave (cw) Doppler (Pedof) [1]. Tricuspid regurgitation (TR) was diagnosed when reverse flow in systole, originating at the tricuspid orifice, could be followed back into the right atrium (RA) (Figure 1). With significant tricuspid regurgitation, forward flow across the valve increases, and assessment of the degree of regurgitation was attempted from the velocity of forward flow across the valve, the intensity of the Doppler signal from the regurgitant jet (increases with increased flow) and the extension of the TR in the right atrium. From these Doppler data the patients were divided in three groups, mild, moderate and severe regurgitation.

Maximal velocity in the regurgitant flow in TR will depend upon the right ventricular (RV) to right atrial pressure difference in systole, the higher this pressure difference the higher the velocity. Even with normal RV pressure

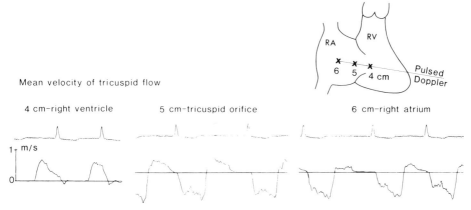

Figure 1. Velocity of tricuspid flow recorded noninvasively with pulsed Doppler. In the right ventricle, flow is towards the transducer (positive) in diastole. Reverse flow during systole is recorded at the valve area and in the right atrium. At the valve, velocity of forward flow in still recorded as in the ventricle, in the atrium it is decreased or no longer recorded. The sound of valve movements, together with flow signals, are used to localise the valve area; tricuspid valve opening is best recorded in the right ventricle, the closing movement best at the orifice. Tricuspid and mitral flow are distinguished by the different location and by the respiratory variation present in tricuspid flow velocity.

Rijsterborgh H, ed: Echocardiology, p 299-304. All rights reserved.
Copyright © 1981 Martinus Nijhoff Publishers, The Hague/Boston/London.

this may be above the limit for the pulsed Doppler. With the cw mode, the audio signal was used to find the highest frequency shift and velocity in the TR in 29 patients. From maximal velocity, RV-RA pressure drop in systole was calculated as in obstructions [2] and compared to the pressure drop recorded at catheterization.

PATIENTS

Tricuspid regurgitation was diagnosed in 85 patients during a 2½ year period. Seventy of the patients were catheterized. In the 31 patients where a right ventricular angiogram or contrast echocardiography (3 cases) was done, the diagnosis was confirmed in all. In another 8 patients, a pathological V-wave in the RA pressure curve indicated TR. Twelve of the patients died and an autopsy was done in all cases. Age was from 6–86 years (mean 52). The diagnoses are seen in Table 1. The patients with secundum atrial septal defects (ASD II) were either elderly with dilated right ventricles (3 cases), or young with combined ASD II and pulmonary stenosis (PS). Among the patients with coronary heart disease, 3 had acute myocardial infarctions. One died and autopsy showed involvement of the right ventricle and papillary muscles. Pulmonary heart disease included 2 patients with acute pulmonary emboli and 4 with primary pulmonary hypertension. A primary lesion of the tricuspid valve or valve apparatus was present in 8 (Ebsteins malformation in 2, a malformed tricuspid valve in one with ASD II and PS, combined tricuspid stenosis and regurgitation in 3 and ASD I in 2) and possibly in another 8 (repair of congenital heart disease in 7 and papillary muscle infarction in one). In the 69 others, the tricuspid regurgitation was most likely secondary to pulmonary hypertension or right ventricular dilatation. Forty-nine patients were in RV failure. A clinical diagnosis of TR was based on one or more of the following: visible systolic pulsations of neck veins, palpable systolic pulsations of the liver and a systolic murmur over the lower

Table 1. Cause of tricuspid regurgitation in 85 patients.

Valvular heart disease		37
mitral	29	
aortic	4	
combined	4	
Congenital heart disease		22
ASD II, ASD II+PS	7	
ASD I	2	
PS, Fallot	5	
Other	8	
Coronary heart disease/cardiomyopathy		17
Pulmonary heart disease		7
Constrictive pericarditis		2

third of the sternum, or at the lower left sternal border, with increase during inspiration.

A clinical diagnosis was made in 32 of the 85 patients (38%), the frequency of a clinical diagnosis was not influenced by the presence of RV failure. Table 2 shows the frequency of clinical signs related to severity assessed by Doppler and to presence of abnormal V-waves in the RA pressure curve. A clinical diagnosis was made in only 1 of the 35 patients with a mild lesion, it also failed in nearly half of those with moderate TR and in 2 of 11 with severe TR. In the 2 with severe TR, contrast echocardiography also indicated pronounced regurgitation. Both had large right atria, which might have decreased the effect of TR on the peripheral veins. Pathological V-waves were seen in 82% of patients assessed as having severe TR and in 59% of those with moderate TR. The clinical diagnosis of systolic pulsations in neck veins and/or liver correlated well with the presence of V-waves in the RA pressure tracing; pulsations were noted in 22 out of 27 cases.

The murmur of TR was in most cases soft and low grade and, since many patients had louder murmurs from other lesions, the respiratory variations of the former might not have been possible to detect. In several patients no systolic murmur could be heard despite auscultation following the Doppler diagnosis. Five patients had a harsher murmur, grade III-IV, 3 of these had severe pulmonary hypertension with hypertrophic non-dilated right ventricles, the other two had Ebstein's malformation. A systolic murmur with inspiratory increase was the only sign of TR in 6 patients.

Table 2. Tricuspid regurgitation (TR), diagnosis and assessment by Doppler compared to clinical diagnosis.

		Severity of TR		
	Total	mild	moderate	severe
No. of patients	85	35	39	11
Clinical diagnosis	32 (38%)	1	22	9
systolic venous pulsations	23	1	15	7
systolic hepatic pulsations	20	0	13	7
murmur of TR	18	0	12	6
No. catheterized *	62	22	29	11
Abnormal V-waves	27 (44%)	1	17	9
Systolic venous pulsations	22	0	15	7

* In close relation to the clinical and Doppler examination.

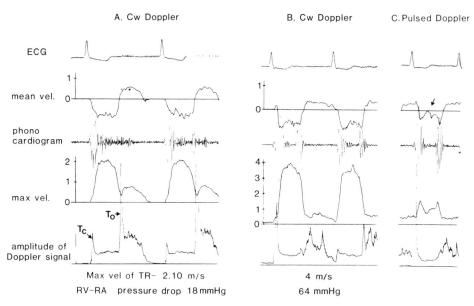

A. Cw Doppler   B. Cw Doppler   C. Pulsed Doppler

Max vel of TR- 2.10 m/s   4 m/s
RV-RA   pressure drop 18 mmHg   64 mmHg

Figure 2. With cw Doppler, high velocities in the tricuspid regurgitation can be recorded and used to calculate the right ventricular (RV) – right atrial (RA) pressure difference in systole. A, maximal velocity (non-directional) indicates a RV pressure within the normal range. In B, maximal velocity indicates a RV pressure about 70 mm Hg (with normal RA pressure) or higher (raised RA pressure). C = pulsed Doppler at the valve area in the same patient. With the pulsed mode, high velocities cannot be recorded and the mean velocity curves shows a midsystolic artefact due to velocities above the limit for the pulsed mode. In the amplitude curve valve movements are clearly seen. T_c = tricuspid valve closure. T_o – tricuspid valve opening.

Maximal velocity of forward tricuspid flow was 0.61 m/s (range 0.34–0.90) in mild TR, 0.79 m/s (0.46–1.25) in moderate and 1.02 m/s (0.64–1.50) in severe TR (normal range 0.35–0.80 m/s, unpublished data). With reduced cardiac output, as in heart failure, lower velocities are found and may then be within the normal range, even in the presence of severe TR. With normal cardiac output, velocities up to 1.5 m/s were found indicating a peak pressure drop from RA to RV of 9 mmHg in early diastole in the absence of tricuspid stenosis.

Figure 2 shows maximal velocity in the TR in one patient with normal and one with raised RV pressure. Panel C shows the limitations of the pulsed mode when high velocities are present. The amplitude curve indicates the intensity of the Doppler signal. Maximal velocity in TR ranged from 1.32–4.04 m/s – with calculated RV-RA pressure drops of 7–65 mmHg. In Figure 3 the calculated and recorded RV-RA pressure drops are compared. In patients with raised RV pressures, the high velocities in the TR were easy to find and the good correlation with recorded pressures indicates that small angles to the regurgitant jet could be obtained in most. With a noninvasive estimate of the RV-RA pressure difference in systole available, RV systolic

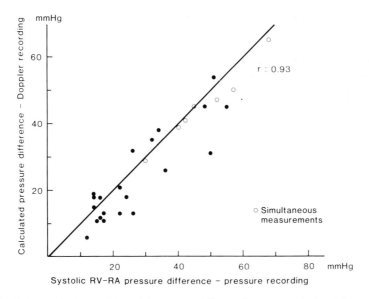

Figure 3. Right ventricular − right atrial pressure difference in systole calculated from maximal velocity in tricuspid regurgitation recorded noninvasively with Doppler and compared to the pressure difference recorded at catheterization.

pressure can also be estimated if the level of RA pressure can be judged from the neck veins.

CONCLUSION

Diagnosis of TR with Doppler is an easy and sensitive method as compared to the clinical diagnosis, which could be missed even in significant regurgitation. The lack of clinical signs in many of the patients with TR could mostly be explained by lack of abnormal RA pressure curves and abnormal venous pulsations in many of the patients with mild to moderate TR, and by the presence of systolic murmurs from other lesions. Comparing the attempted grading of the TR to the clinical and hemodynamic data indicates that semiquantitation of the TR may be possible. RV-RA pressure drop in systole can be calculated from cw Doppler recording of maximal velocity in the regurgitant jet.

REFERENCES

1. Brubakk AO, BAJ Angelsen, L Hatle: Diagnosis of valvular heart disease using transcutaneous Doppler ultrasound. Cardiovasc Res 11:461, 1977.

2. Hatle L, A Brubakk, A Tromsdal, B Angelsen: Noninvasive assessment of pressure drop in mitral stenosis by Doppler ultrasound. Brit Heart J 40:131, 1978.
3. Lieppe W, VS Behar, R Scallion, JA Kisslo: Detection of tricuspid regurgitation with two-dimensional echocardiography and peripheral vein injection. Circulation 58:128, 1978.

II. PEDIATRIC ECHOCARDIOLOGY

A. GENERAL APPLICATIONS

35. SEGMENTAL ANALYSIS OF CONGENITAL HEART DISEASE. A CORRELATION BETWEEN PATHOLOGY AND ECHOCARDIOGRAPHY

A. E. BECKER and W. J. GUSSENHOVEN

INTRODUCTION

The segmental analysis of congenital heart disease is at present well established and has proven to be relevant for the echocardiographer [4, 8]. The method consists of a step-by-step analysis of the various "building blocks", which together constitute the heart.

The first step in this procedure is the identification of cardiac chambers, a step in which echocardiographic evaluation may play an important role. Identification of the morphology of the atria is often difficult and may require a particular approach, such as a four-chamber view enabling the identification of the venous connections, or contrast echocardiographic methods. Identification of the ventricular chambers, on the other hand, is often established with plain echographic methods, since the morphological characteristics of the right ventricle are quite distinct from those of the left ventricle. In this paper we will not expand on morphology and chamber identification: for further reading see Anderson and Becker [1] and Tajik et al. [7].

The second step in the process of segmental analysis is the identification of the type and mode of the connection at the atrioventricular and ventriculo-arterial junctions [8]. The main part of this paper is devoted to this aspect in an attempt to correlate anatomy with echographic images and to point out the potential pitfalls that may hamper correct evaluation.

ATRIOVENTRICULAR JUNCTION

In describing the atrioventricular junction, two features should be specified. Firstly, one has to establish which atrium connects to which ventricle. This constitutes the *type* of connection. Secondly, one has to describe the specific morphology of the connections. This feature is known as the *mode* of connection.

Rijsterborgh H, ed: Echocardiology, p 307-321. All rights reserved.
Copyright © 1981 Martinus Nijhoff Publishers, The Hague/Boston/London.

Types of atrioventricular connections

Four basic types of connection can be encountered, i.e. concordant, discordant, double inlet, or absent connection (Figure 1). For the sake of completeness, ambiguous atrioventricular connection should also be considered, although of less clinical significance. This situation is characterized by isomeric atria, in which the right and the left atrium both exhibit the morphological characteristics of either morphological right or left atria. It often concurs with the so-called visceral symmetry syndromes, generally known as the asplenia and polysplenia syndrome [10, 11, 12]. It follows from this description that an ambiguous atrioventricular connection cannot be defined as concordant or discordant. Double inlet and absent connections, however, may coexist with isomeric atria. The main contribution to be expected from echographic evaluation in such cases is the identification of valve morphology relative to the underlying chamber morphology.

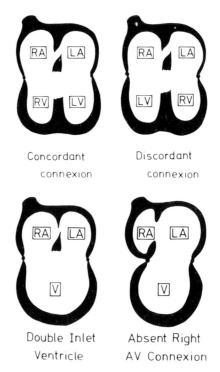

Concordant
connexion

Discordant
connexion

Double Inlet
Ventricle

Absent Right
AV Connexion

Figure 1. The basic types of atrioventricular connection in biventricular (upper panel) and univentricular hearts (lower panel).

Concordant atrioventricular connection

A concordant atrioventricular connection is present when the major part of each atrium connects to the appropriate ventricle irrespective of valve morphology. In other words, the right atrium connects to the right ventricle and the left atrium to the left ventricle (Figure 1). A concordant atrioventricular connection can occur with situs solitus or with situs inversus.

Concordancy thus represents the usual type of atrioventricular connection. Its presence can be established on the basis of the distinct features that characterize the morphological right and left atrioventricular valves. The tricuspid valve is characterized by septal chordal insertions and a large mobile anterior leaflet. Single beam techniques usually fail to demonstrate the septal attachments, but this feature is clearly recognized with two-dimensional techniques. The mitral valve lacks septal connections, but is guarded by two firm papillary muscle groups. The mitral valve, furthermore, is in direct continuity with the posterior great artery. These features are usually amenable to two-dimensional as well as single beam techniques.

Four-chamber views may be used to ascertain the existence of a concordant atrioventricular connection by visualizing the right and left atrioventricular valves in the same image. The sound beams pass through the inlet part of the ventricular septum and display the tricuspid valve insertion at a slightly lower level than that of the mitral valve (Figure 2). Moreover, the

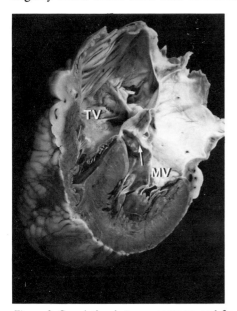 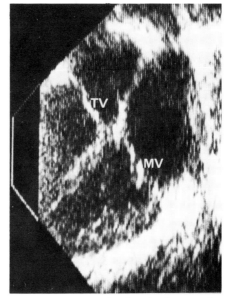

Figure 2. Correlation between anatomy and four-chamber echogram, showing the features of a concordant atrioventricular connection. Note the lower attachment of the tricuspid valve (TV) compared to the mitral valve (MV). The latter is in direct contact with the aortic root (arrow).

insertion of the atrial septum into the central fibrous body (the echocardiographical crux) is somewhat to the left of the insertion of the ventricular septum.

Discordant atrioventricular connection

A discordant atrioventricular connection is present when the two atria connect to *in*appropriate ventricles, irrespective of valve morphology. In other words, the morphological right atrium connects to the morphological left ventricle and the morphological left atrium connects to the morphological right ventricle (Figure 1). In a patient with situs solitus, therefore, the mitral valve is right-sided and anterior and the tricuspid valve is left-sided and posterior.

Generally speaking, the initial echographic pictures are confusing because of the abnormal spatial relationship of the valves and the ventricular septum. In itself this may already suggest the presence of a discordant connection. Positive identification, however, is primarily based on the recognition of valve morphology and of the abnormal spatial orientation of the ventricular septum. The latter presents as a more or less straight shelf and thus lacks the distinct curvatures of the normal ventricular septum. Hence, the septum is not readily identified in a conventional parasternal long-axis approach and the echocardiographer is often tempted to diagnose a univentricular heart on

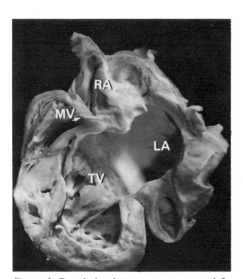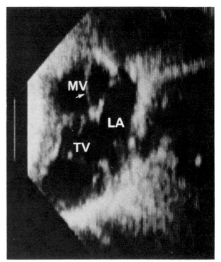

Figure 3. Correlation between anatomy and four-chamber echogram, showing the features of a *dis*cordant atrioventricular connection. The mitral valve (MV) is right-sided and the tricuspid valve (TV) is left-sided. The lower insertion of the tricuspid valve as compared to that of the mitral valve does not indicate the presence of Ebstein's malformation. The morphological right (RA) and left atria (LA) show situs solitus.

these grounds. Two-dimensional techniques and, in particular, four-chamber views should resolve this potential problem (Figure 3).

Double inlet atrioventricular connection

In double inlet atrioventricular connection the two atria connect to a sole main chamber (Figure 1). By definition, hearts with this type of atrioventricular connection are classified as univentricular [2].

The heart with a double inlet atrioventricular connection is morphologically characterized by absence of the inlet septum, which usually separates the two atrioventricular inlets. This feature also forms the basis for echographic recognition. In a classical case single beam and two-dimensional techniques will reveal two atrioventricular valves, which during diastole meet in the middle without an intervening septum (Figure 4). However, the position of the heart and the internal relations may be such that initially only one valve is imaged, instead of two. Deliberate attempts to visualize a second atrioventricular valve usually will reveal the features outlined above. Two-dimensional techniques are particularly helpful when the M-Mode is inconclusive and for specifying additional features, such as abnormalities in atrioventricular valve morphology and the presence or absence of an abnormally positioned septal structure within the ventricular mass.

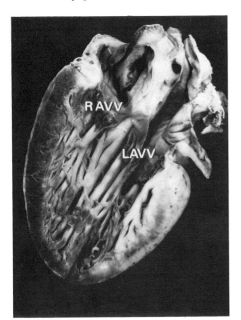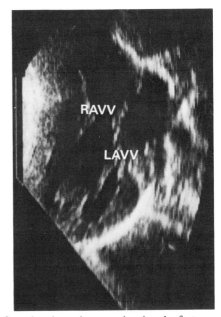

Figure 4. Correlation between the anatomy of the four-chamber echogram showing the features of a *double-inlet* atrioventricular connection. There is no intervening septum between the right (RAVV) and left (LAVV) atrioventricular valves.

Absence of an atrioventricular connection

Absent atrioventricular connection is characterized by the presence of only one atrial outlet, while the contralateral atrium possesses no ventricular connection (Figure 1). Dissection of the atrioventricular groove at the site of the absent connection will reveal that the "blind" atrium is completely separated from the underlying ventricular mass by fibro-fatty tissue. The central fibrous body is the only site where atrial and ventricular musculature come into contact. Absence of an atrioventricular connection thus typifies the situation where the "blind" atrium possesses not even a potential connection with the underlying chamber. As such, absent connection needs differentiation from hearts with an imperforate atrioventricular valve, in which a potential connection does exist [2]. From a functional point of view this distinction may not always be obvious, but from a morphological point of view important consequences ensue that relate in particular to the topographic anatomy of the atrioventricular conduction tissues [2].

It follows that echographic identification of an absent atrioventricular connection is difficult. Two-dimensional techniques are the ones most apt to give the correct diagnosis (Figure 5). Nevertheless, an unidentified atrioventricular valve may still be present, since the plane of sectioning may pass beyond the valve or because of its diminished size. Moreover, echographic identification of only one atrioventricular valve necessitates further differen-

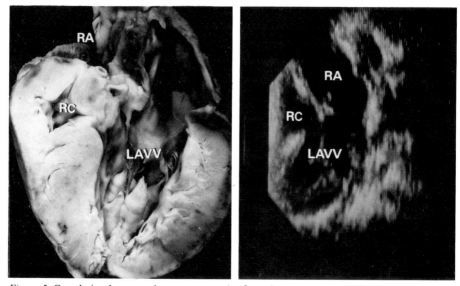

Figure 5. Correlation between the anatomy and a four-chamber echogram showing the features of *absent* atrioventricular connection. In this example the right atrium (RA) has no potential connection with an underlying rudimentary chamber (RC). The only atrial outlet is through a left-sided atrioventricular valve (LAVV).

tiation between an absent connection, on the one hand, and a connection characterized by a common valve, on the other hand. The distinction between the latter two options can be made with four-chamber views, visualizing both atrial and ventricular septa in the same plane.

MODES OF ATRIOVENTRICULAR CONNECTIONS

The mode of an atrioventricular connection is determined by the specific morphology of the valve apparatus through which the atria connect to the ventricles. Thus, a connection can be established through two perforate valves, one perforate and one imperforate valve or through a common atrioventricular valve (Figure 6). Moreover, each of these morphologies can be associated with an overriding or straddling atrioventricular valve (Figure 7).

Different morphologies may occur with almost any type of atrioventricular connection described above.

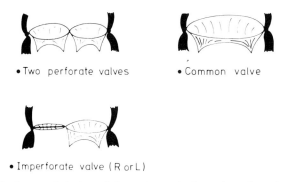

•Two perforate valves   •Common valve

• Imperforate valve (R or L)

Figure 6. Three basic morphologies of the atrioventricular valves through which the atria connect to the ventricles; the so-called *mode* of connection.

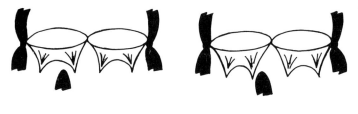

Straddling valve (R or L)   Overriding valve (R or L)

Figure 7. Overriding versus straddling atrioventricular valves. In case of a straddling valve part of the tension apparatus is attached to the contralateral chamber.

Imperforate atrioventricular valve

This is the rare condition in which an imperforate membrane-like structure is substituted for a perforate atrioventricular valve, be it right or left. It needs to be differentiated from "absent atrioventricular connection" (see above). Thus, an imperforate atrioventricular valve may complicate a concordant, discordant or double inlet connection.

Identification of an imperforate atrioventricular valve is difficult, but two-dimensional echocardiography seems to be the best method thus far. With single beam techniques, positive identification of an imperforate valve is almost impossible. When of moderate or large size the imperforate valve can be seen as an undulating membrane at the site of the anticipated atrioventricular valve. Usually, even with two-dimensional methods, contrast studies are necessary to ascertain the diagnosis.

Common atrioventricular valve

In this situation the two atria drain through a common atrioventricular valve, so that the right and the left atrioventricular ostia are no longer separated. This situation may thus occur in combination with a concordant,

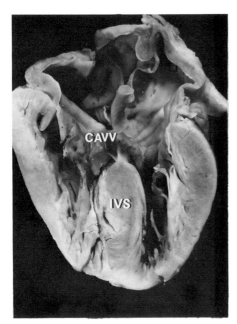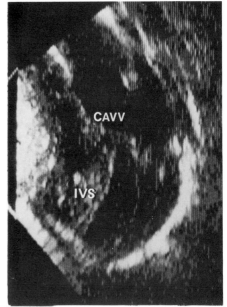

Figure 8. Correlation between anatomy and four-chamber echogram showing the features of a *common* atrioventricular valve. Note the common leaflet (CAVV) attached only by chordae to the top of the interventricular septum (IVS).

discordant or double inlet type of atrioventricular connection. Since the morphology is dominated by valve leaflets which extend along the anterior and posterior circumferences of the common ostium, the echocardiogram is usually highlighted by large valve excursions. The leaflets appear free-floating and their motion pattern is not restricted by a septal structure (Figure 8). Single beam techniques may suggest the diagnosis, but the actual demonstration of the common valve requires the use of two-dimensional systems.

Straddling atrioventricular valve

A distinction should be made between a straddling atrioventricular valve and an overriding ostium (Figure 7). In the latter situation the atrioventricular ostium overrides the underlying ventricular septum, but the valve apparatus is still confined to the appropriate ventricle. In the case of a straddling atrioventricular valve, part of the tension apparatus originates in the inappropriate ventricle. At present, echocardiographic techniques appear to be the most reliable tools for diagnosing a straddler.

The morphology of the straddling valve may vary considerably. In some cases only a minute papillary muscle originates from the contralateral chamber with only minimal or no override of the ostium. In other instances, however, a major part of the tension apparatus originates from the contralateral chamber, usually associated with marked ostial override.

Single beam techniques may detect an overriding or straddling atrioventricular valve, because the leaflet is seen to move beyond the septal boundary. Two-dimensional methods are necessary to ascertain this diagnosis and, in particular, to differentiate a posterior (left-sided) straddling atrioventricular valve from a common atrioventricular valve. Positive identification of the abnormally situated tension apparatus is mandatory in order to make such a distinction. However, even with the most sophisticated techniques the distinction between these two morphologies remains as yet difficult.

Straddling atrioventricular valves may be associated with concordant, discordant, double inlet and absent atrioventricular connections as well as with almost every possible valve morphology. Since the degree of straddling may vary, the inlet component may also vary. This creates a problem in nomenclature since hearts with overriding and straddling valves constitute a spectrum that ranges from biventricular hearts with concordant or discordant atrioventricular connections to univentricular hearts with a double inlet connection [8]. The degree of commitment will largely determine the basic flow pattern through the atrioventricular connection and it seems logical and practical, therefore, to assign an overriding atrioventricular valve by definition to the underlying chamber that receives more than half of its circum-

316

ference. This chamber is then designated a ventricle. The remaining chamber, receiving less than 50% of the straddling atrioventricular orifice, is no longer regarded a ventricle, but is termed a rudimentary chamber. The "50% rule" is only a decision making device, useful in situations which require a solution [8].

VENTRICULO–ARTERIAL JUNCTION

In describing the ventriculo-arterial junction we will first consider the different types of connections, prior to a brief consideration of the possible modes of arterial connections.

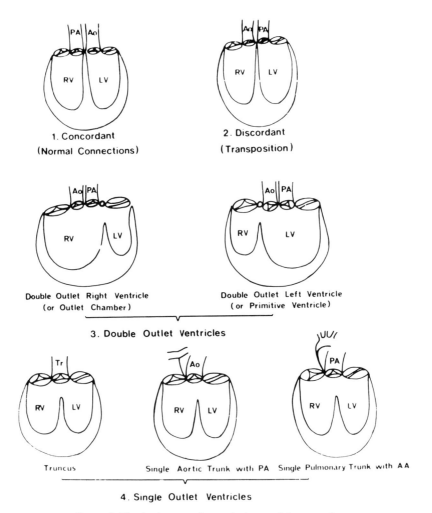

Figure 9. The basic type of ventriculo-arterial connections.

There are basically four types of arterial connections, i.e. concordant, discordant, double outlet and single arterial trunk (Figure 9).

Concordant ventriculo-arterial connection

In this condition the great arteries arise from their appropriate ventricles, or their derivatives, as in univentricular hearts. Concordancy represents the usual anatomical configuration. However, the term concordant only specifies the connection and it does not necessarily indicate that the relations of the great arteries are normal. Despite a concordant connection the aorta may be positioned anterior to the origin of the pulmonary trunk and, hence, the relations of the great arteries are highly abnormal.

Discordant ventriculo-arterial connection

A discordant arterial connection is characterized by an aorta arising from the morphological right ventricle and a pulmonary trunk arising from the morphological left ventricle, or their remnants (Figure 9). This type of arterial connection is often referred to as "transposition", although usage of the latter term has led to considerably debate [3, 9, 13]. It is important, therefore, to state that the term "discordant ventriculo-arterial connection" only describes the aforementioned type of connection. It does not encompass the heart as a whole and, hence, cannot lead to a misconception regarding the cardiac condition under discussion.

Echographic identification of a discordant arterial connection is based on the fact that the abnormal connection is almost always associated with an abnormal relation of the great arteries. Instead of the usual "cross-over" of the two great arteries at the base of the heart, a discordant arterial connection usually exhibits two great arteries arising from the heart in parallel fashion although the position of the aorta relative to that of the pulmonary trunk may vary considerably. In other words, identification of two chambers and two parallel great arteries arising from two separate ventricles suggests a discordant arterial connection (Figure 10). It is important to know that in neonates and very young infants, with normally connected and normally related great arteries, similar parallel images may occasionally be obtained.

Two-dimensional echocardiographic systems will yield the best results in identifying a discordant arterial connection.

318

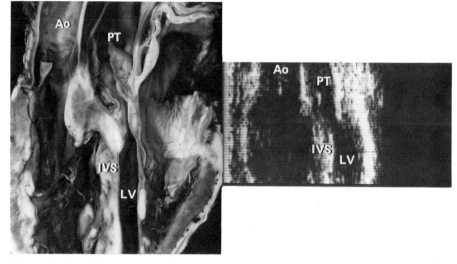

Figure 10. Correlation between anatomy and a long-axis echogram showing the features of a discordant ventriculo-arterial connection. The aorta (Ao) and pulmonary trunk (PT) arise in almost parallel fashion. Note the slight override of the pulmonary trunk over the interventricular septum (IVS), although the greater part of the trunk is confined to the left ventricle (LV).

Double outlet ventriculo-arterial connection

A double outlet connection is characterized by the major parts of both great arteries arising from one ventricle, be it morphologically right or left (Figure 9). The term "double outlet" thus defines a specific type of connection, irrespective of relations and other morphological features. This is an important point, since the term "double outlet right ventricle" is often considered to typify hearts in which the mitral and aortic valves are seperated by a muscle bar. Experience has taught that double outlet connections may occur both with and without such a specific morphology (Figure 11).

The main problem in classifying a connection as double outlet relates to overriding ostia (see modes of ventriculo-arterial connections). M-mode techniques may facilitate the recognition of an overriding valve, but there are serious drawbacks regarding its reliability. Two-dimensional methods are more helpful in estimating the degree of override, although again one has to be extremely cautious in interpreting the precise position of the arterial valve in relation to the underlying septum. Despite many pitfalls the two-dimensional approach definitely helps in differentiating a double outlet connection from a concordant or discordant connection.

It is important to emphasize that the relationship between the two great arteries is of no help in differentiating between double outlet or discordant connection.

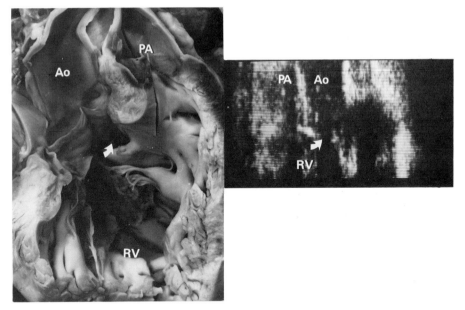

Figure 11. Anatomical and echocardiographic display of a *double-outlet* connection. The cases shown exemplify double outlet from the right ventricle (RV). The aorta (Ao) overrides a ventricular septal defect (arrow). Note that the greater part of the aorta arises to the right of the interventricular septum (IVS) from the RV. PA = pulmonary artery.

Single arterial trunk

In this situation only one great artery arises from the heart. It comprises a heterogenous group of conditions, which encompass truncus arteriosus, single aortic trunk in the presence of pulmonary atresia, and single pulmonary trunk in the presence of aortic atresia (Figure 9).

Echographic techniques usually enable the identification of the sole trunk, although its nature may remain speculative (Figure 12). The investigator is almost always left in doubt whether a second great artery is still present. It is for these situations, in particular, that the term "single outlet heart" has been introduced, which of course should be further specified when possible. For a precise diagnostic evaluation, invasive techniques are usually indicated.

MODES OF ARTERIAL CONNECTIONS

The only specific morphology of the arterial junction that needs a brief comment is overriding arterial ostium. Following the precedent set by Kirklin et al. [6] an arterial valve is assigned to the chamber that supports at

320

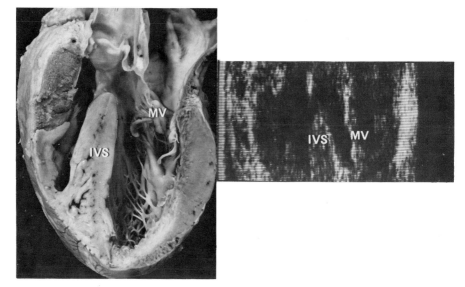

Figure 12. Correlation between anatomy and a long-axis echogram showing the features of *single outlet* heart. There is one main trunk arising from the base of the heart, which in this case overrides the interventricular septum (IVS). MV = mitral valve.

least 50% of its circumference. A similar "50% rule" is used for the atrioventricular valve morphologies. We fully accept that it is not always definable with certainty, but it at least creates a pragmatic approach to the problem of overriding arterial valves. As with atrioventricular valves, the estimated degree of override should always be stated.

SUMMARY

Segmental analysis of the heart in congenital heart disease is at present widely accepted, particularly in cases of complex malformations. The step-by-step analysis of the various junction sites of the heart is also amenable to echocardiographic investigation. Analysis of the atrioventricular and ventriculo-arterial junctions takes into account the type of connection and the specific morphology of the valve apparatus through which the connection is established. Echographic recognition of these parameters largely depends on the identification of the morphological features of ventricles and atrioventricular valves. Careful evaluation will usually enable the correct diagnosis regarding the type and mode of the connections at both the atrioventricular junction and the ventriculo-arterial junction.

Echocardiography may thus greatly contribute to the understanding of the complexity of the malformed heart as a whole.

REFERENCES

1. Anderson RH, AE Becker: Cardiac Anatomy. An integrated text and colour atlas. Gower Medical Publishing, London, 1980.
2. Anderson RH, AE Becker, RM Freedom, M Quero-Jimenez, FJ Macartney, EA Shinebourne, JL Wilkinson, M Tynan: Problems in the nomenclature of the univentricular heart, Herz 4:97, 1979.
3. Becker AE: Introductory remarks. In: Embryology and Teratology of the Heart and the Great Arteries. (Van Mierop LHS, A Oppenheimer-Dekker, CLDCh Bruins, Eds), Leiden University Press, Leiden 1978.
4. Becker AE, MJ Tynan, RH Anderson: Cardiac anatomy in congenital heart disease. In: Echocardiology (Bom N, ed.) p 113. Martinus Nijhoff, The Hague, 1977.
5. Becker AE, JL Wilkinson, RH Anderson: Atrioventricular conduction tissues in univentricular hearts of left ventricular type. Herz 4: 166, 1979.
6. Kirklin JW, AD Pacifico, LM Bargeron, B Soto: Cardiac repair in anatomically corrected malposition of the great arteries. Circulation 48:153, 1973.
7. Tajik AJ, JB Seward, DJ Hagler, DD Mair, JT Lie: Two-dimensional real-time ultrasonic imaging of the heart and great vessels. Mayo Clin Proc 53:271, 1978.
8. Tynan MJ, AE Becker, FJ Macartney, M Quero-Jimenez, EA Shinebourne, Rh Anderson: Nomenclature and classification of congenital heart disease. Br Heart J 41:544, 1979.
9. Van Mierop LHS: Transposition of the great arteries. I. Classification or further confusion? Am J Cardiol 28:735, 1971.
10. Van Mierop LHS, IH Gessner, GI Schiebler: Asplenia and polysplenia syndrome. In: Birth Defects: Original Article Series 8:(no 1) 74, 1972.
11. Van Mierop LHS, IH Gessner, GI Schiebler: Asplenia and polysplenia syndrome. In: Birth Defects: Original Article Series 8:(no 5) 36, 1972.
12. Van Mierop LHS, RR Patterson, RW Reynolds: Two cases of congenital asplenia with isomerism of the cardiac atria and the sinoatrial nodes. Am J Cardiol 13:407, 1964.
13. Van Praagh R: Transposition of the great arteries. II. Transposition Clarified. Am J Cardiol 28:739, 1971.

36. ERRONEOUS INTERPRETATION OF ECHOCARDIOGRAMS IN CONGENITAL CARDIAC ABNORMALITIES CONSEQUENT TO ANATOMIC VARIABILITY

W. J. GUSSENHOVEN and A. E. BECKER

INTRODUCTION

The introduction of ultrasound techniques had proved a major step forward in the field of the noninvasive diagnosis of congenital cardiac abnormality. M-mode echocardiography has now been largely superseded for this purpose by two-dimensional (2D) real-time techniques, with their ability to visualize the cardiac anatomy directly.

It is well known that cardiac anatomy can display wide variability. Even hearts falling in the same broad diagnostic classification (the same "name") may display considerable variation in their individual features. Fallot's tetralogy, which is characterized by an anterior deviation of the infundibular septum, a ventricular septal defect and an overriding aorta, is a good example of this phenomenon. The infundibular septum may be nearly normal or it may be small or even absent, while the ventricular septal defect may be perimembraneous or muscular and the degree of override of the aorta may vary markedly.

It should not come as a surprise, therefore, that anatomical variants may give rise to confusing echographic images, introducing a potential for fallacious interpretation, which may be additionally enhanced by variations in transducer position and the specific limitations of two-dimensional echocardiography.

ATRIAL SITUS

Echocardiography has its place in identifying atrial structures, such as the interatrial septum, and may be of help in establishing atrial situs. Moreover, echographic images of the left atrium are often taken as a means of measuring left atrial size. Identification of cardiac chambers is based on morphological criteria. In the usual situation the morphological right atrium receives the systemic veins and the coronary sinus, while the morphological left atrium receives the pulmonary veins. Positive identification of these venous connections can be obtained with two-dimensional techniques, thus allowing one to state atrial situs based on echographic grounds. It is

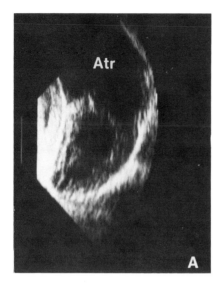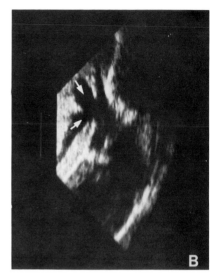

Figure 1. Echogram of a univentricular heart with absent right atrio-ventricular valve. *A* shows an image in which there appears to be only a single atrium (Atr). No interatrial septum can be identified. *B* shows an image taken from a different transducer position, which clearly reveals the interatrial septum. Note the hepatic veins (arrows) entering the right atrium.

necessary, however, that both atria be clearly recognized. This may create a problem for the echocardiographer, since identification of the atrial septum is usually difficult because of the position of the septum. Moreover, the greater part of the atrial septum is extremely thin. In most 'echographic cuts' the thin atrial septum will thus run parallel to the ultrasound beam and, hence, dropout artefacts may occur. Since the septum is thinnest in the area of the fossa ovalis, such artefacts may lead to a false diagnosis of a fossa ovalis type atrial septal defect. Another consequence is that occasionally no septum can be identified. which may lead to the erroneous conclusion that 'single atrium' is present and, hence, the possibility of situs ambiguous (Figure 1A). Careful manipulation of the transducer will almost always reveal the presence of an atrial septum (Figure 1B).

Left atrial dimensions

The left ventricular long-axis view visualizes the relation between the aortic and mitral valves and an atrium, which is generally considered to be the morphological left atrium. In the vast majority of instances this will indeed be true, but occasionally one may come across a case where the left ventricular long-axis view transects the right atrium (Figure 2). This is important since there are no means to distinguish on these images between

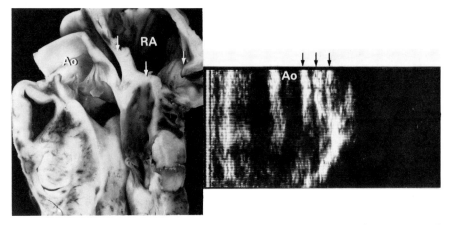

Figure 2. Correlation between the anatomy and a long-axis echogram showing that the main atrial cavity located posterior to the aorta (Ao) is the right atrium (RA) rather than the left atrium. The situation also classifies the occasional occurrence of several echo lines, which most likely relate to the right and left atrial free walls and the interatrial septum all coming into the plane of sectioning (compare arrows).

right and left atria. Nevertheless, the cardiologist is accustomed to measure 'left atrial' dimensions from these particular cross-sections without any hesitation. A slight tilt of the transducer in the parasternal long-axis position may occasionally produce an image of both left and right atrium (Figure 2). This phenomenon might also explain the occasional finding of unidentified echoes in the posterior atrium, which probably derive from the interatrial septum.

ATRIOVENTRICULAR JUNCTION

Echocardiography plays an important role in establishing the type of atrioventricular connection and the morphology of the valve apparatus through which the atrium connects to the underlying ventricle. With these techniques one is usually able to distinguish between biventricular hearts with either a concordant or discordant atrioventricular connection and univentricular hearts with either a double inlet connection or an absent connection. The latter type, of which classical 'tricuspid atresia' is a perfect example (Anderson et al. 1979), needs to be differentiated from the situation where one valve is perforate while the other valve is imperforate, although still located between an atrium and an underlying main chamber. Distinguishing between these options can be extremely difficult, even with the most sophisticated techniques.

On the other hand, making the differential diagnosis between absent connection and double inlet is generally considered easy, since the latter

326

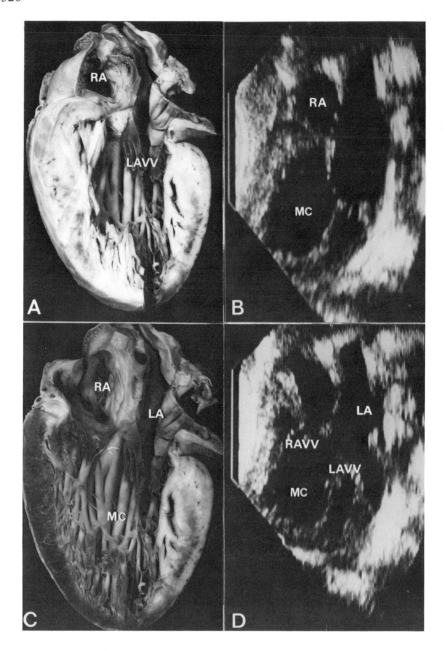

Figure 3. Correlation between anatomy and echograms showing the potential problem in differentiating absent atrioventricular connection from a double inlet connection. *A* and *B* show a plane through the heart which mimics a right sided absent connection. The right atrium (RA) appears to be completely isolated from an underlying main chamber (MC), which receives only one atrioventricular valve (LAVV). *C* and *D* show that a different plane, in the same heart, reveals a second, right-sided atrioventricular valve (RAVV). Thus, the right (RA) and left (LA) atria both connect to the main chamber (MC).

situation is characterized by the presence of two distinct valves. However, the internal anatomy of a double inlet univentricular heart may be such that the second valve is not at all easily detected and the images that are then obtained mostly suggest absent connection (Figure 3). The echocardiographer should thus be aware of this pitfall, knowing that quite different transducer positions may be indicated in order to identify the second atrioventricular valve. This statement applies to every instance where only one atrioventricular valve is recognized, be it in a biventricular or in a univentricular heart.

CHAMBERS

Generally speaking, it is possible using 2D echocardiography, and particularly the so-called four-chamber views, to enable identification of a heart as either biventricular or univentricular in nature. There are circumstances, however, in which the echogram may fail to visualize a chamber although it is definitely present. There are two main factors that play a part: the size and the position of the chamber. When a chamber is extremely small, despite a

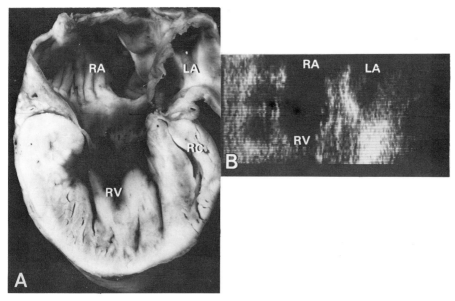

Figure 4. Correlation between anatomy and a long-axis echogram showing the problems in resolution encounteres in cases where a rudimentary chamber is minute and "embedded" within hypoplastic myocardium. *A* shows the small rudimentary chamber (RC) posterior in the heart in a case of univentricular heart of right ventricular type (RV). Note the slit-like appearance of the cavity. *B* shows an echogram of a patient with a similar malformation. At the site of the anticipated rudimentary chamber a clear picture is not obtained because of multiple blurring echoes.

LA = left atrium; RA = right atrium.

normal position, the 2D technique may have limitations. Due to limited axial and lateral resolution the echoes from such a small chamber may completely blur the cavity, which makes recognition virtually impossible in the beating heart. But even when the wall of the chamber is perpendicular to the transducer beam, the resolution of the ultrasound machine may be insufficient to produce an image on which a reliable diagnosis can be based. Secondly, these problems may increase when the small chamber is in an unusual position. Univentricular hearts with rudimentary chambers are examples of this (Figure 4). In univentricular hearts of left ventricular type, the rudimentary chamber, whether acting as an outlet chamber or not, is usually positioned in the anterior aspect of the ventricular muscle mass. It may be left-sided, anterior or right-sided, independent of the atrioventricular or arterial connections. To identify such a rudimentary chamber echographically may thus be difficult, except in the case of an anterior location. The rudimentary chamber in univentricular hearts of right ventricular type is less likely to be diagnosed, since it is usually in a posterior location (Figure 4). One should be aware of both the anatomical details and the limitations of all the aspects of the echographic technique, in each instance when only one chamber is imaged. The inherent limitations of both M-mode and 2D echography, together with the complexities of possible cardiac anatomy, thus makes it virtually impossible to diagnose an univentricular heart of the indeterminate type, i.e. without rudimentary chamber, using echographic techniques alone.

ARTERIAL JUNCTION

Echocardiography is a helpful tool in establishing ventriculo-arterial connections.

Concordant versus discordant

In concordant arterial connection the aorta arises from the morphological left ventricle. In the normal heart this concordant connection is further characterized by a particular relationship of the great arteries. At the base of the heart, the aorta and the pulmonary trunk are twisted round each other. Because of this, the usual right ventricular long-axis views of the arterial pedicle show one great artery (the pulmonary trunk) as a tube arising from the heart and one great artery (the aorta) as a circular structure.

In hearts with a *dis*cordant arterial connection the two great arteries, arising from *in*appropriate ventricles, usually run parallel to one another. Consequently, the same long-axis views show two parallel great arteries and

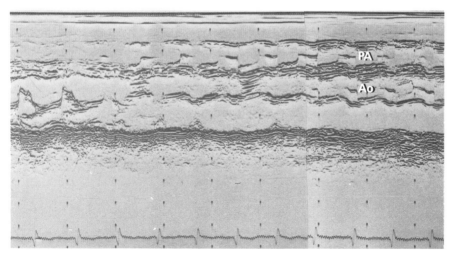

Figure 5. M-mode echogram showing a parallel arrangement of the great arteries. This tracing suggests a discordant connection but in fact the connections were completely normal.
Ao = aorta; PA = pulmonary artery.

it is customary to diagnose "transposition" of the great arteries on these grounds. There are two major objections to this simple approach. Firstly, the parallel position of the great arteries cannot be interpreted as diagnostic for transposition, where the latter term is used to indicate complete transposition of the great arteries. A similar arterial relationship can occur with many other congenital malformations, such as univentricular hearts and hearts with double outlet arterial connections. In other words, the parallel arrangement indicates the likelihood of an abnormal arterial relationship, but it does *not* specify arterial connections, nor does it specify a particular cardiac entity. Secondly, one has to consider another pitfall, namely that in neonates and young infants both the M-mode and the two-dimensional echogram may show the great arteries in parallel, arising from the base of the heart, although the actual topography is actually absolutely normal (Figure 5). Indeed, one may also envision that pathological processes, in themselves unrelated to the heart, may lead to torsion of the heart and arterial pedicle, which may then yield M-modes similar as seen in complete transposition on the echogram.

Overriding arterial valves

The overriding arterial valve poses a problem in classifying the connection. An artery may be assigned to one ventricle or to the other, depending on the exact degree of override. From a surgical point of view it is often important to be well informed about the degree of override prior to the surgical

330

procedure. For these reasons the clinician will have to be precise when judging the overriding arterial valve.

In order to make it possible to assign an artery to a ventricle in such cases, Kirlin et al. formulated the 50% rule. If more than 50% of the circumference of an overriding arterial valve is supported by the given ventricle then the artery is assigned to that ventricle. The 50% rule is also important for

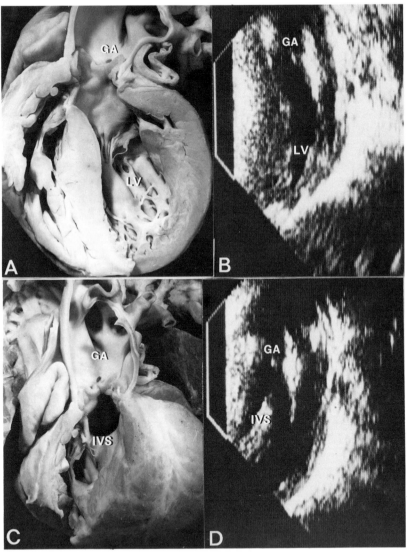

Figure 6. Correlation between anatomy and long-axis echograms showing the problems in ascertaining the degree of override of a great artery. *A* and *B* show a position in which a great artery (GA) is positioned almost exclusively over the left ventricle (LV). *C* and *D* show the same heart and the same patient now studied from a different transducer position so that the artery has a biventricular origin, overriding the interventricular septum (IVS).

establishing the type of connection. A double outlet connection is defined on the basis that more than 50% of the circumference of each of the great arteries arises from one chamber. It is presently widely accepted that echocardiography is the most suitable technique for evaluating the problem of overriding arterial valves. Despite this, one should realize that there are major pitfalls in using either M-mode or two-dimensional techniques for this. In the case of M-mode tracings, the precise position of the transducer in relation to the underlying arterial junction is vital. The technique may display an artery which appears to arise predominantly from the right ventricle but in the same heart may display exactly the reverse when a slightly different transducer position is used. M-mode tracings are, therefore, unreliable for determining the degree of override.

Two-dimensional techniques are more useful for this, but the exact positioning of the transducer is still important. In order to evaluate override, the arterial ostium must be related to the outflow part of the ventricular septum. Two-dimensional methods should, therefore, aim primarily at visualizing this particular structure. Four chamber-views usually portray the inlet and trabecular part of the ventricular septum and, hence, are usually not ideal for judging arterial override. In such views, even when one of the great arteries is seen to arise from a ventricle, its precise position in relation to that ventricle remains questionable (Figure 6). In the case of overriding arterial valves one has to be meticulous in evaluating the arterial junctions using many different transducer positions, in order to obtain a three-dimensional impression of the actual topography at the base of the arterial pedicle.

SUMMARY

Echocardiography plays an important role in evaluating the various "building blocks" that constitute the congenitally malformed heart. This applies in particular to the different types of connections that can occur. Difficulties arise from the anatomical variations that can occur within a given entity. These variations relate primarily to variable relations in morphological features. Echocardiography may detect these variations, but at the same time may lead to faulty interpretations.

Examples have been shown of erroneous interpretations of M-mode and two-dimensional echograms where the possible misinterpretation is caused by anatomic variation, with or without faulty or inadequate transducer positioning. Moreover certain aspects of the shortcomings of the echographic techniques have been demonstrated.

It follows that the investigator should be well acquainted with the marked anatomical variability that forms an integral part of congenital heart disease.

REFERENCES

1. Anderson RH, JL Wilkinson, LM Gerlis, A Smith, AE Becker: Atresia of the right atrioventricular orifice. Brit Heart J 39:429, 1979.
2. Kirklin JW, AD Pacifico, LM Bargeron, B Soto: Cardiac repair in anatomically corrected malposition of the great arteries. Circulation 48:153, 1973.
3. Tynan MJ, AE Becker, FJ Macartney, M Quero-Jimenez, EA Shinebourne, RH Anderson: Nomenclature and classification of congenital heart disease. Brit Heart J 41:544, 1979.

37. QUANTITATIVE ASSESSMENT OF CONGENITAL HEART DISEASE BY TWO-DIMENSIONAL ECHOCARDIOGRAPHY

NORMAN H. SILVERMAN, A. REBECCA SNIDER, and NELSON B. SCHILLER

M-mode echocardiography has been useful for evaluating the dimensions of various cardiac chambers and for assessing left ventricular function. However, the ability of M-mode echocardiography to evaluate cardiac size and function is limited by the narrow field which can be viewed at any given time. Because of its ability to visualize larger areas of the heart, two-dimensional echocardiography has recently been used to assess cardiac size and function. Quantitative assessment of the heart by two-dimensional echocardiography has been especially useful in the evaluation of children with congenital heart disease.

TECHNICAL CONSIDERATIONS FOR VOLUME ANALYSIS BY TWO-DIMENSIONAL ECHOCARDIOGRAPHY

For volume analysis, a two-dimensional system with excellent resolution throughout its range is desirable. Throughout the two-dimensional image, the axial and lateral resolutions vary considerably (Figure 1). The lateral resolution, which is always poorer than the axial resolution, is best in the center of the field [1]. In order to maximize lateral resolution the cardiac chamber undergoing volume analysis should be positioned as close to the center of the fan as possible.

Gain setting is an important consideration. At high gain settings, the targets appear enlarged and closer to each other (Figure 1). The gains should be turned to the lowest possible setting at which the endocardium can be seen clearly.

Calibration

For volume analysis, calibration of the image in the vertical and horizontal directions is necessary. Unfortunately, some two-dimensional systems provide calibration markers in the axial direction only. For these systems, a test target must be available to calibrate in both the vertical and horizontal directions.

Rijsterborgh H, ed: Echocardiology, p 333-344. All rights reserved.
Copyright © 1981 Martinus Nijhoff Publishers, The Hague/Boston/London.

334

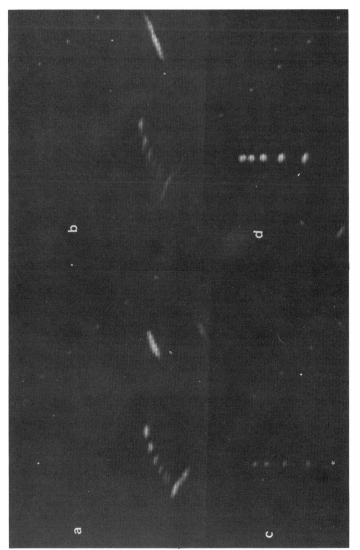

Figure 1. A two-dimensional scan of a target test block with markers. Frames (a) and (b) test the lateral resolution. The preselected range focus is appropriate in (a) and inappropriate in (b). The resolution is better towards the center of the fan. Frames (c) and (d) show differences in axial resolution. With the gains set low in (c), the front marker is barely discernible but separation of the targets is accurate. In (d) the gain setting is higher and the distance between the markers less. The same manipulations of gain can be applied to the test markers in frames (a) and (b).

Optimizing the image for tracing its outline

The image should be magnified as much as possible in order to trace it more accurately. Tracing an image directly from the video screen by means of a light pen system is the most accurate method. With this system, the inaccuracies of tracing with a wax crayon and plastic overlay or from a small photographic record are eliminated. In addition, the area outline of the endocardium can be inspected directly for accuracy and adjustments can be made in the tracing. Even under optimal conditions, small errors in estimation of the chamber size cannot be completely avoided because the area outline of the chamber utilizes the inner edges rather than the leading edges [2, 3].

Precise demonstration of the entire endocardial outline from a particular frame is generally not possible, and areas of echo dropout, related to technical factors or to true anatomic defects, require that extrapolation be made between the points. The outline can be completed by drawing a straight line between the adjacent endocardial echoes with reference to the pattern of contraction of the preceding and succeeding beats.

Timing

Selection of the appropriate frames for measurements at end-diastole and end-systole is important. Although the electrocardiogram present on most two-dimensional systems is useful for timing events in the cardiac cycle, end-diastolic and end-systolic measurements should be made from frames representing maximum and minimum chamber size. An electronic clock and frame counter should be displayed on the image so that the frame selected for analysis can be recalled.

LEFT VENTRICULAR VOLUME ANALYSIS

Recent studies suggest that the left ventricular volumes and ejection fraction can be calculated accurately by two-dimensional echocardiography from infancy to adulthood [4, 5, 6, 7, 8, 9, 10, 11]. Also, left ventricular mass can be evaluated using two-dimensional echocardiography [11, 12]. Some of these studies suggest that two-dimensional echocardiography is more accurate than M-mode echocardiography for determining these indices of left ventricular function. In 20 consecutive patients undergoing cardiac catheterization, we compared the left ventricular volume and ejection fraction predicted by M-mode and two-dimensional echocardiography to those predicted by angiography. The patients, who ranged in age from 2 months to

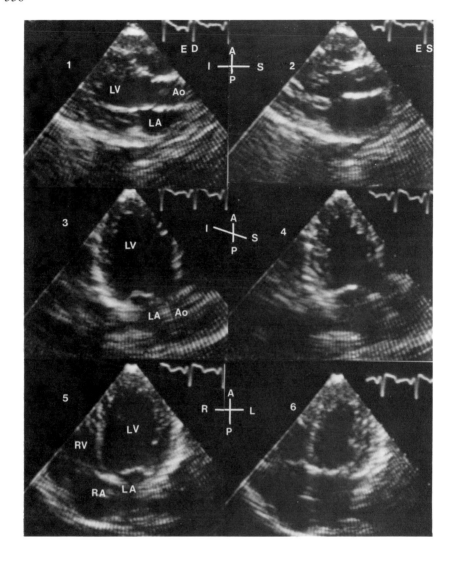

Figure 2. End-diastolic (ED) frames (left) and end-systolic frames (ES) (right) used to calculate chamber volumes. Orientation: A = anterior; P = posterior; R = right; L = left; S = superior; I = inferior. Abbreviations: LV = left ventricle; RV = right ventricle; RA = right atrium; LA = left atrium; AO = aorta. Frames 1 & 2 are parasternal long-axis views used to calculate left atrial volume. The parasternal view is oriented higher than usual in order to display the roof of the left atrium. Frames 3 & 4 are apical long-axis views used to calculate the left ventricular and left atrial volumes. Frames 5 & 6 are apical four-chamber views used to calculate left ventricular and left atrial volumes. In addition, these views were used to estimate right ventricular and right atrial size. Biplane measurements of left ventricular and left atrial volumes are possible from the combination of 3 & 5 and 4 & 6.

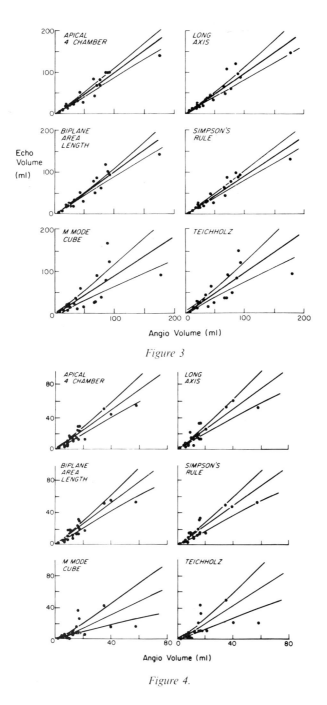

Figure 3

Figure 4.

Figure 3 and 4. Comparisons between the various echocardiographic methods and angiography for estimating end-diastolic and end-systolic volume. The regression line, the weighted 95% confidence limits for the line, and the data points are shown for each comparison. Published with permission from Circulation [8].

18 years, weighed between 3.5 and 70 kg and had body surface areas between 0.24 and 1.86 m². No specific cardiac geometry influenced our results as the patients had a wide variety of congenital defects.

The two-dimensional views used to calculate left ventricular volumes were obtained from the cardiac apex (Figure 2, frames 3-6). For the apical four-chamber view, the transducer was positioned over the cardiac apex in a plane passing through the mitral and tricuspid valves, the ventricular and atrial septa, and the pulmonary veins posteriorly. To obtain the apical long-axis view, the transducer was rotated 90° counterclockwise from the apical four-chamber view. In the apical long-axis view, the plane passes through the mitral and aortic valves and the left atrium posteriorly. In order to ensure a reproducible plane, we include the aortic root in the apical long-axis view as an additional internal cardiac reference point. The apical four-chamber and long-axis views were used because they are orthogonal views around the major axis of the left ventricle and, therefore, satisfy requirements for biplane volume analysis.

A light pen interfaced to a microprocessor was used to draw the endocardial outline in the apical planes at end-diastole and end-systole. The papillary muscles were excluded from the volume calculations by drawing the endocardial outline through their bases. The longest length of the ventricle from the closed mitral valve to the cardiac apex was used to calculate left ventricular volume by the area-length method. Single plane area-length estimates of the ventricular volume at end-diastole and end-systole and the ejection fraction were calculated for both of the apical views. The area outlines obtained from these views were subsequently combined, and ventricular volumes and ejection fraction were calculated using a biplane area-length method and Simpson's rule method. The end-diastolic and end-systolic volumes and the ejection fraction calculated from cineangiograms were compared to those calculated from the M-mode echocardiogram using cube [13] and corrected cube [14] methods and were also compared to those calculated from the two-dimensional sector scan (Figures 3–5, Table 1).

In estimating the end-diastolic and end-systolic volumes and the ejection fraction the two-dimensional echocardiographic correlations with angiography were superior to the M-mode echocardiographic correlations with angiography. In general, the biplane methods for calculating volume from the two-dimensional sector-scan were superior to the single plane methods.

End-diastolic volumes from the various two-dimensional techniques correlated well with the angiographic end-diastolic volumes (Figure 3, Table 1); however, end-systolic volumes calculated from the two-dimensional methods correlated less well with the angiographic end-systolic volumes (Figure 4, Table 1). The end-systolic volumes calculated from two-dimensional and M-mode echocardiography overestimated the angiographic end-systolic volumes (Table 1).

Table 1. Linear regression equations (y = slope·x+intercept) for comparison between angiographic (x) and echocardiographic (y) volumes.

Technique	Slope	Intercept	r
End-Diastolic Volumes (ml)			
A4C	1.01	−4.15	0.97
ALA	0.98	−2.15	0.96
BAL	1.05	−3.64	0.96
SR	0.95	−3.31	0.97
Cube	0.93	−4.60	0.83
Corr Cube	0.98	−0.41	0.86
End-Systolic Volumes (ml)			
A4C	1.29	−1.67	0.92
ALA	1.35	−0.82	0.88
BAL	1.37*	−1.37	0.91
SR	1.25	−1.59	0.89
Cube	0.84	−1.83	0.74
Corr Cube	1.17	−1.97	0.78
Ejection Fraction (%)			
A4C	0.85	+0.30	0.73
ALA	0.95	−0.80	0.77
BAL	0.87	0.00	0.82
SR	0.66*	+0.16	0.68
Cube	0.78	+0.22	0.67
Corr Cube	0.76	+0.18	0.63

* Slope significantly different from 1 at 5% level by Student's t-test. Abbreviations: A4C = apical four-chamber method; ALA = apical long-axis method; BAL = biplane area-length method; SR = Simpson's rule; Cube = M-mode cube method; Corr Cube = corrected cube method; r = correlation coefficient.

The overestimation of angiographic end-systolic volume was the major source of error in the two-dimensional assessment of ejection fraction (Figure 5). This error may be related to improper selection of the frame used to measure the end-systolic volume. At rapid heart rates, a frame rate of 32 frames/second may be insufficient to locate end-systole as accurately as end-diastole.

Other investigators have also found that the biplane techniques provide the closest estimates of ventricular volume. In a recent study in children, a formula using the area of the left ventricle in the short-axis view at the level of the papillary muscles and the major length of the left ventricle in the apical long-axis view provided the best approximation of angiographic ejection fraction. However, a method utilizing a single area outline would not predict ventricular volume and function as accurately as a biplane method in patients with dyskinesis.

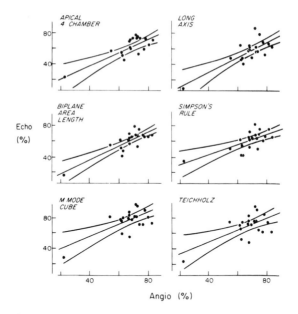

Figure 5. Comparisons between various echocardiographic methods and angiography for estimating the ejection fraction. The regression line and nonweighted 95% confidence limits for the line are shown for each comparison. Published with permission from Circulation [8].

Left atrial volume

M-mode echocardiography has been used to estimate left atrial size in the antero-posterior direction [16]. Left atrial enlargement may occur not only in the antero-posterior directions but also in the superior-inferior and right-left directions [16, 17]. Estimation of left atrial size by two-dimensional echocardiography is more accurate than by M-mode echocardiography because the left atrium can be measured in several planes.

We estimated the left atrial volume by two-dimensional echocardiography in 12 patients, aged from 6 months to adulthood, with a variety of congenital and acquired heart diseases [18]. The estimates of left atrial volume by M-mode and two-dimensional echocardiography were compared to angiographic estimates of left atrial volume. The parasternal long-axis view, the apical four-chamber view, and the apical two-chamber view were used individually to measure the left atrial size (Figure 1, frames 1–6). Also, the left atrial size was calculated from the combined apical areas using Simpson's rule method. In each view, the maximum and minimum left atrial sizes were measured at the downslope of the T-wave and the peak of the R-wave on the electrocardiogram. Using the light pen, the area of the left atrium was drawn along the inner border of the atrium. When there was dropout of echoes in

Table 2. Comparisons between two-dimensional echocardiography and angiography for estimating left atrial volume.

Algorithm	2D echo window and view	Regression equation	r	s.e.e.
Single plane area-length method	Precordial long-axis	y = 0.81x + 4.5	0.85	± 13.8
	Apical long-axis	y = 1.3x + 1.9	0.86	± 20.8
	Apical four-chamber	y = 1.2x + 8.8	0.78	± 26.6
Biplane simpson's rule method	Paired apical views	y = 1.0x + 6.3	0.86	± 16.5

y = volume (ml) from echocardiogram; x = volume (ml) from angiogram; r = correlation coefficient; s.e.e. = standard error of the estimate.

the atrial septum in the apical four-chamber view, the area outline was completed by drawing a straight line between the visualized portions of the atrial septum. The pulmonary veins were excluded from the area outline by drawing the line through their origins. For the area-length method, the major axis of the left atrium was drawn from the mid-mitral plane to the posterior atrial wall.

For each of the three individual echocardiographic planes and for the combined apical views, comparisons were made between the echocardiographic and angiographic estimates of the end-systolic and end-diastolic volumes. In each of the four sets of data, covariance analysis showed no significant difference between the slopes of the regression lines for the end-systolic and end-diastolic volumes; therefore, for each of the three individual planes and for the combined apical views, the measurements at end-systole and end-diastole were combined and compared as a single function (left atrial volume) against angiography. The correlations between left atrial volume measured by two-dimensional echocardiography and angiography are shown in Table 2. All the two-dimensional estimates of left atrial volumes correlated closely with the angiographic estimates of left atrial volume.

The best estimate of left atrial volume was obtained from the apical views using Simpson's rule method (Figure 6). This biplane technique slightly overestimated the angiographic measurement of left atrial volume. Of the single planes, the parasternal long-axis view provided the best estimate of left atrial volume (Figure 7). The parasternal long-axis view slightly underestimated the angiographic measurement of left atrial volume.

Other investigators have compared the left atrial area from the apical four-chamber view with the body surface area in children [9]. Using this method, left atrial areas falling outside the 95% confidence limits for body surface area correlated well with increases or decreases in left atrial volume seen on angiography.

342

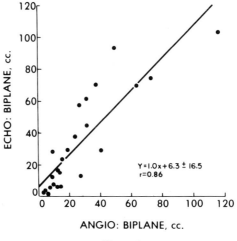

Figure 6

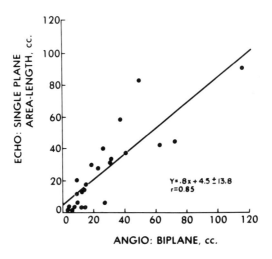

Figure 7

Figure 6 and 7. Comparison of two-dimensional echocardiography and angiography in calculating left atrial volume. In Figure 6, Simpson's Rule method combining the apical long-axis and four-chamber views was used. In Figure 7, a single plane area-length method using the parasternal long axis view was used. The equation for the line, the standard error of the estimate, and correlation coefficient for these data are shown.

Right-side heart measurements

Because of the irregular shape of the right ventricle, it is difficult to estimate the right ventricular size. Right atrial and right ventricular areas obtained from the apical four-chamber view in normal children have been measured.

Normal values have been established with respect to body surface area [9]. These data are still preliminary but the results are encouraging. Enlargements in right atrial and right ventricular areas on the two-dimensional echocardiogram have correlated well with right atrial or right ventricular enlargement on angiography [19].

These studies do not provide a reliable means of estimating right atrial and right ventricular volumes or ejection fraction. It is probable that biplane techniques will provide more accurate assessment of right heart chamber volumes and function.

CONCLUSIONS

Because of its ability to image large areas of the atria and ventricles, two-dimensional echocardiography is a valuable technique for estimating atrial and ventricular volumes. Current studies suggest that the left ventricular volumes and the ejection fraction can be determined reliably by two-dimensional echocardiography in children and adults. Also, left atrial volumes can be predicted by two-dimensional echocardiography using biplane techniques. The ability of two-dimensional echocardiography to quantitatively assess right heart chambers has not been adequately investigated; however, preliminary studies are encouraging. With the use of transducers of higher frequency and better resolution, digital scan converters, and more sophisticated computer facilities, even better quantitative information will be available from the two-dimensional echocardiogram in the future.

REFERENCES

1. Anderson WA, JT Arnold, LD Clark, WT Davids, WJ Hillard, WJ Lehr, LT Ziteli: A new real-time phased-array sector-scanner for imaging the entire adult human heart. Ultrasound Med 3B:1547, 1977.
2. Bom N, CT Lancée: Current Instrumentation. In: Echocardiology (Lancée CT, ed.), pp 373–378. Martinus Nijhoff The Hague, 1980.
3. Roelandt J, W Van Dorp, N Bom, JD Laird, PG Hugenholtz: Resolution problems in echocardiography: a source of interpretation errors. Am J Cardiol 37:256, 1976.
4. Gehrke J, S Leeman, M Raphael, RB Pridie: Noninvasive left ventricular volume determination by two-dimensional echocardiography. Br Heart J 37:911, 1975.
5. Carr KW, RL Engler, JR Forsythe, AD Johnson, B Gosink: Measurement of left ventricular ejection fraction by mechanical cross-sectional echocardiography. Circulation 59:1196, 1979.
6. Schiller NB, H Acquatella, TA Ports, D Drew, RJ Goerke, H Ringerts, NH Silverman, B Brundage, EA Botvinick, R Boswell, E Carlsson, WW Parmley: Left ventricular volume from paired biplane two-dimensional echocardiography. Circulation 60:547, 1979.

7. Folland D. AF Parisi, PF Moynihan, DR Jones, CL Feldman, DE Tow: Assessment of left ventricular ejection fraction and volumes by real-time two-dimensional echocardiography. Circulation 60:760, 1979

8. Silverman NH, TA Ports, AR Snider, NB Schiller, E Carlsson, DC Heilbron: Determination of left ventricular volume in children: echocardiographic and angiographic comparisons. Circulation 62:548, 1980.

9. DiSessa TG, JH Kirkman, CT Ching, AD Hagan, SE Kirkpatrick, WF Friedman: Evaluation of cardiac chamber size and left ventricular function in children using two-dimensional apex echocardiography. Amer J Cardiol 56:468, 1980.

10. Mercier JC, TG DiSessa, T Nakanishi, JB Isabel-Jones, JM Jarmakani, WF Fredman: Two-dimensional echocardiographic assessment of left ventricular volumes and ejection fraction in children. Circulation 62:III-72, 1980.

11. Wyatt HL, MK Heug, S Meerbaum, JD Hestenes, JM Cobo, RM Davidson, E Corday: Cross-sectional echocardiography: analysis of mathematic models for quantifying mass of the left ventricle in dogs. Circulation 60:1104, 1977.

12. Schiller NB, C Skiolderbrand, E Schiller, C Mavroudis, N Silverman, S Rahimtoola, M Lipton: In vivo assessment of left ventricular mass by two-dimensional echocardiography. Circulation 60:II-58, 1979.

13. Pombo JF, BL Troy, RO Burrell Jr: Left ventricular volumes and ejection fraction by echocardiography. Circulation 43:480, 1971.

14. Teichholz LC, T Kreulen, MV Herman, R Gorlin: Problems in echocardiographic volume determinations in the presence or absence of asynergy. Am J Cardiol 37:7, 1976.

15. Hirata H, SB Wolfe, RL Popp, CH Helmen, H Feigenbaum: Estimation of left atrial size using ultrasound. Am Heart J 78:43, 1969.

16. Allen HD, DJ Sahn, SJ Goldberg: New serial contrast technique for assessment of left-to-right shunting patent ductus arteriosus in the neonate. Amer J Cardiol 41:288, 1978.

17. Schabelman SE, NB Schiller, RA Anschuetz, NH Silverman: Comparison of four two-dimensional echocardiographic views for measuring left atrial size. Amer J Cardiol 41:391, 1978.

18. Schabelman SE, NB Schiller, TA Ports, NH Silverman, WW Parmley: Left atrial volume by two-dimensional echocardiography. Cirulation 57 & 58:II-188, 1978.

19. Bommer W, L Weinert, A Newmann, J Neef, DT Mason, A DeMaria: Determination of right atrial and right ventricular size by two-dimensional echocardiography. Circulation 60:91, 1979.

38. THE SPECTRUM OF ATRIOVENTRICULAR VALVE ATRESIA: A TWO-DIMENSIONAL ECHOCARDIOGRAPHIC/PATHOLOGICAL CORRELATION

G. R. Sutherland, M. J. Godman, R. H. Anderson, and S. Hunter

INTRODUCTION

The clinical picture of tricuspid or mitral atresia may be due either to absence of an atrioventricular connexion or to the presence of an imperforate membrane [1]. The distinction between these types may in itself have clinical significance and for this cross-sectional two-dimensional (2D) echocardiography should provide the ideal tool. In this study we have investigated 46 patients known to have right or left atrioventricular valve atresia, and correlated our 2D echocardiographic findings with a study of similar autopsy material.

DEFINITION AND TERMS

In the normal heart, the atrial and ventricular chambers on each side of the septum communicate via the right and left atrioventricular connexions (Figure 1a). Morphologically atrial and ventricular myocardial tissues are continuous both parietally and septally. Parietally, the two tissues are contiguous at the insertion of the valve leaflets, but are indented to a limited degree by the atrioventricular sulcus. The indentation is more pronounced on the right side where sulcus tissue partially separates the two myocardial masses, since there is not a well developed tricuspid valve annulus. In contrast, on the left side the mitral annulus is better formed, with the sulcus indentation being less obvious. Septally the atrioventricular junction lies obliquely, since the tricuspid valve attachment is more apical than the attachment of the mitral valve. In this area, the fibrous tissue separating the valve annuli becomes thickened anteriorly to form the central fibrous body.

Echocardiographically, the atrioventricular connexions are best profiled in the so-called four-chamber projection [2], using either the parasternal or subcostal echocardiographic windows (Figure 1b). On the parietal side distinct atrial and ventricular muscle masses can be identified, which are contiguous at the insertion of the mitral and tricuspid valve leaflets. It is also possible to distinguish pinched-in sulcus tissue from myocardium, this being more prominent on the right side and bounded on the outside of the heart by

Rijsterborgh H, ed: Echocardiology, p 345-353. All rights reserved.
Copyright © 1981 Martinus Nijhoff Publishers, The Hague/Boston/London.

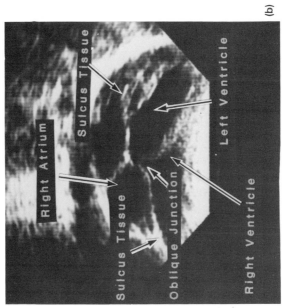

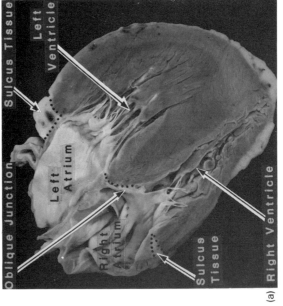

Figure 1

a distinct layer of pericardial echoes. Septally, the atrial septum is recorded as a thin band of tissue with the mitral leaflet originating from its base. An echo-dense area can be seen between the septal mitral attachment and the more apical tricuspid attachment. This echo-dense area separates left ventricle from right atrium. In the posterior aspect of the four-chamber view this is the muscular portion of the atrioventricular septum. Scanning anteriorly, but still in the four-chamber view, the atrioventricular septum is seen to expand, to be continuous with the central fibrous body. Echocardiographically it is usually possible to distinguish the thinner muscular from the thicker fibrous atrioventricular septum in a normal heart. Apically, the inlet muscular part of the ventricular septum is seen beyond the atrioventricular septum supporting the septal tricuspid leaflet.

From the standpoint of atrioventricular valve atresia, an atrioventricular connexion can be formed as described above but can be blocked by an imperforate membrane [1] (Figure 2a). This must be distinguished from the alternative situation in which one atrioventricular connexion is absent and where there is no continuity between atrial and ventricular myocardium [1] (Figure 2b). Here the atrioventricular sulcus tissue extends in to the area of the central fibrous body/atrioventricular septum, interposing between the pinched-in segments of the two myocardial masses (Figure 2b). Thus when an atrioventricular connexion is absent, the blind-ending atrium has no potential connexion with its corresponding ventricular chamber, (sulcus tissue interposing) but may have a potential connexion with the remaining ventricular chamber via the atrioventricular septum.

MATERIALS AND METHODS

Forty-six patients were studied who were known angiographically to have no direct communication between one of the atrial chambers and the ventricular mass. All patients had situs solitus. In 37 patients the morphologically right atrium was blind-ending, the left atrium being blind in the remaining nine. The patients had 2D echocardiograms recorded with either a Toshiba phased-array sector-scanner (2.4 MHz) or an ATL mechanical sector-scanner (5MHz).

Standard four-chamber views were scanned and recorded in each patient from the parasternal, apical and subcostal echocardiographic windows. Other views were recorded, but for the purposes of the investigation all the required information was provided by the four-chamber approach. Clearly other planes are necessary for elucidation of ventriculoarterial connexions and associated malformations. Following the echocardiographic examination, autopsy specimens of comparable malformations were sectioned to simulate the echocardiographic planes.

348

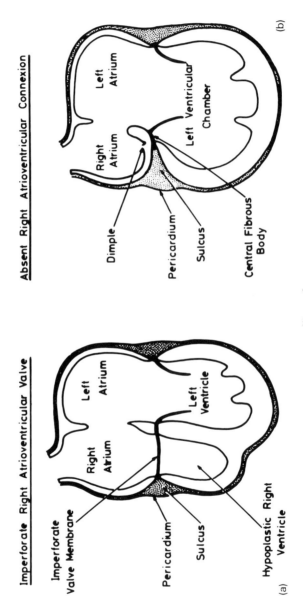

Figure 2

a) Right atrioventricular valve atresia (37 patients).

Thirtythree patients (89%) were found to have absence of the right atrioventricular connexion; in all cases the left atrium connecting to a morphologically left ventricular chamber. A broad band of thick, immobile echoes was found extending from the pericardial echoes to the area of the atrioventricular septum/central fibrous body. In 13 patients (35%) this broad band, shown by sectioning to be the atrioventricular sulcus tissue, separated the right atrium from the rudimentary right ventricular chamber (Figure 3a and b). In the remaining 20 patients (65%) the right atrial chamber bore no spatial relationship to the rudimentary right ventricular chamber. By sectioning of autopsy specimens it can always be shown that the right atrium is separated from the left ventricular chamber by the atrioventricular membranous septum, which is the classical "dimple" [3]. From the standpoint of echocardiography, it is not possible to identify this "dimple" as a distinct entity. This is because the atrial septum primum is deficient in a significant number of patients, making it difficult to distinguish the components of the central fibrous body, the atrioventricular septum and their precise junction with the left atrioventricular valve. An area of dense echoes can usually be seen in this position where the sulcus tissue joins the central fibrous body at the same level as the left atrioventricular valve. This broad band of echoes also obscures the presice insertion of the atrial and ventricular myocardial masses into the central fibrous body.

In four patients a totally different pattern was recorded. A thin, mobile, diaphragm-like structure was identified between the right atrial and right ventricular chambers. A normal parietal atrioventricular myocardial contiguity was recorded, with the usual pinched area containing sulcus tissue overlain by pericardial echoes. The diaphragm extended from this area to insert into the central fibrous body/atrioventricular septal region. It bulged into the ventricular cavity with atrial systole and in the opposite direction with ventricular systole. In all cases it was seen best from the subcostal echocardiographic window.

b) Left atrioventricular valve atresia (nine patients). Three patients (33%) were studied with absence of the left atrioventricular connexion; in all three the right atrium was connected via a right atrioventricular valve to a right ventricular chamber. On the left side, a broad band of echoes separated the blind-ending left atrium from an underlying rudimentary left ventricular chamber, the broad band extending from the pericardium to the region of the central fibrous body/atrioventricular septum. Sectioning again showed this band to be atrioventricular sulcus tissue. In the remaining six patients, an imperforate left atrioventricular membrane was found between the left atrium and a hypoplastic left ventricle (Figure 4a). This membrane showed

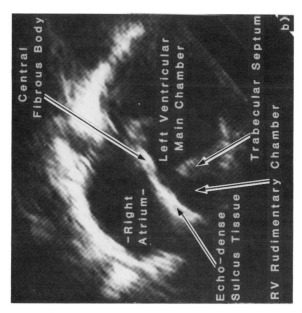

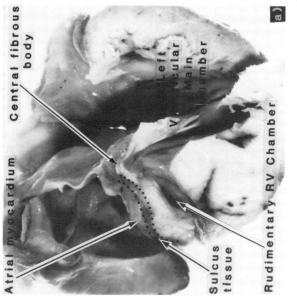

Figure 3

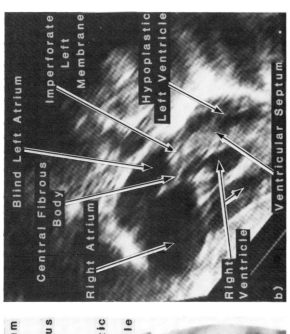

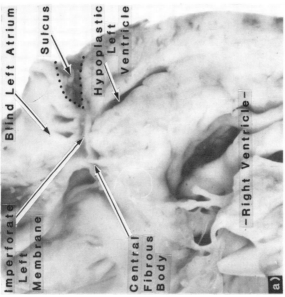

Figure 4

identical motion to the comparable membranes found with right atrioventricular valve atresia. Sectioning of comparable autopsy material illustrated the presence of an imperforate atrioventricular connexion (Figure 4b).

Our study has confirmed that "valve atresia" can be produced by either an imperforate membrane or an absent atrioventricular connexion, and more importantly has shown that the distinction can be made with total confidence using high resolution two-dimensional echocardiography. In the setting of right atrioventricular valve atresia, the majority of cases encountered in our series had absence of the right atrioventricular connexion. Echocardiographically this was not initially easy to perceive, as the floor of the right atrium overlaid the cavity of the rudimentary right ventricle in 35% of these cases, suggesting that right atrial to right ventricular communication might be potentially possible. It was only after careful anatomical study that we appreciated the fact that sulcus tissue was interposed between the atrial and ventricular myocardial masses, there being no direct atrioventricular connexion. The distinction between absent connexion and imperforate membrane in our cases was academic since, even in the cases of "tricuspid atresia" with imperforate membrane, the diaphragm and the right ventricle were hypoplastic, precluding surgical "correction". However, cases of imperforate membrane associated with a right ventricular cavity of normal size do exist [4] and in this situation precise diagnosis could lead to corrective surgical treatment. In the setting of "mitral atresia", the distinction between absent connexion and imperforate membrane is rarely of practical significance, since the left ventricle, or the rudimentary left ventricular chamber, is nearly always grossly hypoplastic.

Although echocardiographic characterisation of the types of valve atresia is of limited therapeutic significance, the distinction improves our understanding of the nature of the malformation. When one connexion is absent, only one ventricular chamber has an atrial connexion. Such hearts are, in this respect, comparable to those with double inlet ventricles, and for this reason we group these anomalies together as univentricular hearts. In contrast, those with imperforate valve membranes have both ventricular chambers connected to separate atrial chambers, and should be considered to be biventricular hearts. thus, from the standpoint of classification, atrioventricular valve atresias can conveniently and simply be divided into the biventricular and univentricular varieties, with each type consistently identified by 2D echocardiography.

REFERENCES

1. Shinebourne EA MJ Tynan, RH Anderson, FJ Macartney: Atrioventricular connections. In: Paediatric Cardiology (Anderson et al., eds.), p 27, 1977.
2. Tajik AJ, JB Seward, DJ Hagler, DD Mair, JT Lie: Two-dimensional real-time ultrasonic imaging of the heart and great vessels: Technique, image orientation, structure identification and validation. Mayo Clin Proc 53:271, 1978.
3. Anderson RH, JL Wilkinson, LM Gerlis, A Smith, AE Becker: Atresia of the right atrioventricular orifice. Br Heart J 39:414, 1977.
4. Bharati S, HA McAllister, CJ Tatooles, RA Miller, M Weinberg, HG Bucheleres, M Lev: Anatomic variations in underdeveloped right ventricle related to tricuspid atresia and stenosis. J Thorac Cardiovasc Surg 72:383, 1976.

39. THE DETECTION AND ASSESSMENT OF STRADDLING AND OVERRIDING ATRIOVENTRICULAR VALVES BY TWO-DIMENSIONAL ECHOCARDIOGRAPHY

J. F. SMALLHORN, G. TOMMASINI, and F.J. MACARTNEY

ABSTRACT

Sixteen patients with a straddling tricuspid and two with a straddling mitral valve were identified by two-dimensional echocardiography. In all but one the atrioventricular valves (AV) appeared at the same level indicating absence of the ventriculo-atrial septum.

Straddling was determined by identifying subvalvular apparatus from one AV valve in both chambers. Overriding was greater than 50% in 12, and less than 50% in 5, with one having no detectable overriding.

INTRODUCTION

A straddling AV valve is one whose tensor apparatus arises from both chambers in the ventricular mass [1]. These two chambers may either be two ventricles, or a main chamber and a rudimentary chamber. In many cases straddling is associated with overriding of the valve annulus. The diagnosis has important surgical implications and in the past angiocardiography and M-mode echocardiography have not provided a complete assessment of the straddling and associated overriding [2]. The aims were to determine the reliability of two-dimensional echocardiography in detecting straddling and overriding and in delineating the precise relationships of the tensor apparatus and annuli to the septum dividing the chambers in the ventricular mass.

METHODS

The cases were drawn from the routine work with patients at the Hospital for Sick Children, Great Ormond Street, London, over a nine month period. Ventricles, main chambers and rudimentary chambers are defined as suggested by Tynan and colleagues [3]. This study includes sixteen patients with a straddling right AV valve, associated with a biventricular heart in five and univentricular in eleven. Two further patients had a straddling left AV valve, one with a univentricular and the other a biventricular heart. In all but one,

Rijsterborgh H, ed: Echocardiology, p 355-361. All rights reserved.

straddling was associated with overriding. For purposes of comparison, a further group of seven patients with two perforate, non-straddling valves were studied. Five had a univentricular and two a biventricular heart with an inlet ventricular septal defect (VSD). The patients were studied using an Advanced Technology Laboratory mechanical sector-scanner with a 3.5 or 5 MHz transducer. The level of the AV valves and type of VSD were studied. To determine the degree of overriding, the relationship of the central fibrous body to the tip of the interventricular septum was assessed.

RESULTS

In the four-chamber view, two AV valves at the same level were identified in twenty-four cases whatever the ventricular morphology (Figure 1), with one

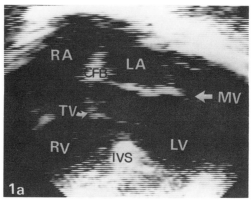

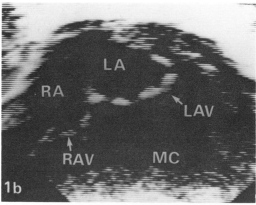

Figure 1. Apical four-chamber view showing AV valves at the same level, a) in a biventricular, b) in a univentricular heart.

Abbreviations: RA = right atrium, RV = right ventricle, LA = left atrium, LV = left ventricle, TV = tricuspid valve, MV = mitral valve, IVS = interventricular septum, CFB = central fibrous body, RAV = right atrioventricular valve, LAV = left atrioventricular valve, MC = main chamber.

further case with a straddling right atrioventricular valve having a ventriculo-atrial septum visualised (Figure 2). Fifteen cases had evidence of overriding involving the right AV annulus and two the left. In twelve the overriding was greater than 50% (Figure 3) and in six it was less than 50% (Figures 1 and 4). In one case no overriding was seen (Figure 2), and at surgery a VSD in the trabecular septum through which a tricuspid valve straddled was seen. In seventeen patients with univentricular hearts, the rudimentary chamber was posterior and to the left of the main chamber in one patient and anterior and to the right in fifteen. The remaining patient had no identifiable rudimentary chamber and therefore no straddling or overriding.

In all biventricular hearts the affected valve moved through the VSD (Figure 5). In the two cases without straddling, the valves were clearly shown to open into the appropriate chamber in one and, in the other, chordae were attached to the crest of the ventricular septum where a rudimentary chamber was present; identification of papillary muscles and chordae helped to confirm the presence of a straddling AV valve.

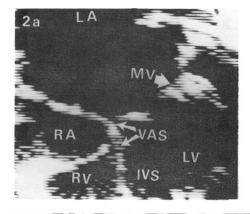

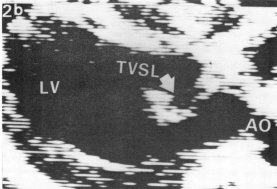

Figure 2. Subxiphoid long-axis views showing an intact ventriculo-atrial septum (VAS) and straddling tricuspid valve.

The same abbreviations as in Figure 1; TVSL = tricuspid valve septal leaflet.

358

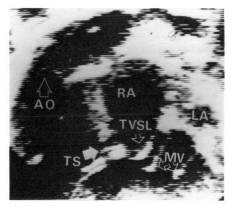

Figure 3. Subxiphoid view showing straddling tricuspid valve in a univentricular heart. An overriding greater than 50% is shown.
The same abbreviations as in Figure 1. TVSL = tricuspid valve septal leaflet, TS = trabecular septum.

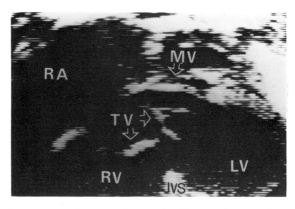

Figure 4. Apical view with transducer rotation to visualize mainly tricuspid annulus, straddling tricuspid valve is noted.
The same abbreviations as in Figure 1.

A four-chamber view in three patients with a straddling right AV valve gave the appearance of a common anterior leaflet as seen in complete atrioventricular defects (Figure 4). This represented the anterior leaflet of the right AV valve with tensor apparatus in both chambers.

The morphology of the straddling AV valve was correctly identified in all those cases with biventricular hearts. Surgical confirmation of a straddling AV valve was possible in two, with one further case having chordal attachments to the crest of the interventricular septum identified. Autopsy confirmation was possible in only one case with a straddling left AV valve and a biventricular heart. When the overriding was greater than 50%, a four-chamber view reliably detected its presence but when it was less than 50% other views were necessary. The most helpful was one in which only the

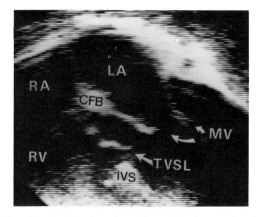

Figure 5. Apical four-chamber showing the tricuspid septal leaflet moving through the VSD in a biventricular heart.

The same abbreviations as in Figure 1. CFB = central fibrous body, TVSL = tricuspid valve septal leaflet.

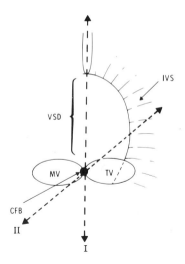

Figure 6. Diagram indicating view necessary to visualize the more posterior part of the interventricular septum. Plane I straight four-chamber. Plane II with transducer rotation.

The same abbreviations as in Figure 1. VSD = ventricular septal defect, CFB = central vibrous body.

tricuspid annulus and interventricular septum are visualized. In this position the most posterior part of the septum is visualized and hence the degree of overriding can be determined. This view is necessary since in a straddling right AV valve (tricuspid) the septum does not run to the crux of the heart (Figure 6).

DISCUSSION

Demonstration of a straddling valve in association with a univentricular heart is of little importance, but in biventricular hearts foreknowledge of the presence of straddling is of great importance to the surgeon. Simple closure of a ventricular septal defect can render the atrioventricular valve incompetent, hence necessitating replacement by another valve [4]. Furthermore, the presence of straddling also affects the disposition of the conduction tissue, most importantly in hearts with atrioventricular concordance. In contrast to all other hearts with this atrioventricular connexion, the atrioventricular node may be situated posterior to its anticipated site in the triangle of Koch [1]. The conduction tissue continues from this abnormal postero-lateral node onto the posterior rim of the ventricular septal defect.

In a straddling tricuspid valve, the ventricular septal defect is usually posterior and roofed by the two atrioventricular valves in continuity. In this situation one should expect to see them at the same level, as was the case with two-dimensional echocardiography. If they appear at different levels it indicates the presence of a ventriculo-atrial septum and hence the defect is most likely to exist in the trabecular septum with its total circumference bordered by muscle. In this case the atrioventricular node is normally situated.

In the rare case of straddling mitral valve, the defect is normally anterior so, unless the defect excavates posteriorly to a considerable degree, one might expect to find the valves at a different level.

The relationship of the central fibrous body to the tip of the interventricular septum was used to assess the degree of overriding. If it was greater than 50% then a straight four-chamber view was adequate, but when it was less than 50% a cut to view just the tricuspid annulus and interventricular septum was necessary (Figure 6). This view was necessarily due to the absence of a posterior interventricular septum in a straddling right (tricuspid) atrioventricular valve.

Normally during diastole the atrioventricular valve leaflets oppose the interventricular septum when the subvalvular apparatus is contained in the appropriate ventricle. If some of the tensor apparatus is inserted in the opposite chamber then the particular leaflet involved moves in that direction and the free edge of the leaflet flies through the septal defect.

To conclude, two-dimensional echocardiography can reliably detect the presence of straddling and determine the degree of annular overriding, which provides valuable information for the surgeon when deciding the feasibility of surgical intervention.

REFERENCES

1. Milo S, SY Ho, FJ Macartney et al.: Straddling and overriding atrioventricular valves: Morphology and classification. Am J Cardiol 44:1122, 1975.
2. La Corte MA, KE Fellows, RG Williams: Overriding tricuspid valve: echocardiographic and angiocardiographic features. Am J Cardiol 37:911, 1979.
3. Tynan M, AE Becker, FJ Macartney et al.: Nomenclature and classification of congenital heart disease. Br Heart J 41:544, 1979.
4. Tabry IF, DC McGoon, GK Danielson et al.: Surgical management of straddling atrioventricular valve. J Thorac Cardiovasc Surg 77:191, 1979.

40. TWO-DIMENSIONAL ECHOCARDIOGRAPHY FOR PRE- AND POST-SURGICAL EVALUATION OF ATRIOVENTRICULAR CANAL MALFORMATIONS

A. MAGHERINI and G. AZZOLINA

In our experience, traditional M-mode echocardiography has proven of limited usefulness in the diagnosis of atrioventricular canal (AVC) malformations, as it cannot provide specific information about the anatomical details typical of these disorders. Differential diagnosis between partial and complete forms, or the definition of the anatomical types of complete AVC, is not possible with this technique.

This paper refers to our experience in the diagnosis of AVC, using a phased-array sector-scanner on a group of patients in which the diagnosis was confirmed at surgery.

1. MATERIAL AND METHODS

Twenty-four patients were studied using a phased-array sector-scanner (Varian V3000). The echocardiographic investigation was routinely carried out using three approaches: parasternal (long-axis and short-axis views) and apical/subcostal (four-chamber view). In 14, the echocardiographic images were compared with the actual anatomy at surgery (all patients routinely underwent cardiac catheterization and angiocardiography). Twelve patients showed partial and twelve complete AVC malformations.

2. RESULTS

In normal subjects the four-chamber view (by the apical/subcostal approach) allows visualization of both the atrial and ventricular cavities, separated respectively by the atrial and ventricular septa and by the atrioventricular (AV) valves. Although the lowermost portion of the atrial septum (septum primum) is clearly visualized, this technique usually cannot demonstrate the uppermost portion (septum secundum).

Rijsterborgh H, ed: Echocardiology, p 363-370. All rights reserved.
Copyright © 1981 Martinus Nijhoff Publishers, The Hague/Boston/London.

364

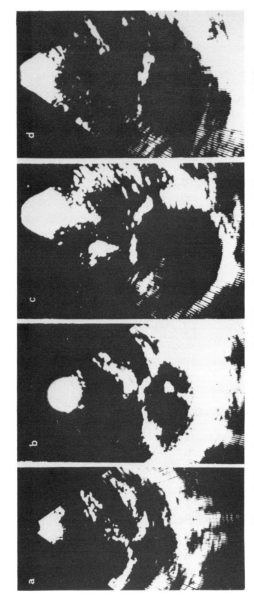

Figure 1. Four-chamber view. a: partial AVC malformations. b, c, d: Types of complete AVC malformations.

2.1. Partial atrioventricular canal malformations

2.1.1. Four-chamber view

In all patients with AVC malformations this technique demonstrated the absence of the septum primum well. The septum secundum, which cannot usually be visualized in normal patients, could be demonstrated in these patients, with its free margin somewhat thickened (later confirmed at surgery). Thus the location and extent of the ostium primum can be approximately determined. A photographic image taken in the late systolic phase gives a morphological definition of the insertion of the medial portion of the anterior mitral cusp. When no "typical" interventricular septal defect (VSD) exists, this structure appears to be directly inserted into the interventricular septum. This image can be found in a partial AVC (Figure 1a), but also in the case of simple "ostium primum" atrial septal defect (ASD).

A differential diagnosis can be achieved by means of the long-axis and short-axis views, demonstrating the morphology of the left ventricular outflow tract and the presence of a cleft of the anterior mitral cusp respectively.

2.1.2. Short-axis view

At the level of the atrioventricular valves it is possible to study the relative positions of the anterior cusp of the mitral valve and the tricuspid leaflet. The mitral valve axis appears more oblique than normal, due to the septal insertion. The opening movement of the valve is in the median-lateral rather than in the postero-anterior direction. Moreover, by this approach the mitral cleft can be demonstrated, a finding of specific diagnostic value. The anterior mitral cusp appears to be split into two half cusps, which tend to move away from each other in diastole. However, in seven of our patients we found a lack of continuity in the echoes arising from the anterior mitral leaflet but the diastolic separation movement could not be visualized (Figure 2b, c). On surgical inspection these patients' valves showed only a minor split with no loss of substance.

2.1.3. Long-axis view

By this approach anomalies of the left ventricular outflow tract can be studied. Multiple echoes originate from the anterior mitral cusp. The diastolic opening movement is of reduced amplitude, directed toward the interventricular septum, so that the anterior mitral cusp almost touches the left endocardium in diastole (Figure 2a).

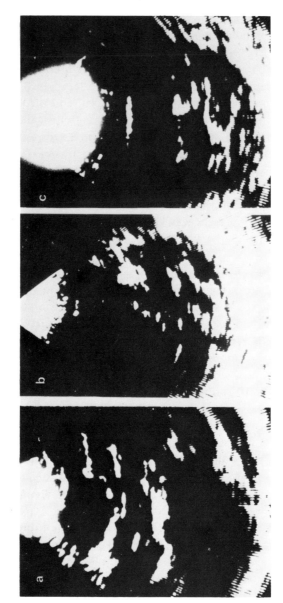

Figure 2. a: Long-axis view; anomalies of the left ventricular outflow tract. b, c: Short-axis view: mitral cleft.

2.2. Complete atrioventricular canal malformations

Among AVC malformations, two-dimensional echocardiography has proven useful in the characterization of "typical" VSD's, even when small. Using the four-chamber, late systolic view, a VSD appears as an echo-free area, closed during systole, between the AV valves and the interventricular septum. Obviously no diagnostic problems rise in identification of VSD's in advanced complete forms of AVC. However, differential diagnosis between partial AVC malformations and complete forms with small VSD's can be difficult. In these cases, systolic closure movement of the AV valve must be detected as a further diagnostic feature. In the partial forms of AVC, the various portions of the AV valve are visible on different circular sections with the concavity facing anteriorly during systole. In complete forms, the valvular components lie on the same circular section with the concavity facing posteriorly. This different systolic closure movement in partial and complete AVC forms is due to different insertion of medial portion of the anterior mitral leaflet. Only in partial AVC is it directly inserted into the interventricular septum; existence of this situation demonstrates the characteristic presence of two separate valvular ostia and absence of a typical VSD. Using these diagnostic criteria, we were able to distinguish partial from complete forms, to demonstrate the presence of "typical" VSD and to evaluate its dimensions in all patients observed (Figure 1a, b, c).

Once the diagnosis of complete AVC malformations is made, it is necessary to obtain further information in order to define the anatomical type. In our experience, two-dimensional echocardiography can define the split level of the anterior leaflet of the common AV valve. We use the term "divided at the level of the interventricular septum" when in early diastole the anterior leaflet of the common AV valve splits into a left and a right component, each moving toward their respective ventricles. This feature is due to the presence of the commissure aligned with the plane of the interventricular septum. We use the term "undivided at the level of the interventricular septum" when the commissure is displaced to the right: that is, the left anterior portion of the common valve is not divided at the point where it crosses the plane of the interventricular septum. This intact portion of the anterior leaflet appears, during the cardiac cycle as a single linear echo, which moves freely above the margin of interventricular septum (Figure 1d). Two-dimensional echocardiography has not always been able to define the insertion of medial portion of the anterior valvular leaflet. Important surgical information can also be obtained on interatrial and interventricular septal anatomy and their development. We express the degree of development of the atrial septum by the following ratio:

"The distance from the posterior atrial wall to the free margin of the septum secundum" divided by "the distance from the posterior atrial wall to

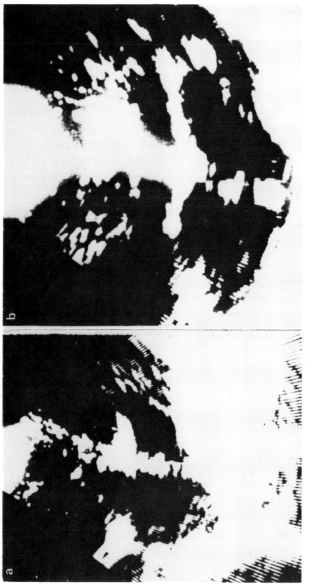

Figure 3. Postoperative remarks.

the plane of the AV valve (closed, in systole)". The degree of development of the interventricular septum may also be expressed by a ratio:

"The distance from the cardiac apex to the free margin of the ventricular septum" divided by "the distance from the cardiac apex to the plane of the AV valve (closed, in systole)." The data were in accord with the surgical findings.

In complete forms, especially, the size of the VSD must be determined during preoperative evaluation in order to define a specific operative program. When the VSD is small, it is not necessary to use a septal patch for its closure and the medial portion of the anterior leaflet of the common AV valve can be directly sutured onto the interventricular septum, without resulting in any important reduction in the ventricular capacity. When the VSD is large, it is important to determine, preoperatively, the distance between the apex and the plane of the AV valve (closed, in systole). In these cases the surgeon has to know at what level the medial portion of the AV valve must be sutured on the prosthetic patches. Too low a suturing level would induce a disproportion in the ventricular chamber capacity, while too high a one would result in shortening of the chordae tendineae, with consequent valvular insufficiency.

It is possible to obtain the information previously described for partial forms by using the precordial approaches (short-axis and long-axis views).

3. POSTOPERATIVE REMARKS

In the postoperative controls using the short-axis view, the disappearance of the discontinuity and of the diastolic movement of separation in the anterior leaflet of the mitral valve, which now appears as a single, thickened linear echo, may be remarked. In the four-chamber view, patches on the septal defects are visualized and characterized by a high-density, linear echo. The anterior mitral leaflet appears thickened (an indirect image of the sutured cleft). In complete AVC malformations, the medial portion of the anterior mitral leaflet appears sutured directly to the free margin of the interventricular septum or into the patch used to close the septal defects (Figure 3).

4. CONCLUSIONS

From the foregoing discussion on the evaluation of AVC malformations by two-dimensional echocardiography, the following conclusions were reached:
  – The diagnosis of AVC is based on the echocardiographic demonstration of the characteristic anatomical malformations: the ostium primum, the

370

cleft anterior mitral leaflet and the anomalies of the left ventricular outflow tract.
- In all cases, in our experience, two-dimensional investigation provided diagnosis of AVC malformations; it was also possible to differentiate the partial from the complete forms.
- In the complete forms, the level of splitting of the anterior leaflet of the common AV valve, together with the development of the atrial and ventricular septa, can be demonstrated. Both these anatomical findings are particularly important with regard to preoperative typing.
- In postoperative controls, it is possible to demonstrate the prosthetic atrial and ventricular septa, the thickening of the anterior mitral leaflet in relation to the sutured cleft and the division of the common AV valve into two separate valvular apparatus.

Two-dimensional echocardiography has greatly improved the performance of ultrasound for patients with AVC malformations [1, 2, 3] by the high sensitivity and specificity of its information.

REFERENCES

1. Hagler DJ, AJ Tajik, JB Seward, DD Mair, DG Ritter: Real-time wide-angle sector echocardiography: atrioventricular canal defects. Circulation 59:1944, 1979.
2. Magherini A, G Azzolina, V Wiechmann, F Fantini: Pulsed-Doppler echocardiography for diagnosis of ventricular septal defects. Br Heart J 43:143, 1980.
3. Magherini A, G Azzolina: L'ecocardiografia bidimensionale nella valutazione pre- e post-chirurgica dei difetti del canale atrioventricolare. G Ital Cardiol 10:984, 1980.

II. PEDIATRIC ECHOCARDIOLOGY

B. APPLICATIONS OF CONTRAST ECHOCARDIOLOGY
   AND DOPPLER ECHOCARDIOLOGY

41. CONTRAST M-MODE ECHOCARDIOGRAPHY, THE SUPRASTERNAL NOTCH APPROACH

STEWART HUNTER and GEORGE R. SUTHERLAND

1. INTRODUCTION

The combination of contrast echocardiography and the suprasternal approach offers a very reliable method for the evaluation of right to left shunts and ventriculoarterial connections in infants and children with complex congenital heart disease to the clinician who does not have real-time two-dimensional echocardiography.

In our institution, contrast echocardiography was initially used at cardiac catheterisation to establish the origin of unidentified M-Mode echoes [1, 2]. Subsequently, we concentrated on peripheral vein contrast echocardiography with the suprasternal approach before catheterisation in infants and children with complex congenital heart disease. The combination of the two techniques has been invaluable in the assessment of the level of right to left shunts and of the ventriculoarterial connections in complex congenital heart disease.

1.1. Echocardiographic and anatomic considerations

Normally in the M-Mode echocardiogram cardiac structures are identified by characteristic patterns of movement associated with the varying phases of the cardiac cycle. The morphology of the individual cardiac structures has also to be inferred from their antero-posterior relationships, although there is some additional evidence from lateral relationships. It is thus assumed that anterior structures are part of the right heart and posterior structures part of the left. Of course, this is frequently very misleading in complex congenital lesions, because of changes in spacial orientation of the heart within the chest and in antero-posterior and lateral relationships of the cardiac structures. In particular, the semilunar valves in the neonate may be identical in appearance from the parasternal M-Mode approach.

The reliability of the underlying anatomical relationships of the aortic arch, right pulmonary artery and left atrium provides the suprasternal approach with an enormous advantage (Figure 1). The arch always lies closer to the transducer than the pulmonary artery, thus allowing the two individ-

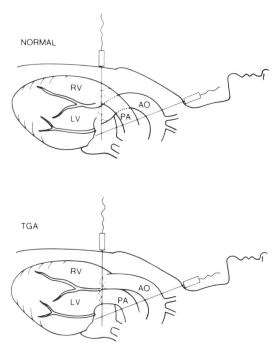

Figure 1. These diagrams illustrate the route of the ultrasonic beam from the parasternal and suprasternal approaches in the normal heart and in transposition of the great arteries. They demonstrate the constant relationship of aorta and pulmonary artery from the suprasternal approach.

AO = aorta; PA = pulmonary artery; LV = left ventricle; RV = right ventricle; TGA = transposition of the great arteries.

ual great arteries to be reliably differentiated. A bolus of ultrasonic indicator injected into the peripheral systemic venous system is observed suprasternally to provide the necessary diagnostic information.

2. METHODS

We usually place an intravenous cannula in the vein on the back of the hand or in the leg. It is preferable not to use a scalp vein as the injection tends to cause discomfort, making the child move and spoiling the echo. Babies are done shortly after feeding when they are quiet and settled, older children on the other hand may require sedation. The transducers used depend empirically on which gives the best definition.

The transducer is directed downwards through the suprasternal notch and slightly posteriorly to cut the underlying cardiac structures at right-angles to their walls. If parts of either semilunar valve are seen, then the beam is not angled through the appropriate part of the aortic arch and the right pulmonary artery. This is crucial, particularly in the diagnosis of ventriculoarterial discordance. 5% Dextrose is used as the contrast medium and is injected rapidly through a 1 ml syringe as a bolus. Quantities of gaseous microbubbles in the bolus reflect ultrasound intensely and the blood-filled cavities are opacified on the echocardiogram. In the normal heart, peripheral systemic venous injection is followed by opacification of the right ventricle and pulmonary artery in the parasternal and suprasternal views. The microbubbles are then filtered out in the lungs and none appear in the left heart. When a right to left shunt is present or an abnormality of ventriculoarterial connections, contrast also appears in the left heart. Several cardiac cycles are recorded before the injection so that the initial timing of opacification is clear. The recording is then continued until the contrast effect has disappeared. In the normal heart, contrast disappears within five to six cardiac cycles, but in the presence of right sided valvular regurgitation it may persist for as long as a minute. Such contrast injections are always made by hand and as a result there is a wide spread of intensity of opacification between individual injections and no attempt is made to compare the intensity and persistence of opacification in sequential injections. However, it is possible, as will be discussed later, to compare the relative opacification of two structures during the same injection.

3. RESULTS

3.1. Identification of the great arteries from the suprasternal approach

In the great majority of cases we have been able to identify the aortic arch and the right pulmonary artery. With increasing confidence in the technique, inability to record the right pulmonary artery strongly suggests that it is either abnormal in situation or absent. Although Allen et al. [3] have reported ranges of echo dimensions for the three structures in the suprasternal view in normal children, we confined ourselves to the relative size of the pulmonary artery and aorta. It is occasionally impossible to record the three cardiac structures in the presence of abnormalities of the aortic arch.

3.2. Detection of right to left atrial shunts

In our initial study we validated the detection of right to left atrial shunts by suprasternal contrast echocardiography in a large series of children who underwent cardiac catheterisation. We accepted only patients who at cardiac catheterisation had definite right to left shunts in the presence of full pulmonary venous saturation. In all of these contrast echocardiography

376

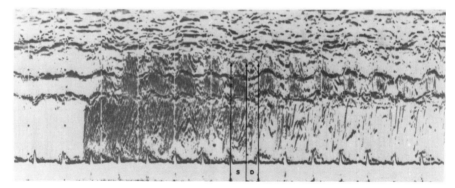

Figure 2. The aorta, pulmonary artery and left atrium are demonstrated in this suprasternal echocardiogram. Following peripheral venous injection of contrast the left atrium opacifies during diastole and subsequently both aorta and pulmonary artery opacify.
S = systole; D = diastole.

demonstrated opacification of the left atrium following peripheral venous injection, confirming a right to left atrial shunt.

Left atrial opacification was always associated with opacification of both great arteries (Figure 2). If a large amount of contrast appeared in the left atrium it was usually only possible to diagnose a right to left atrial shunt and not possible to infer the presence of an additional right to left ventricular shunt. However, on some occasions the great arteries opacified very intensely but the left atrium was barely opacified and in these we were able to demonstrate at catheterisation that the major right to left shunt was at the ventricular level and that there was a small atrial shunt.

3.3. Detection of right to left ventricular shunts

Again in the initial validatory study, the detection of right to left ventricular shunts was compared using catheterisation and contrast echocardiography. Again there was 100% correlation between the two methods. The left atrium remained unopacified while the great arteries opacified strongly (Figure 3).

3.4.. Assessment of ventriculoarterial connections

In the normal heart, or in the absence of right to left shunting, contrast from the peripheral circulation will only appear in the right pulmonary artery in the suprasternal view. With the exception of the rare isolated ventricular inversion, it is possible for all clinical purposes to infer that the ventriculoarterial connections are normal (Figure 4). In the presence of a right to left shunt at atrial or ventricular level, it is still usually possible to determine that

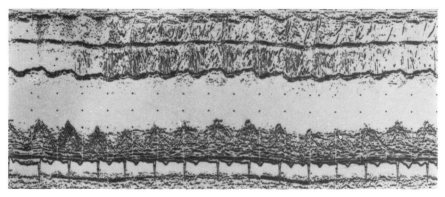

Figure 3. A suprasternal echocardiogram with following selective peripheral venous injection of contrast. The left atrium does not opacify, but both great arteries do with about equal intensity. Only a right to left ventricular shunt was noted at cardiac catheterisation.

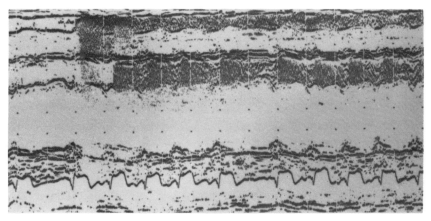

Figure 4. Selective peripheral venous injection in the left hand demonstrates the left innominate vein lying anterior to the aorta in the suprasternal view. Contrast appears first at this site and there is no constant relationship to ventricular systole, as judged on the ECG.

Later, the pulmonary artery, only, opacifies, establishing normal ventriculoarterial connections. At the start of opacification of the innominate vein, artefactual smearing of contrast occurs across the boundaries of the innominate vein and the aorta.

one great artery opacifies more persistently and more intensely, suggesting that it receives most of the systemic venous return (Figure 5). If this is the pulmonary artery, then, with the previously mentioned exception, it can be inferred that most of the systemic venous return goes to the pulmonary artery and hence ventriculoarterial connections are normal. In cases of ventriculoarterial discordance (Transposition of the Great Arteries), the pattern of opacification from the suprasternal approach is very different [6]. The aorta receives most of the systemic venous return and is thus opacified more intensely and persistently than the pulmonary artery. However, usually the left atrium and pulmonary artery will receive some opacification in view

378

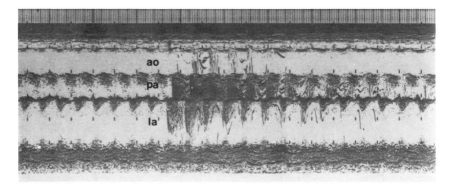

Figure 5. Selective peripheral venous injection into the right hand. The left atrium opacifies first in diastole and then the pulmonary artery and aorta also opacify. Both great arteries opacify most intensely in systole but the pulmonary artery receives most of the systemic venous return and opacifies most intensely and persistently.

of the obligatory intracardiac shunting which is required for the baby to survive.

Transposition differs from other cyanotic congenital heart disease in that the greater the right to left shunt at atrial or ventricular level, the higher the effective pulmonary blood flow will be and the higher the systemic arterial oxygen saturation. By comparing aortic percentage oxygen saturation in children with transposition to the relative opacification (at each injection) of

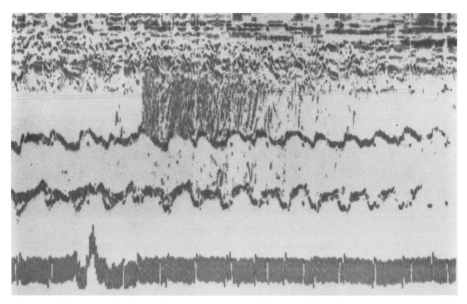

Figure 6. Suprasternal echocardiogram in a case of transposition of the great arteries with minimal interatrial shunting. Very little contrast appears in the pulmonary artery and most of the contrast is seen in the aorta.

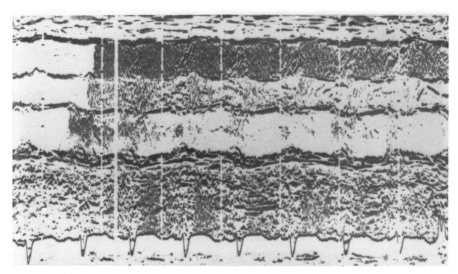

Figure 7. This suprasternal echocardiogram is from a patient with transposition of the great arteries. The left atrium opacifies followed by both great arteries. The aorta is more persistently and intensely opacified, suggesting that it receives most of the systemic venous return.

both great arteries, some comment can be made about the approximate effective pulmonary blood flow. When aortic saturation is less than 40%, the amount of contrast appearing in the left atrium on suprasternal echocardiogram is minimal and the aorta opacifies for more than twice as many cycles as the pulmonary artery (Figure 6). When the aortic saturation lies between 40% and 60%, the pulmonary artery opacifies more than half as many cycles as the aorta, although there is usually still sufficient differential opacification to make the diagnosis of ventriculoarterial discordance (Figure 7). When aortic saturation is greater than 60%, both great arteries opacify equally intensely and for the same number of cardiac cycles and accurate assessment of ventriculoarterial connections becomes impossible (Figure 8). Under these

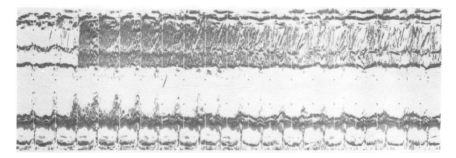

Figure 8. In this suprasternal echocardiogram both great arteries opacify with equal intensity and persistence, and it is not possible to assess accurately the ventriculoarterial connections. This patient had a very small right to left shunt which was not picked up on this echocardiogram. The major shunting occurred at ventricular level.

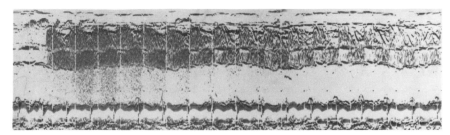

Figure 9. In this suprasternal echocardiogram the aorta and the pulmonary artery opacify in systole with similar intensity and little contrast reaches the left atrium. These findings suggest a right to left ventricular shunt which was present. In the later cardiac cycles the aorta opacifies more intensely in systole and the pulmonary artery in diastole. Indicating the presence of co-existing transposition of the great arteries and persistent ductus arteriosus.

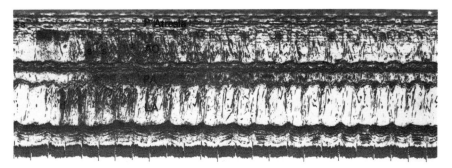

Figure 10. A suprasternal echocardiogram in a case of pulmonary atresia following systemic injection of contrast. The large aorta opacifies first, followed by left atrial opacification and finally by opacification of the pulmonary artery. The aorta is most intensely opacified in systole while the pulmonary artery initially shows a flat non-cyclical opacification, indicating that it is not connected to the heart directly by a semilunar valve but receives its blood supply from the aorta.

P. Atresia = pulmonary atresia; AO = aorta; PA = pulmonary artery; LA = left atrium.

circumstances, at cardiac catheterisation there is usually less than 10% difference between aorta and pulmonary artery oxygen saturation.

In children with Transposition of the Great Arteries and persistent ductus arteriosus, a unique type of cyclical opacification of the pulmonary artery is seen. The aorta is cyclically opacified with each systole, but the pulmonary artery, even in the presence of a co-existing ventricular septal defect, shows mainly diastolic opacification (Figure 9). This suggests that most of the contrast reaches the pulmonary artery through an aortopulmonary communication in diastole and that blood with less contrast reaches the pulmonary artery in systole through the pulmonary valve, causing momentary clearing. This curious phenomenon disappears when the ductus is closed surgically or spontaneously.

In pulmonary valve atresia with ventricular septal defect and persistent ductus arteriosus, the aorta opacifies cyclically in systole. The pulmonary artery opacifies initially in diastole and later than the aorta. Thereafter, there is a flat, non-cyclical opacification of the pulmonary artery, suggesting that it is receiving none of its blood from the heart directly but rather through the persistent ductus arteriosus (Figure 10).

3.5. Visualisation of systemic veins

When contrast is injected into the left hand or arm, it is frequently possible to see an opacified space anterior to the aorta (Figure 4). This opacifies very early and without any cyclical change and almost certainly represents the left innominate vein. Again with increasing experience, the absence of this opacification following left hand or arm injection strongly suggests absence of the left innominate vein. Occasionally it is possible to diagnose a left superior vena cava draining to the coronary sinus, by suprasternal contrast echocardiography. In these circumstances, the left innominate vein does not opacify after a left hand injection, but the coronary sinus opacifies behind the left atrium.

4. CONCLUSION

Most infants admitted as emergencies to paediatric cardiological units undergo an extensive work-up, including clinical examination, chest X-ray blood/gas analysis and electrocardiography. It is now common practice to include in this pre-catheterisation diagnostic cascade M-Mode echocardiography. The use of the suprasternal technique and contrast echocardiography gives a great deal of diagnostic information, which is not only qualitative but can sometimes be semi-quantitative. The undoubted advantages of real-time two-dimensional echocardiography over M-Mode in such children is not available to all units because of cost. M-Mode contrast echocardiography from the suprasternal approach in our experience greatly enhances the diagnostic possibilities of the single probe technique.

REFERENCES

1. Goldberg BB: Ultrasonic measurement of aortic arch, right pulmonary artery and left atrium. Radiology 101:383, 1971.
2. Mortera C, M Tynan, A Goodwin, S Hunter: Infradiaphragmatic total anomalous pulmonary venous connection to the portal vein. Diagnostic implications of echocardiography. Brit Heart J 39:685, 1977.
3. Allen HD, SJ Goldberg, DJ Sahn, TW Ovitt, BB Goldberg: Suprasternal notch echocardiography. Assessment of its clinical utility in paediatric cardiology. Circulation 55:605, 1977.
4. Mortera C, S Hunter, M Tynan: Contrast echocardiography and the suprasternal approach in infants and children. European J of Cardiology 9/6:437–454, 1979. Elsevier/North-Holland Biomedical Press.

42. EVALUATION OF RIGHT-TO-LEFT INTRACARDIAC SHUNTING IN NEWBORNS BY CONTRAST ECHOCARDIOGRAPHY

E. J. Meijboom, M. H. Gewitz, D. C. Wood, and W. W. Fox

1. INTRODUCTION

Echocardiography has an established role in the evaluation of the cyanotic newborn. Its value for the recognition of an abnormal intracardiac anatomy is well published and widely accepted.

Contrast echocardiography has less often been used to document and localize the exact level of right-to-left shunting. It can add substantially to the information about anatomic malformations already recognized by standard echocardiography, but it has unique features in cyanotic patients with normal intracardiac relations [9, 11, 12], for instance patients with persistent fetal circulation syndrome [1, 2, 3, 4, 5, 6, 7, 8]. This syndrome remains a complicated perinatal management problem and is associated with a high incidence of mortality, due to intractable hypoxemia. The right-to-left shunting in these patients is based on severely elevated pressures in the pulmonary artery system. An early diagnosis and initiation of therapy in these patients is important. The purpose of this paper is to describe our experience with contrast echocardiography as a tool for both, evaluation and management of such patients.

2. MATERIALS AND METHODS

The twenty-two newborns studied by contrast echocardiography were divided into two groups.

The control group of eleven newborns *without* persistent fetal circulation comprised four patients with congenital heart disease (three d-Transpositions of the Great Arteries (d-TGA) and one cor triatriatum), three with mild meconium aspiration, three with transient cyanotic episodes without underlying cardiopulmonary disease and one with mild respiratory distress syndrome. Four of these patients required ventilatory assistance and five needed only supplemental oxygen. The three infants with d-TGA had contrast echocardiography performed before and after cardiac catheterization and balloon atrioseptostomy.

The eleven patients *with* persistent fetal circulation, all of whom required extensive ventilatory support [1, 3, 7], ten of them at a very early stage. Five of the ten succumbed, four as a result of hypoxemia and one from a late complication (necrotizing enterocolitis).

Contrast studies were carried out according to previously described methods [9, 11, 12, 13]. The transducer (5.0 MHz) was positioned to view the right ventricular outflow tract, the aortic root at valvular level and the left atrium, from a standard M-mode transducer position, with the recorder set at a paper speed of either 100 mm per second or 50 mm per second [14]. A bolus of 5% dextrose/water was administered via an indwelling venous line in either the umbilical vein or a peripheral vein of a lower extremity. Approximately $\frac{1}{4}$–$\frac{1}{2}$ cc/kg of fluid was rapidly injected, the total never exceeding 2 cc. Each study was recorded at least twice and, for recording, the reject control was set to eliminate the overload phenomenon described by others [9]. If contrast was visualized in both the right ventricular outflow tract and the left atrium (and subsequently in the aortic root), the presence of a right-to-left intracardiac shunt was confirmed. In these patients, the time interval (in milliseconds) between the appearance of contrast in the right ventricular ourflow tract and its first appearance in the left atrium was measured and was recorded as the LA-RV difference. LA-RV difference measurements greater then zero milliseconds indicate that contrast was noted first in the left atrium and subsequantly in the right ventricular outflow tract, consistent with a large right-to-left shunt at the atrial level (Figure 1).

LA-RV difference measurements less than zero milliseconds indicate that contrast was noted first in the right ventricular outflow tract and later in the left atrium and was considered to be consistent with a relatively smaller degree of righ-to-left shunting (Figure 2).

On three occasions, the M-mode studies were confirmed using two-dimensional echocardiography, enabling more specific determination of the level of intracardiac shunting.

For this study, M-mode echocardiograms were obtained with an Irex Continuetrace System II echocardiograph and the two-dimensional echocardiograms were performed using an ATL Mark V System.

3. RESULTS

Figure 3 shows an M-mode tracing of a control patient in which contrast is only seen in the right ventricular outflow tract while the left atrium and the aorta remain echo free. Figure 4 demonstrates a typical contrast echocardiogram as obtained from a patient with persistent fetal circulation, contrast fills the left atrium, followed by the aortic root and the right ventricular outflow tract, indicating a marked degree of right-to-left shunting.

LA-RV differences were measured as previously described. For example in

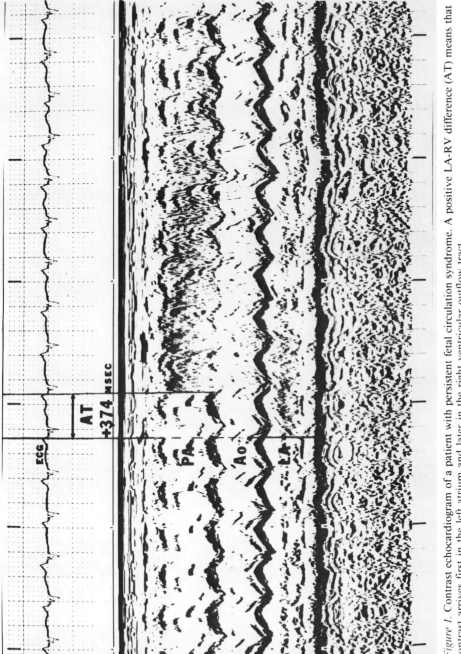

Figure 1. Contrast echocardiogram of a patient with persistent fetal circulation syndrome. A positive LA-RV difference (AT) means that contrast arrives first in the left atrium and later in the right ventricular outflow tract.

386

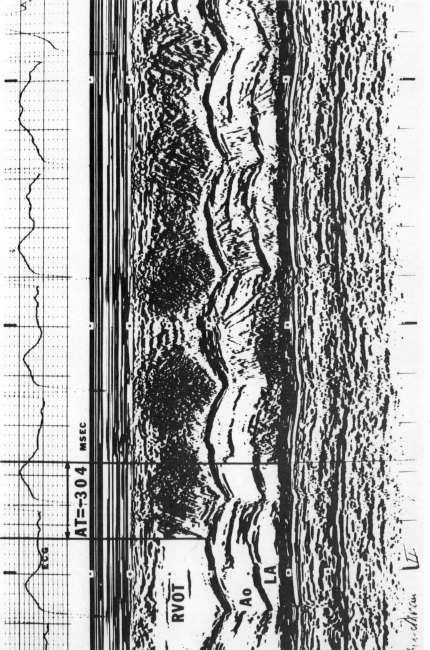

Figure 2. Contrast echocardiogram of a patient with persistent fetal circulation syndrome. A negative LA-RV difference (AT) means that contrast arrives first in the right ventricular outflow tract and later in the left atrium.

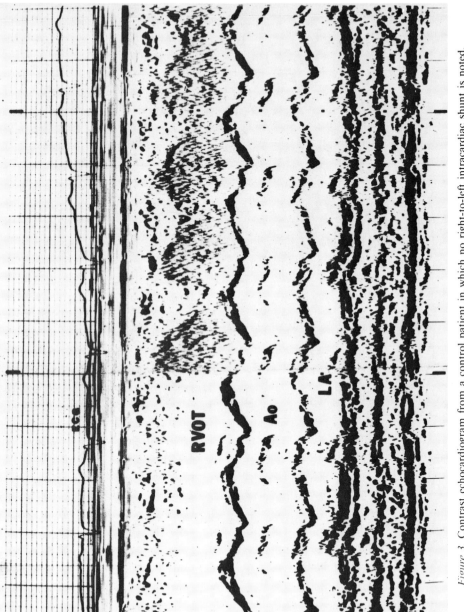

Figure 3. Contrast echocardiogram from a control patient in which no right-to-left intracardiac shunt is noted.

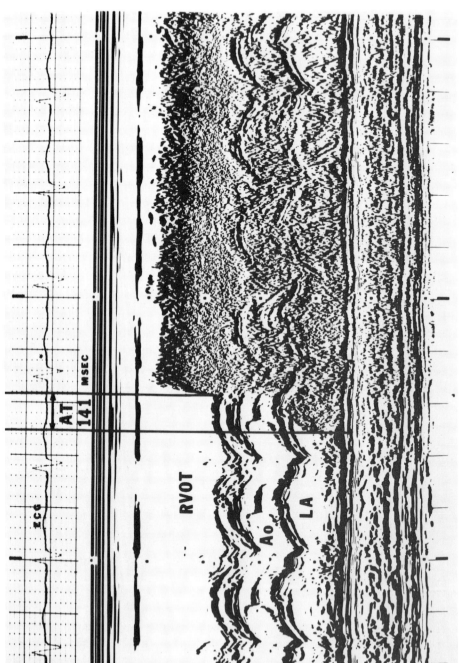

Figure 4. Initial contrast echocardiogram of a patient with persistent fetal circulation syndrome. Contrast is seen first in the left atrium and subsequently in the right ventricular outflow tract. LA-RV difference (AT) is calculated in milliseconds.

Figure 4, the time interval between the appearance of contrast in the left atrium and its first appearance in the right ventricular outflow tract is approximately 141 milliseconds.

In ten of the eleven control patients no right-to-left shunting was seen on the contrast echocardiogram, although contrast was clearly identified in the right ventricular outflow tract in all cases. In one control patient, later proven at cardiac catheterization to have cor triatriatum, contrast was apparent in the well defined inferior part of the left atrium. Thus this child did have right-to-left shunting at atrial level, but only in a part of the left atrial chamber below an atrial membrane, and this membrane had already been recognized as an anatomical abnormality.

In the three control patients with d-TGA, contrast echocardiography showed no right-to-left shunting before septostomy. After catheterization and balloon atrioseptostomy these contrast echocardiograms became positive, indicating that a satisfactory atrial communication had been established.

Ten of the eleven patients with persistent fetal circulation demonstrated right-to-left shunting on their initial contrast echocardiogram. In one patient no right-to-left shunting was present in the initial study, but was subsequently noted on the second contrast echocardiogram one day later. For the group, the LA-RV difference, on the inital contrast echocardiograms, varied from $+755$ milliseconds to -320 milliseconds, mean $= +300$ milliseconds. As indicated earlier, these values represented right-to-left shunting, with negative values being found in the smaller shunts.

Assessment of both highest (positive) and lowest (negative) LA-RV difference did not yield any specific correlation between either LA-RV difference and clinical indices of disease or LA-RV difference and prognosis.

As shown in Figure 5, the appearance times in eight of the eleven patients with persistent fetal circulation were followed serially over the first nine days of their illness. In the six surviving patients the pattern of LA-RV difference was seen to follow a consistently decreasing trend, which corresponded to an improving clinical picture. In one other infant a decresing LA-RV difference was recorded, which paralleled the patient's clinical course, but this infant ultimately succumbed to severe necrotizing enterocolitis despite improvement in the underlying persistent fetal circulation syndrome. Of the four infants who succumbed of intractable hypoxemia, three lived only long enough for one contrast echocardiogram and the fourth demonstrated an increasing LA-RV difference until he died.

Two-dimensional contrast echocardiography was performed in two patients with persistent fetal circulation and clearly localized the shunt to the atrial level while confirming the absence of other intracardiac abnormalities. A completely different picture was seen in the two-dimensional contrast study of the child with a cor triatriatum, where the membrane and the

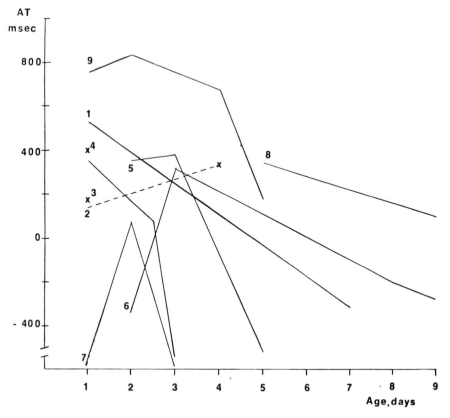

Figure 5. Serial changes in LA-RV difference over clinical course in patients with persistent fetal circulation.

AT = LA-RV difference, msec = milliseconds, x = expired.

contrast flow, which was confined to the lower left atrium, provided clear differentiation from the other patients.

4. DISCUSSION

These data demonstrate the usefulness of contrast echocardiography in establishing the diagnosis of intracardiac right-to-left shunting in newborns suspected of having persistent fetal circulation. In addition, serial evaluation of these patients with contrast echocardiography appears to verify objectively the changing magnitude of the intracardiac right-to-left shunt as the clinical course proceeds.

These results are consistent with previous publications which have demonstrated the ability of contrast echocardiography to evaluate intracardiac right-to-left shunting [9, 11, 12, 13]. Other noninvasive methods of estimating pulmonary artery pressure and pulmonary vascular resistance, such as the use of echocardiographic right ventricular systolic time intervals, have been proposed [15], but recent data have raised questions about the reliability of such techniques [16]. All but one of the persistent fetal circulation patients in this series showed right-to-left shunting on the first contrast echocardiography. In the patient whose contrast echocardiogram showed no intracardiac right-to-left shunting, a repeat study the following day did demonstrate a shunt. This patient followed a clinical course typical of some patients with persistent fetal circulation in whom pulmonary pressures may not be at their highest early in the disease but then gradually increase further over the first few days of life [1]. Thus, in such patients contrast echocardiography can be helpful for following the development of an intracardiac shunt.

The absence of right-to-left shunting on precatheterization contrast echocardiography in the three control patients with d-TGA is consistent with the severe clinical picture associated with negligible bidirectional flow at the atrial level. After successful balloon atrioseptostomy, mixing at the atrial level was demonstrated by contrast echocardiography.

Our findings underscore the point that if the diagnosis of persistent fetal circulation is suspected clinically, right-to-left shunting should be demonstrated on contrast echocardiography. If it is not seen, the diagnosis of persistent fetal circulation is suspect. Of course, right-to-left intracardiac shunting can occur in certain forms of congenital heart disease not necessarily associated with pulmonary hypertension, such as tricuspid or pulmonary atresia, Ebstein's anomaly or right ventricular dysfunction associated with myocardial ischemia. Similarly, the patient in our series with cor triatriatum exemplifies a situation in which congenital heart disease may be associated with pulmonary hypertension and intracardiac right-to-left shunting. In these instances, however, the total clinical picture, chest x-ray, electrocardiogram and standard echocardiogram usually point to a diagnosis other than persistent fetal circulation.

Finally, while the magnitude of the LA-RV difference was not correlated with any specific clinical factor such as blood gas data or ventilatory pressures, changes in the LA-RV difference in both degree and direction may be helpful for evaluation of therapy. Management of these patients often requires hyperventilation [1] which can be associated with serious complications, including pneumothorax and pneumopericardium. Since pCO_2 is often kept at low levels, and pO_2 may be variable, depending on several factors including parenchymal lung problems, measures of LA-RV difference offer a noninvasive means of evaluating changes in the intracardiac shunting pattern. Although in these patients we did not use LA-RV difference for clinical management, our data suggest that a decreasing LA-RV difference would permit the clinician to reduce hyperventilation at a time when other measurements may not clearly suggest improvement. It should be noted, however, that the specific numerical value for LA-RV difference may be related to the timing of injection of contrast, as well as to the level of pulmonary arterial pressure. Thus, contrast arriving in the right atrium in. diastole may produce a shorter LA-RV difference than that produced by contrast reaching the right atrium in systole.

SUMMARY

Contrast echocardiography has been shown to be helpful in clarifying the diagnosis and in following the intracardiac shunting patterns in a group of infants with the clinical picture of persistent fetal circulation. In certain instances, contrast echocardiography can provide enough corroborating evidence to obviate the need for cardiac catheterization in these critically ill newborns. Serial evaluation of these children using contrast echocardiograms may be helpful in following their clinical course and in adjusting therapy.

REFERENCES

1. Peckham GJ, WW Fox: Physiologic factors affecting pulmonary artery pressure in infants with persistent pulmonary hypertension. J Pediatr 93:1005, 1978.
2. Gersony WM: Persistence of fetal circulation, a commentary. J Pediatr 82:1103, 1973.
3. Fox WW, MH Gerwitz, R Dinwiddie, WH Drummond, GJ Peckman: Pulmonary hypertension in the perinatal aspiration syndromes. Pediatrics 59:205, 1977.
4. Haworth SG, L Reid: Persistent fetal circulation; newly recognized structural features. J Pediatr 88:614, 1976.
5. Burnell BH, MC Joseph, MH Lees: Progressive pulmonary hypertension in newborn infants. Amer J Dis Child 123:167, 1972.
6. Siassi B, SJ Goldberg, GC Emmanouilides, SM Higashino, L Elmore: Persistent pulmonary vascular obstruction in newborn infants. J Pediatr 78:610, 1971.
7. Drummond WH, GJ Peckman, WW Fox: The clinical profile of the newborn with persistent pulmonary hypertension: observations in 19 affected neonates. Clin Peds 16:335, 1977.
8. Rowe RD: Abnormal pulmonary vasoconstriction in the newborn. Peds 59:318, 1976.
9. Roelandt J, RS Meltzer, PW Serruys, J McGhie, W Gorissen, WB Vletter: Contrast Echocardiografie (preliminary information).
10. Levin DL, MA Heymann, JA Kitterman, GA Gregory, RH Phibbs, AM Rudolph: Persistent pulmonary hypertension of the newborn infant. J Pediatr 89:626, 1976.

11. Valdez-Cruz LM, DR Pieroni, A Roland, PJ Varghese: Echocardiographic detection of intracardiac right-to-left shunts following peripheral vein injections. Circulation 54:558, 1976.
12. Serwer GA, BE Armstrong, PAW Anderson, et al.: Use of contrast echocardiography for evaluation of right ventricular hemodynamics in the presence of ventricular septum defects. Circulation 58:327, 1978.
13. Serruys PW, M van den Brand, PG Hugenholtz, J Roelandt: Intracardiac right-to-left shunt demonstrated by two-dimensional echocardiography after peripheral vein injection. Br Heart J 42:429, 1979.
14. Meyer RA: Pediatric echocardiography. Lea and Febiger, Philadelphia, 1977.
15. Hirschfeld S, R Meyer, DC Schwartz, J Korfhagen, S Kaplan: Echocardiographic assessment of pulmonary artery pressure and pulmonary vascular resistance. Circulation 82:642, 1975.
16. Silverman MD, RA Snider, AM Rudolph: Evaluation of pulmonary hypertension by M-mode echocardiography in children with ventricular septal defect, Circulation 61:1125, 1980.

43. CONTRAST ECHOCARDIOGRAPHY IN UNIVENTRICULAR HEARTS

G. LUTFALLA, M. TOUSSAINT, FL. DE VERNEJOUL, and F. GUERIN

The term univentricular heart has been proposed by Anderson to define a form of congenital heart disease which includes only one ventricle. A normal ventricle is composed of three components; it can be divided into inlet, trabecular and outlet components. A chamber which does not possess both an inlet and trabecular component is termed a rudimentary chamber. There are two forms of rudimentary chamber. The first possesses a trabecular component and an outlet component; it is termed an outlet chamber. The second possesses a trabecular component alone and is termed a trabecular pouch.

Eight patients with univentricular hearts underwent contrast echocardiography: three primitive ventricles with double inlet, four primitive ventricles with absent right atrioventricular connexion and one primitive ventricle with overriding tricuspid valve. Their ages ranged from 3 to 40 years.

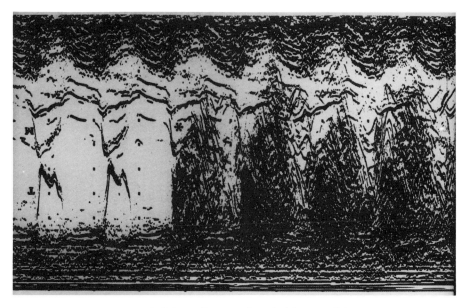

Figure 1. Echocardiogram of a primitive ventricle.

Rijsterborgh H, ed: Echocardiology, p 395-398. All rights reserved.
Copyright © 1981 Martinus Nijhoff Publishers, The Hague/Boston/London.

The patients underwent peripheral venous injections of contrast before cardiac catheterization as well as injection through a catheter positioned in the left atrium during catheterization. An injection of 20 mg of indocyanine green dye diluted in 2 ml of isotonic saline solution was used to produce the contrast effect. The results of our study are summarized below.

1. *Primitive ventricle* with normal atrioventricular connexion ("single ventricle") is defined as an univentricular heart with double inlet.

We studied two cases of primitive ventricle with outlet chamber and one case without an outlet chamber.

In echocardiography, the simultaneous recording of the echoes of two atrioventricular valves without an intervening septal echo is characteristic of a primitive ventricle; moreover, the recording of a small outlet chamber anterior to the atrioventricular valves and of a ventricular septal remnant echo suggests a primitive ventricle with an outlet chamber.

After a peripheral injection of indocyanine green dye, a "cloud of echoes" fills the ventricle. After an injection in the left atrium, the ventricle is also completely filled and the presence of echo-dense material posterior to the mitral valve proves that this valve is not atretic (Figure 1). In two-dimensional sector-scan echocardiography, the injection of indocyanine green dye results in a "cloud of echoes" that fills the ventricle from either the tricuspid valve or the mitral valve.

2. *Primitive ventricle with an outlet chamber and absent right atrioventricular connexion* ("tricuspid atresia") is defined as an univentricular heart.

We investigated four patients with this malformation.

The echocardiographic features are the absence of tricuspid valve echoes, in association with reduced outlet chamber size. After a peripheral injection, the echo-dense material appears first in the left atrium during the mid-systole, then in the aorta two ventricular systoles later; the "cloud of echoes" appearing posterior to the mitral valve proves that this valve is not atretic; we can also observe an area of negative contrast in the left atrium due to the pulmonary venous return (Figure 2).

3. *Primitive ventricle* with overriding of the tricuspid valve is defined as an univentricular heart if more than 50% of the tricuspid annulus is positioned above the left ventricle and overrides the ventricular septum.

In echocardiography, the apparent movement of the tricuspid valve crossing the plane of the septum in diastole, appearing to override it, strongly suggests the diagnosis. This echocardiographic feature is best viewed on a complete base to apex scan, which can be done during the peripheral venous injection of echo-dense material (Figure 3). After the injection, the cloud of echoes fills the left ventricle and the rudimentary chamber.

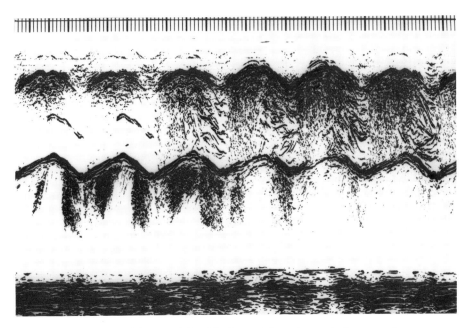

Figure 2. Primitive ventricle with absent right atrioventricular connexion.

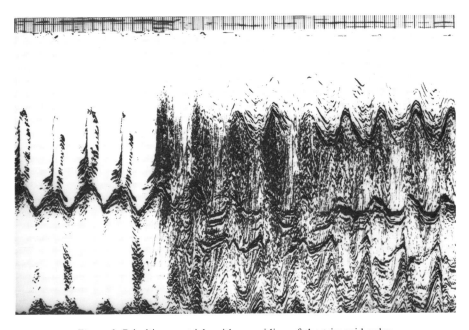

Figure 3. Primitive ventricle with overriding of the tricuspid valve.

The data demonstrate that contrast echocardiography is of great diagnostic value in the identification of patients with univentricular heart.

REFERENCES

1. Anderson RH, EA Shinebourne: Pediatric Cardiology, Churchill Livingstone, Edinburgh, 1978.
2. Seward JB, AJ Tajik, DJ Hagler et al.: Echocardiogram in common (single) ventricle: angiographic-anatomic correlations. Am J Cardiol 39:217, 1977.
3. Seward JB, AJ Tajik, DG Ritter: Echocardiographic features of straddling tricuspid valve. Mayo Clin Proc 50:427, 1975.

44. A TWENTY-MONTH EXPERIENCE COMPARING CONVENTIONAL PULSED-DOPPLER ECHOCARDIOGRAPHY AND COLOR-CODED DIGITAL MULTIGATE DOPPLER, FOR DETECTION OF ATRIOVENTRICULAR VALVE REGURGITATION, AND ITS SEVERITY

J. Geoffrey Stevenson, Isamu Kawabori, and
Marco A. Brandestini

INTRODUCTION

Conventional pulsed-Doppler echocardiographic (PDE) detection of mitral regurgitation has been shown in several series to have a sensitivity and specificity of about 90%, when compared with angiocardiography [1, 2, 3]. We, and others have used PDE for detection of tricuspid valve regurgitation as well [4, 5, 6]. In many centers, including ours, atrioventricular valve regurgitation (AVVR) has been detected through the use of an audio PDE output, with detection of a harsh systolic flow disturbance posterior to the atrioventricular (AV) valve. Though it is not difficult to differentiate smooth, normal flow from rough, disturbed flow on the basis of the audio signal, some remain skeptical about this subjective differentiation. A time interval histographic (TIH) output is commonly used for PDE registration, depicting abnormal flow with dot scatter, and documenting normal flow with the absence of dot scatter. While several centers have enjoyed good sensitivity and specificity for PDE diagnosis of various flow disturbances, even with the several limitations imposed by audio and TIH outputs, there is need for a PDE display format which does not require adjustment during examinations, and which does not have the potential for subjectivity. A 128-channel, digital multigate Doppler (DMD) device, described by Brandestini et al. [7], has the distinct advantage of visual representation of flow, superimposed on a familiar M-mode format. For the question of AVVR, the display format either shows regurgitant flow posterior to the AV valve, or shows no regurgitant flow. The detection and display of the flow characteristics are not under the control or adjustment of the examiner; the only judgement made in the evaluation is the presence or absence of directional flow.

PROCEDURE

We evaluated 99 infants and children, age 1 day to 12 years (mean = 2.6 yr) for the presence or absence of AVVR. Each patient was examined with a conventional 5 MHz single crystal PDE unit (ATL Model 400A, Advanced

Technology Laboratories Bellevue, Washington), and also with the 5 MHz DMD device [8, 9, 10]. Usually the PDE examination preceeded the DMD exam. All examinations were performed by the same examiner. The patients were not routinely sedated for study. Complete examinations were done in all cases but, for the purposes of this study, attention was directed to the presence or absence of AVVR, as described below. Once AVVR was detected, careful attention was paid to the breadth and extent of abnormal flow. Flow disturbances that occupied only a portion of systole, or were present only in the immediate peri-valvar area were considered mild, and more extensive jets moderate. Flow disturbances extending through the atrium to the far atrial wall were considered severe.

In a later experience, we evaluated a subgroup of 24 patients who had been admitted for cardiac catheterization, and whose ventriculograms did not suggest the presence of artifactual, catheter, or arrythmia-induced AVVR. We compared the breadth and extent of the AVVR jet on angio with the PDE and DMD estimations of AVVR severity.

The PDE examinations were performed as previously described [11, 12, 13]. For the detection of AVVR, the sample volume was placed posterior to the AV valve and then carefully moved along the interface of coapted AV valve leaflets. The audio notation of harsh systolic flow was used for initial detection of AVVR. Then the TIH output was adjusted to proper threshold and signal level to record a diagnostic flow record [11, 14]. The presence of systolic dot scatter, with sample volume not touching a solid

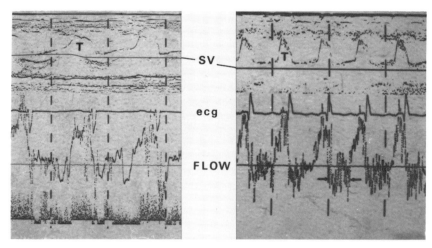

Figure 1. PDE flow record of normal tricuspid valve flow (left) and tricuspid regurgitation (right). The sample volume (SV) is posterior to the tricuspid valve (T) in each panel. In the TIH FLOW record at the bottom, there is systolic dot scatter in the patient with tricuspid regurgitation, and no systolic dot scatter in the normal. The systolic dot scatter is indicative of tricuspid regurgitation.

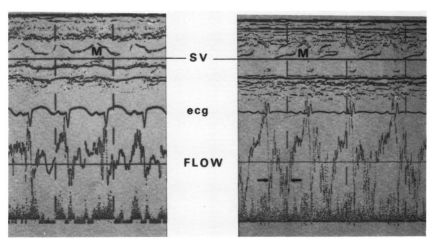

Figure 2. PDE flow record of normal mitral valve flow (left), and mitral regurgitation (right). The sample volume (SV) is posterior to the mitral valve (M) in each panel. In the TIH FLOW record at the bottom, the systolic dot scatter is indicative of mitral regurgitation in the right hand panel; dots are closely grouped in the left hand panel from a normal patient.

structure, was indicative of AVVR. Careful attempts were made to move the sample volume about in the region of the AVVR jet, to assess apparent jet breadth and to assess the greatest depth into the atrium at which AVVR could be detected.

The DMD examinations were performed from a standard precordial approach, similar to that used in PDE. The mitral and tricuspid valves were examined in sequence. Attention was directed to that portion of the M-mode format posterior to the AV valve in systole. The DMD unit does not encode color when there is no directional flow; the portion of the left atrium that is visualized posterior to the mitral valve in systole remains blank, or black, in the normal patient (Figure 3). The directional flow from the vena cavae, in its anterior course to the tricuspid valve, does give a uniform colored flow signal posterior to the tricuspid valve (Figure 4). Flow toward the transducer is coded in blue tones, while flow away from the transducer is coded in red tones. In the color spectrum strip on the left in the DMD records, a white arrow indicates the break in color codes for direction; colors further away from the arrow indicate increasing flow velocities. For each valve, AVVR was diagnosed if blood flow away from the AV valve into the atrium was detected, (Figures 5 and 6). Since the AVVR jet for each valve is directed posteriorly with respect to a precordial transducer, the AVVR jets appear in brilliant red color, at a position where normal flow would be coded black (mitral) or blue (tricuspid); red flow appearing posterior to the AV valve indicated AVVR. Careful attention was directed to the breadth and extent of the red AVVR jet. The severity of AVVR (mild, moderate, severe) was estimated as above. The PDE and DMD results were compared.

Figure 3. Digital Multigate Doppler record of normal mitral valve flow. Blue = mitral inflow. Red = LV outflow. No color-coded flow posterior to mitral valve in systole. See text explanation.

Figure 4. Digital Multigate Doppler record of normal tricuspid valve flow. Blue = Tricuspid inflow. No color-coded flow posterior to the tricuspid valve in systole. B-mode image of tricuspid valve appears at the right. See text explanation.

Figure 5. Digital Multigate Doppler record of tricuspid insufficiency (small jet). At the right, a small red jet appears posterior to the valve in systole, and does not extend to posterior atrial wall, nor into body of ventricle.

Figure 6. Digital Multigate Doppler record of severe mitral insufficiency. Multicolored red/yellow tones appear posterior to the valve in systole, indicating mitral regurgitation, and extend into the body of the ventricle, as well as extending to the wall of the left atrium.

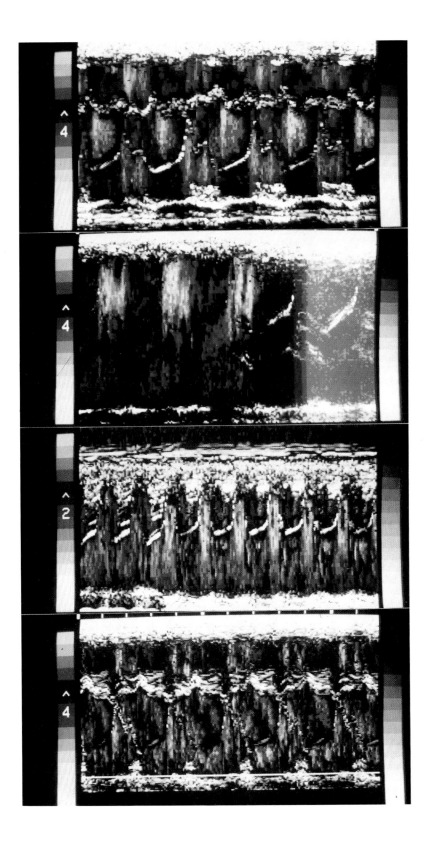

RESULTS

In this series of patients with congenital cardiac defects, not every patient had both a mitral and tricuspid valve. In 92/99 a mitral valve was present, and in 96/99 a tricuspid valve was present. When only a single AV valve was present, its identity was inferred from the ventricular anatomic features noted on angio. Combining the AV valves, a total of 188 AV valves were evaluated by both PDE and DMD.

In evaluations of the mitral valve (N = 92), AVVR was detected by both PDE and DMD in 32, and excluded in 57 (Table 1). Three patients had AVVR visible on DMD and angio, but were equivocal or negative by PDE.

Table 1. Evaluations of the mitral valve.

		Pulsed Doppler echocardiography:	
		MR present	MR absent
Digital multigate Doppler:	MR present	32	3
	MR absent	0	57

In evaluations of the tricuspid valve (N = 96), AVVR was detected in 36 by both PDE and DMD, and was negative by both in 60; there were no discrepancies between PDE and DMD for detection of tricuspid regurgitation.

Table 2. Evaluations of the tricuspid valve.

		Pulsed Doppler echocardiography	
		TR present	TR absent
Digital multigate Doppler:	TR present	36	0
	TR absent	0	60

Of the 24 patients in the ventriculography sub-group, 12 had mild AVVR, 6 had moderate AVVR and 6 had severe AVVR on angio. The PDE and DMD results in these patients are given in Table 3. AVVR was detected by both systems in 11/12 with mild MR, and provided equivocal evidence in 1. Of the 12 patients with moderate to severe AVVR on angio, DMD demonstrated extensive AVVR jets in 12/12; PDE suggested mild AVVR in 1/12, moderate or severe in 11/12. In 6/12 with moderate AVVR on angio, both PDE and DMD demonstrated the AVVR jets extending more than

1 cm into the atrium, but not traversing the atrium. In 6/12 with severe AVVR on angio, with AVVR jets extending to the far atrial wall, DMD demonstrated the jets to the atrial wall in 6/6, while only 3/6 of the jets could be detected near the far atrial walll by PDE.

Table 3. Severity of AVVR by PDE, DMD, and ventriculography.

		PDE correct	DMD correct
Regurgitation	Mild AVVR	11/12	11/12
on	Moderate AVVR	6/6	6/6
ventriculogram	Severe AVVR	3/6	6/6

In patients with mild or moderate AVVR, the regurgitant jets were displayed in one or two color bands, indicating that the velocities detected by the DMD device within the jets were fairly similar (Figure 5). In patients with severe AVVR, several colors were present in the AVVR jets, indicating a greater variety of velocities. Such mixed, multicolored flow disturbances were also noted in the ventricular body in patients with severe AVVR, but not in patients with mild AVVR (Figure 6).

DISCUSSION

It would not be reasonable to have expected a dramatic improvement in sensitivity and specificity from the DMD device, since experienced examiners already enjoy excellent results in the diagnosis of AVVR by PDE, using audio and TIH output. In our series, AVVR was detected by audio output and then displayed on TIH. Had we relied solely on TIH for detection and not taken advantage of the audio output, it is likely that fewer patients with AVVR would have been detected by PDE. In this series the DMD results agreed very well with the PDE results; actually DMD performed more accurately, with detection of proven AVVR in 3 patients whose PDE findings were equivocal. In addition, DMD was more accurate in categorizing the severity of AVVR in the catheterized subgroup.

The ease of detection of AVVR by DMD seems a distinct advantage, but one which is hard to quantitate in a setting where examiners are already proficient in PDE. The detection of AVVR by DMD requires only a "flow-yes" or "flow-no" decision in a dramatic format which is not modified or adjusted by the examiner. In DMD, there is no reliance upon the audio output, and false positive diagnosis of flow disturbances is less likely with DMD since each of the 128 channels codes for structure *or* flow, not both.

In addition to the ease of detection, the DMD format would seem to have considerable potential in estimation of severity of AVVR by visualization of the AVVR jet per se. With PDE we have relied on M-mode echo for assessment of left atrial and left ventricular dimensions, and for an estimation of left ventricular function, in order to make a judgement about AVVR severity. Such combination of PDE and M-mode information has served us well in cases of isolated AVVR, but is limited when AVVR coexists with other lesions which could contribute to M-mode dimensions. In this series the DMD estimation of severity correlated very well with the angio demonstration of severity, even in the presence of mixed lesions. In patients with mixed lesions, it may prove useful to assess severity of AVVR by DMD, and enter that assessment into the interpretation of M-mode dimensions. For example, in a patient with ventricular septal defect and mitral regurgitation, and M-mode signs of left ventricular volume overload, a mild AVVR jet on DMD would lead one to interpret the majority of the M-mode dimension abnormalities as being due to the ventricular septal defect, with a smaller contribution from AVVR. The same may be attempted with PDE, but would probably be less accurate, and would be fraught with the disadvantages of TIH.

We noted that all patients with severe AVVR had regurgitant jets comprising multiple colors, and that the flow disturbance was also carried downstream into the body of the ventricle. One interpretation of these findings is that severe regurgitant volumes have less uniform flow characteristics, contain a greater variety of directions and velocities, and hence lead to a mixture of colors on DMD. The ventricular findings may result from transmission of turbulence downstream, or from the increased diastolic flow associated with severe AVVR states. Either formulation would be consistent with the clinical notation of diastolic murmur in severe AVVR states; we favor the former. The mixed color findings in severe AVVR may not be fully compatible with the PDE/TIH experience, where smaller jets often seem most harsh, and severe regurgitant volumes may seem only mildly turbulent, however diffuse or extensive. Whether DMD color mixture corresponds to TIH dot scatter and turbulence was not evaluated in this series.

SUMMARY

In this series with experienced examiners, there was good agreement between PDE and DMD for detection of AVVR. The DMD system seems advantageous because of ease of detection, dramatic depiction of AVVR jets with quantitative implications, and lack of reliance upon audio output for AVVR detection or on TIH for flow recording. These advantages may reduce the potential for false negative Doppler results, lessen the suspicions of subjectivity, and suggest further application for quantitation of intracardiac and intravascular flow.

REFERENCES

1. Dooley TK, SA Rubenstein, JG Stevenson: Pulsed-Doppler echocardiography: The detection of mitral regurgitation. In: Ultrasound in Medicine, Vol. 4, (White D, EA Lyons, eds.) p 383. Plenum Press, New York, 1978.
2. Stevenson JG, I Kawabori, WG Guntheroth: Differentiation of ventricular septal defect from mitral regurgitation by pulsed-Doppler echocardiography. Circulation 56:14–18, 1977.
3. Abbasi AS, MW Allen, D DeCristofaro, I Ungar: Detection and estimation of the degree of mitral regurgitation by range-gated pulsed-Doppler echocardiography. Circulation 61:143–147, 1980.
4. Waggoner AD, MA Quinones, MS Verani, RR Miller: Pulsed-Doppler echocardiographic detection of tricuspid insufficiency: diagnostic sensitivity and correlation with right ventricular hemodynamics. Circulation 58–2:40, 1978.
5. Stevenson JG: Pulsed-Doppler echocardiography 2 – Applications in pediatric cardiology. In: Pediatric Echocardiography, Cross Sectional, M-Mode and Doppler (Lundstron, N-R, ed.), pp 269–292. Elsevier/North Holland Press, Amsterdam, 1980.
6. Sakakibara H, K Miyatake, M Okamoto, N Kinoshita, Y Nimura: Noninvasive assessment of severity of tricuspid regurgitation with a combined use of the ultrasonic pulsed-Doppler technique and two-dimensional echocardiography. Circulation 62–3:250, 1980.
7. Brandestini MA, MA Eyer, JG Stevenson: M/Q mode echocardiography – the synthesis of conventional echo with digital multigate Doppler. In Echocardiology (Lancée CT, ed.), pp 441–446. Martinus Nijhoff, The Hague, 1980.
8. Brandestini MA, EA Howard, M Eyer, JG Stevenson, T Weiler: Visualization of intracardiac defects by M/Q mode echo/Doppler ultrasound. Circulation 60–2:12, 1979.
9. Stevenson JG, MA Brandestini, T Weiler, EA Howard, M Eyer: Digital multigate Doppler with color echo and Doppler display – diagnosis of atrial septal defect and ventricular septal defect. Circulation 60–2:205, 1979.
10. Stevenson JG, I Kawabori, TK Dooley, WG Guntheroth: Diagnosis of ventricular septal defect by pulsed-Doppler echocardiography: Sensitivity, specificity and limitations. Circulation 58:326, 1978.
11. Stevenson JG: Pulsed Doppler echocardiography 1: Basic Principles. In: Pediatric Echocardiography, Cross Sectional, M-Mode and Doppler. (Lundstrom N-R, ed.), pp 259–268. Elsevier/North Holland Press, Amsterdam, 1980.
12. Stevenson JG, I Kawabori, WG Guntheroth, SA SA Rubinstein, DW Baker: Pulsed-Doppler echocardiography, applications in pediatric cardiology. In: Echocardiology (Lancée CT, ed.), pp 349–354. Martinus Nijhoff, The Hague, 1980.
13. Stevenson JG, I Kawabori, WG Guntheroth: Pulsed-Doppler echocardiographic diagnosis of patent ductus arteriosus- sensitivity, specificity, limitations and technical features. Cathet Cardiovasc Diagnosis 6:255–263, 1980.
14. Nelson CE: A Note regarding the 400A/500A spectral controls. D21584, Advanced Technology Laboratories, Bellevue, Washington.

45. A COMBINED DOPPLER ECHOCARDIOGRAPHIC INVESTIGATION IN PREMATURE INFANTS WITH AND WITHOUT RESPIRATORY DISTRESS SYNDROME *

O. Daniëls, J.C.W. Hopman, G.B.A. Stoelinga, H.J. Busch, and P.G.M. Peer

Premature infants often develop the Respiratory Distress Syndrome (RDS). In the traditional view, this is due to a lack of surfactant causing a collapse of lung alveoli. In a number of cases of RDS, a Patent Ductus Arteriosus (PDA) with Left to Right (L-R) shunt is diagnosed during the recovery phase of the syndrome from the presence of a murmur, bounding pulses and an increased Left Atrium/Aorta ratio (LA/Ao). This diagnosis of the PDA has wrongly led to the conclusion that this L-R shunt first arises in the recovery phase; perhaps because routine clinical examination is not always sufficient to detect a PDA, since a large PDA with L-R shunt is not always acompanied by a heart murmur and even the echocardiographic demonstration of an increase in LA dimension or LA/Ao ratio is not conclusive evidence for the existence of a PDA with L-R shunt. Theoretically, a PDA with L-R shunt can cause respiratory problems, especially in small infants, as a result of pulmonary vessel engorgement, leading in turn to surfactant deficiency due to anoxaemia. So we have the situation indicated below:

$$\text{SURFACTANT DEFICIENCY} \leftrightarrow \text{RDS} \leftrightarrow \text{PDA}$$

In our investigation we demonstrated the existence of a PDA with L-R shunt in premature infants by means of a combined Doppler echocardiographic (DE) technique. The moment of closure of the ductus could be estimated from successive measurements. We also measured the LA/Ao ratio by means of echocardiography to determine the magnitude of the L-R shunt.

METHODS

The flow pattern (velocity as a function of time) in the Main Pulmonary Artery (MPA) can be detected by means of a two-dimensional real-time sector-scanner combined with a Doppler unit (ATL Mark V). Normally, there is no diastolic flow in the MPA but, in the case of a PDA with L-R shunt, there is a systolic backward or turbulent flow and a pandiastolic backward or forward flow, depending on the location in the vessel [7]. As the

* This research was sponsored by the Dutch Heart Foundation.

Rijsterborgh H, ed: Echocardiology, p 409-415. All rights reserved.

410

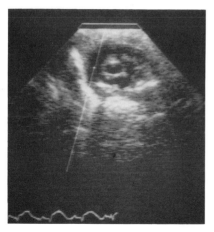

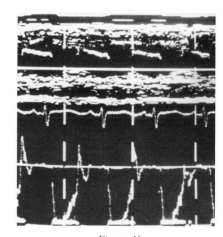

Figure 1a

Figure 1b

Figure 1a. Sector-scan of a longitudinal section through the MPA. The aorta is visible in cross-section. The straight line indicates the M-mode direction. The dot on the line is the depth marker for the Doppler sample volume.

Figure 1b. M/Q-mode registration, as taken from the line indicated in Figure 1a, for a normal patient. Upper part: the M-mode recording with the depth marker for the Doppler sample volume (solid line). Middle trace: the ECG. Lower part: Time Interval Histogram [1] (Q-mode), indicating a systolic forward flow and no diastolic flow (no L-R ductal shunt present).

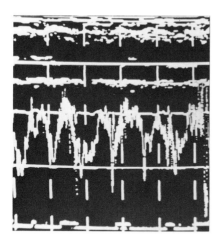

Figure 1c

Figure 1c. Systolic and diastolic backward flow, measured high in the MPA near the ductus in a case of L-R shunt.

measurement of very fast flow as found in systole with a pulsed-Doppler unit can lead to wrong interpretation of the direction of flow, due to frequency ambiguity [2], we used the existence of continuous, diastolic backward *and* forward flow (Figure 1) as the criterion for the existence of a PDA with L-R shunt [3, 7].

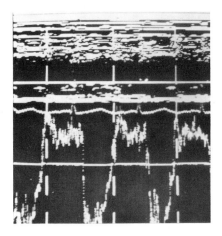 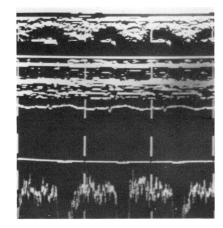

Figure 1d   Figure 1e

Figure 1d. Pandiastolic backward flow on the ventral side of the MPA in a case of PDA with L-R shunt.

Figure 1e. Pandiastolic forward flow on the dorsal side of the MPA in a case of PDA with L-R shunt.

Together with the Doppler investigation, we measured the left atrial size from a parasternal position (LAz) and from a suprasternal position (LAy). The size of the left atrium was calculated as $\overline{LA} = (LAz + LAy)/2$. This was done because this measure is less sensitive to the effects of sternal retraction or to anatomical structural variation (e.g. 'pancaking') [4]. The diameter of the aorta (Ao) was measured from a parasternal position. In all measurements we used the leading edge method, as recommended by the ASE [5]. The $\overline{LA}$/Ao ratio is regarded as an index of the magnitude of the L-R shunt [6].

MATERIAL

In 71 preterm infants, a DE examination was carried out to determine the flow pattern in the MPA. The first measurement was done shortly after birth, in general within 18 hours. The measurements were repeated daily, unless the child showed such respiratory distress that therapy with continuous airway pressure or artificial ventilation was necessary. In that case the measurement was repeated earlier, as soon as the distress became apparent. Measurements were continued until the ductus closed spontaneously, or until the clinical course was interrupted by surgical (ligation) or pharmacologic (Indomethacine) closure of the ductus or by death of the infant.

412

Nearly all preterm infants showed a L-R shunt shortly after birth. Eight children did not have a L-R shunt in the first examination. Five of these subjects showed a shunt in a subsequent examination. Possibly this phenomenon was due to persistent high pulmonary vascular resistance for some hours after birth. This theory is supported by the fact that in some of these cases a patent ductus was seen on the sector-scan before a shunt flow could be measured. Assuming a lognormal distribution for the ductal closure times, the spontaneous closure time was calculated by means of maximum likelihood estimation. Table 1 shows the estimated closure time for different groups. We also included the 30 normal healthy newborns we published earlier [7]. Figure 2 shows the cumulative lognormal distribution of closure times for different gestational age categories. It is clear that the ductus remains patent for a time which is directly related to the degree of prematurity of the infant. In all infants who developed respiratory problems, a PDA with L-R shunt was still present at the onset of clinical illness, except in three children in whom in the first measurement there was not yet a L-R shunt, as mentioned earlier. As can be seen from Table 2, children with a PDA in whom respiratory problems increase have an increase in $\overline{LA}/Ao$ ratio and in children in whom respiratory problems decrease the $\overline{LA}/Ao$ ratio

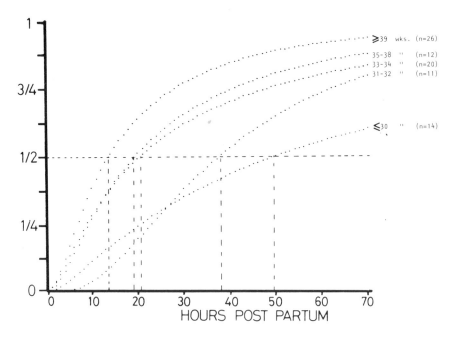

Figure 2. Cumulative lognormal distribution of spontaneous ductal closure times for different gestational age groups. The vertical axis displays the probability that the ductus is closed spontaneously.

Table 1. Estimated closure time of the Ductus Arteriosus for different clinical groups.

	Term	Preterm		
		No resp. problems	Resp. problems	
	Spontaneous closure	Spontaneous closure	Spontaneous closure	Artificial closure or death
Number of children	30	40	13	18
Gest. age in wks.	37–42	26–36	25–36	26–34
median	39	33	31	29
Closure time in hours				
median (P_{50})	14	24	56	all open
5th percentile (P_5)	3	4	8	
95th percentile (P_{95})	72	166	374	

Table 2. Changes in the mean value of $\overline{LA}$/Ao ratio, $\overline{LA}$ and Ao in relation to changes in respiratory (resp.) problems between two successive measurements, analysed by applying a t-test for paired samples. 'n' is the number of patients.
a) increasing resp. problems; on measurement B there was a proven ductal shunt.
b) decreasing resp. problems; on measurement C there was a proven ductal shunt.

a.	A no essential resp. problems	B evident or severe resp. problems	n	P-value
$\overline{LA}$/Ao	1.65	2.04	5	0.054 **
$\overline{LA}$ (mm)	11.7	12.7	5	0.21
Ao (mm)	7.1	6.2	5	0.07 **

b.	C severe or evident resp. problems	D no essential resp. problems	n	P-value
$\overline{LA}$/Ao	1.66	1.52	12	0.006 *
$\overline{LA}$ (mm)	12.3	11.9	12	0.17
Ao (mm)	7.4	7.8	12	0.03 *

* = significant (p $<$ 0.05), ** = indication for significance.

414

Table 3. Changes in the mean value of $\overline{LA}$/Ao-ratio, $\overline{LA}$ and Ao in relation with ductal closure, analysed by a t-test for paired samples. 'n' is the number of patients. On measurement A there was a proven ductal L-R shunt. Measurement B was always made more than 36 hours after disappearance of the shunt.

	A last measurement with ductal L-R shunt	B more than 36 hours no ductal shunt	n	P-value
$\overline{LA}$/Ao	1.61	1.47	41	0.000 *
$\overline{LA}$ (mm)	11.7	11.0	41	0.005 *
Ao (mm)	7.3	7.6	42	0.02 *

* = significant (p<0.05).

decreases. We also tested the ratio before and after ductal closure and found a significant decrease in the $\overline{LA}$/Ao ratio after the disappearance of the L-R shunt (Table 3). On the aorta a two-sided test was applied, because in theory there should be no change.

Nine of the forty-two children involved showed respiratory problems on the last measurement with PDA and L-R shunt. In six of them these problems disappeared within 36 hours after ductal closure.

The results support the concept that the ductal L-R shunt has an influence on the respiratory problems. However, the changes in the parameters are relatively small. The significant change in the $\overline{LA}$/Ao ratio is due to the simultaneous (not significant) change in the $\overline{LA}$ and the (significant) change in the Ao (Table 2). The changes in the $\overline{LA}$ size are smaller than expected. But we have to keep in mind that in the clinical situation of these infants the L-R shunt is not the only factor responsible for changes in $\overline{LA}$ size. Other factors such as fluid balance, digoxin, diuretics, left ventricular performance, positive airway pressure exert a direct or indirect influence [8, 9, 10]. The change in the aortic diameter is more difficult to explain. Until now this size was regarded as being constant [6, 10]. One may speculate that the aortic root dilates somewhat as the afterload on the left ventricle increases. However, since the absolute differences are very small, the relevance of this result would need to be demonstrated by futher research.

CONCLUSIONS

1. With DE techniques, PDA with L-R shunt can be diagnosed even in the absence of a heart murmur.
2. In both term *and* preterm neonates, PDA with L-R shunt exists from shortly after birth.

3. The moment of ductal closure is inversely related to gestational age and tends to occur yet later when in combination with respiratory distress.
4. In nearly all infants who developed respiratory problems, a PDA with L-R shunt was still present at the onset of clinical illness. The relation between ductal shunt, $\overline{LA}$/Ao ratio and respiratory problems supports the hypothesis that a L-R ductal shunt plays an important role in the development of an RDS. However, a further investigation to quantitate the L-R shunt in these children will be necessary to prove this.

REFERENCES

1. Baker DW, EE Simeon, A Rubinstein, GS Lorch: Pulsed Doppler echocardiography: principles and applications. Amer J Med 63:69–80, 1977.
2. Peronneau PA, JP Bournat, A Bugnon, A Barbat, M Xhaard: Theoretical and practical aspects of pulsed Doppler flowmetry: realtime application to the measure of instantaneous velocity profiles in vitro and in vivo. In: Cardiovascular applications of ultrasound (Reneman RS, ed.). North-Holland Publishing Company, Amsterdam, 1974.
3. Stevenson JG, I Kawabori, WG Guntheroth: Noninvasive detection of pulmonary hypertension in patent ductus arteriosus by pulsed Doppler echocardiography. Circulation 60:355–359, 1979.
4. Goldberg SJ, HD Allen, DJ Sahn: Echocardiographic detection and management of patent ductus arteriosus in neonates with respiratory distress syndrome: two- and one-half year prospective study. J Clin Ultrasound 5:161–169, 1977.
5. Recommendation of the American Society of Echocardiography regarding Quantitation in M-Mode Echocardiography. 7 March 1978.
6. Silverman NH, AB Lewis, MA Heyman, AM Rudolph: Echocardiographic assessment of Ductus Arteriosus Shunt in Premature Infants. Circulation 50:821–825, 1974.
7. Daniëls O, JCW Hopman, GBA Stoelinga, HJ Busch, PGM Peer: Doppler flow characteristics in the main pulmonary artery and left atrial size before and after ductal closure in healthy newborns, Pediatric Cardiology (In revision).
8. Warburton D, EF Bell, W Oh: Pharmacokinetics and echocardiographic effects of digoxin in low birth weight infants with left-to-right shunting due to patent ductus arteriosus. Dev Pharmacol Ther 1:189–200, 1980.
9. Björkhem GE, NR Lundström, NW Svenningsen: Influence of continous positive airways pressure treatment on ductus arteriosus shunt assessed by echocardiography. Arch Disease Childhood 52:659–661, 1977.
10. Sahn DJ, Y Vaucher, DE Williams, HD Allen, SJ Goldberg, WF Friedman: Echocardiographic detection of large left to right shunts and cardiomyopathies in infants and children. Amer J Cardiol 38:73–79, 1976.

46. FETAL CARDIAC ACTIVITY

J.W. WLADIMIROFF, J. MCGHIE, and R. VOSTERS

1. INTRODUCTION

Improvement in both real-time two-dimensional (2D) ultrasonic scanners and M-mode recording systems has led to increasing research into fetal cardiovascular dynamics [1, 2, 3]. Recently, the introduction of pulsed Doppler systems of low MHz frequency has opened up the possibility of studying flow velocity in the umbilical vein and abdominal part of the descending aorta [4] during the last trimester of pregnancy. The studies carried out at our Ultrasound Laboratory have been focussed lately on the geometry and functional behaviour of the cardiac ventricles, as well as the flow distribution to the umbilical vein and descending aorta relative to total cardiac output.

2. MATERIAL AND METHODS

Measurements were carried out in two groups of normal subjects during the last trimester of pregnancy:
  a. real-time two-dimensional estimation of the transverse and longitudinal diameter of the left ventricle in the end-diastolic (ED) and end-systolic (ES) position for calculation of left ventricular cardiac output (n = 50) and measurement of blood flow in the descending aorta (n = 30).
  b. M-mode measurement of the transverse diameter of the left and right ventricle (LV and RV) and blood flow in the descending aorta (n = 39).

The essential part of the scanning technique for both groups is that the ultrasound transducer should be placed at the level of the fetal heart in a plane which is situated at an angle of 45° to the antero-posterior diameter of the fetal chest on a transverse cross-section, and an angle of 50° to the fetal spine on a longitudinal cross-section (Figure 1). This plane will run through the right and left ventricle at right angles to the intraventricular septum.

The largest section through the LV and RV should now be identified by making scans parallel to the scanning plane described, until the following 6

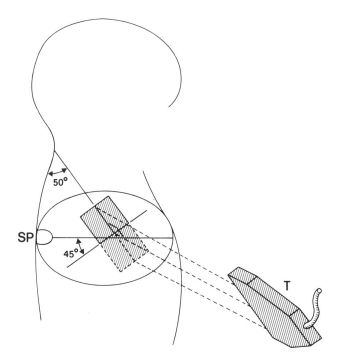

Figure 1. Schematic representation of the transducer position at right angles to the plane through the intraventricular septum (hatched area) of the fetal heart.

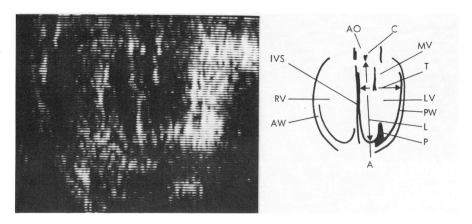

Figure 2. Real-time two-dimensional scan (Fociscan, Organon Teknika) and schematic picture of longitudinal cross-section through LV and RV depicting the right ventricular anterior wall (AW), the intraventricular septum (IVS), the left ventricular posterior wall (PW), the mitral valve leaflets (MV), the aortic root (AO) and the posteromedial papillary muscle (P). T and L represent the largest transverse and longitudinal diameter of the LV.

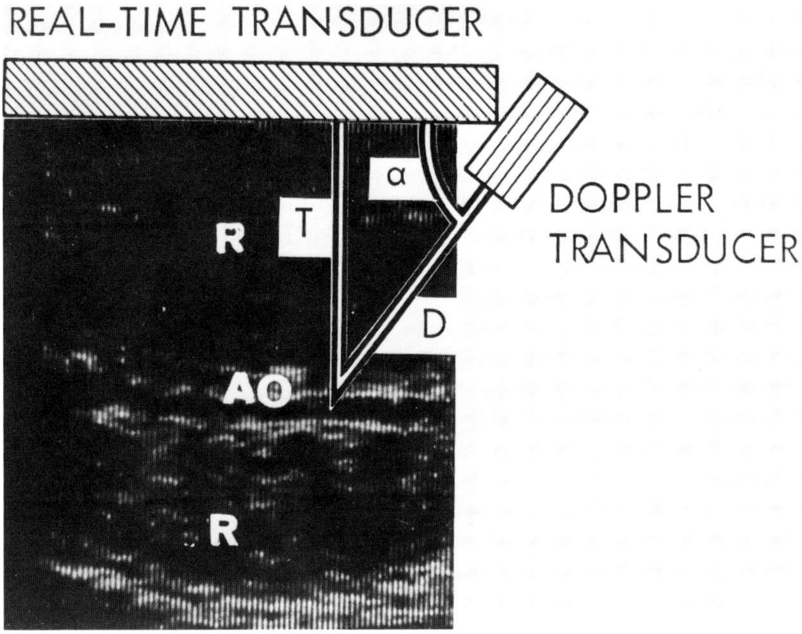

REAL-TIME TRANSDUCER

Figure 3. Positioning of the real-time transducer parallel to the descending part of the fetal aorta (AO).
R = fetal trunk, T = distance between real-time transducer and aorta, α = angle between real-time and Doppler transducer, D = distance between Doppler transducer and aorta.

landmarks are visible on the two-dimensional image (Figure 2): the right ventricular anterior wall; the intraventricular septum; the left ventricular posterior wall; the mitral valve leaflets; the aortic root and the left ventricular apex.

The transverse diameter of the LV is measured at the level of the mitral valve leaflets from the endocardium of the intraventricular septum to the endocardium of the left ventricular posterior wall; the longitudinal diameter of the LV is measured from the base of the aortic root to the left ventricular apex. The longitudinal axis of the RV cannot be measured, since the pulmonary trunk is not visible in this scanning plane.

M-mode recording of the transverse diameter of the LV also allows measurement of the velocity of fractional shortening of the LV. Flow velocity in the descending part of the aorta was estimated by means of a real-time two-dimensional scanner in conjunction with a pulsed Doppler system (PEDOF).

The first step in the measurement of blood flow is the positioning of the real-time transducer parallel to the aorta (Figure 3). The distance (T) between transducer and vessel is now established and with a known angle (α) between real-time and Doppler transducer, the distance (D) between Doppler transducer and vessel can be calculated [4]. The second step involves measurement of the diameter of the vessel.

Blood flow (Q) is now calculated according to the following equation:

$$Q = \frac{V \cdot A}{\cos \alpha} \text{ ml/sec}$$

V = flow velocity (mm/sec); A = vessel lumen area (mm^2); α = angle between the real-time transducer and Doppler transducer.

3. RESULTS

Figure 4 represents the mean and standard deviation for the longitudinal and transverse axis of the LV in the ED and ES position in 50 normal subjects.

Period I represents the gestational period between 27 and 33 weeks and period II between 34 and 41 weeks. There is a significant decrease in both the longitudinal and transverse axis from the ED and the ES positions. There is a

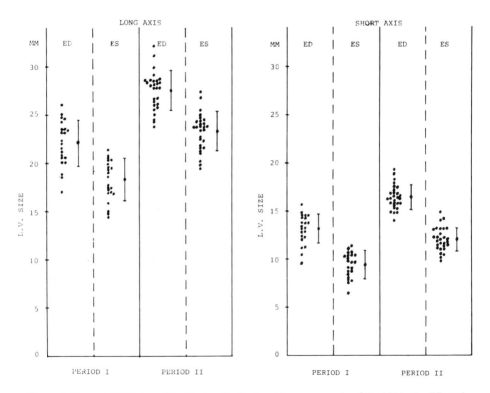

Figure 4. Mean ± 1 S.D. (mm) for the longitudinal and transverse axis of the LV in the ED and ES positions during periods I and II.

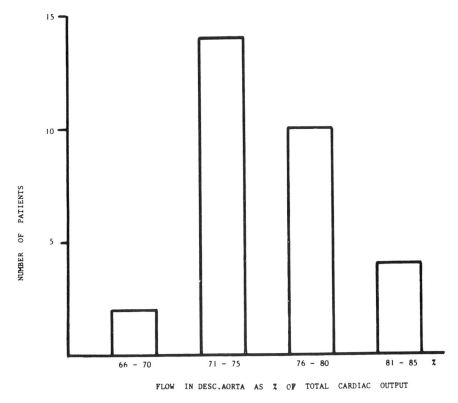

Figure 5. Proportion of total cardiac output being distributed through the descending part of the fetal aorta.

significant increase in the mean longitudinal and transverse axis from period I to period II in both the ED and ES positions. If it is assumed that the antero-posterior axis of the LV which cannot be measured is equal to the transverse axis and the configuration of the LV is similar to a prolate ellipse, an estimation of LV cardiac volume can be made.

The difference between LV cardiac volume in the ED and ES phase of the cardiac cycle represents left ventricular cardiac output (LVCO). In period I, a mean LVCO of 196 ± 52 ml/min and in period II, a mean LVCO of 336 ± 35 ml/min were calculated.

During periods I and II the volume flow in the descending aorta was 365 ± 90 and 490 ± 65 ml/min respectively. This is slightly higher than the figures reported by Eik-Nes et al. [4]. If we compare the aortic flow and LV cardiac output data and assume that LV and RV are equal in output, then the proportion of the combined output which is directed through the descending aorta varies between 70% and 80% (Figure 5).

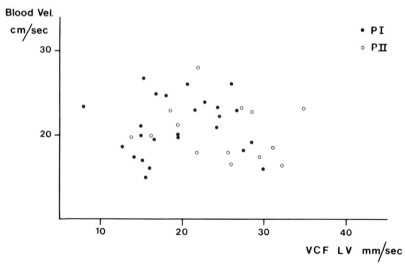

Figure 6. Blood velocity in the descending aorta relative to velocity of fractional shortening (VCF) in LV during period I (●) and period II (○).

From our M-mode study, no relationship between velocity of fractional shortening of LV and RV and flow velocity in the descending part of the aorta could be demonstrated (Figure 6).

4. DISCUSSION

LVCO values in the human fetus are considerably lower than in the fetal lamb, although the distribution of the total cardiac output through the descending fetal aorta is very similar for both species.

The lack of any relationship between the velocity of fractional shortening of LV and RV and flow velocity in the descending aorta is not surprising if one realizes the complexity of flow patterns between both cardiac chambers and the descending aorta such as, the pulmonary circulation, the flow distribution to head and upper extremities as well as the shunting of blood through the patent ductus arteriosus.

REFERENCES

1. Wladimiroff JW: Fetal cardiovascular dynamics. Progress in medical ultrasound. 1, 69–86, (Kurjak A, ed.), Excerpta Medica, Amsterdam, Oxford, Princeton, 1980.
2. Wladimiroff JW, J McGhie, PLJ Custers, P van Hoogdalem: Assessment of human fetal cardiovascular performance by means of two-dimensional real-time and pulsed-Doppler ultrasound. Proceedings first international symposium on

recent advances in prenatal diagnosis (Orlandi C, Rizzo N, eds). John Wiley & Sons Ltd., Chichester, U.K., 1980 (In press).

3. Wladimiroff JW, R Vosters, W Vletter. Real-time assessment of fetal and neonatal cardiac dynamics. Real-time ultrasound in obstetrics (Bennet M, Cambell, eds), pp 79–88. Blackwell Scientific Publications, Oxford, 1980.
4. Eik-Nes SH, AO Brubakk, HK Ulstein: Measurement of human fetal blood flow. Brit Med J 1:283, 1980.

47. FETAL OBSTRUCTION OF THE FORAMEN OVALE DETECTED BY TWO-DIMENSIONAL DOPPLER ECHOCARDIOGRAPHY

D. A. REDEL and M. HANSMANN

1. INTRODUCTION

Premature obstruction of the foramen ovale inevitably leads to right heart failure and imposes serious problems on the fetal circulation. It may cause fetal hydrops of the upper part of the body, universal hydrops and fetal death. The diagnosis of this disease in utero has not been reported previously in the literature.

We present a case of premature obstruction of the foramen ovale that was diagnosed in the 35th week of pregnancy and was treated successfully by delivery by Cesarean section.

2. CASE REPORT

The diagnosis of a fetal hydrops was made in the 35th week of pregnancy by routine ultrasound investigation. It was found that the edema was confined to the upper part of the body and a concomitant right side pleural effusion was detected (Figure 1).

An investigation of the fetus by two-dimensional pulsed-Doppler echocardiography (2D DE) showed no opening movements of the flap of the

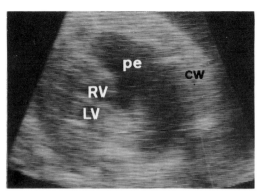

Figure 1. Transverse section through the fetal thorax. A large pleural effusion (pe) occupies the right hemithorax.
cw = chest wall with edema; LV = left ventricle; RV = right ventricle.

Rijsterborgh H, ed: Echocardiology, p 425-429. All rights reserved.

426

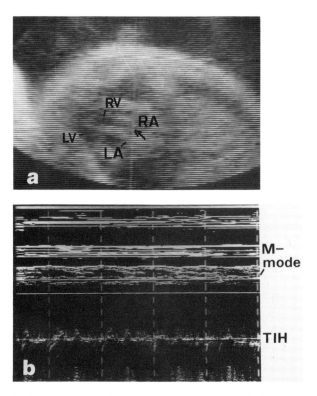

Figure 2. a) The fetal heart in a four-chamber view. The arrow marks the position of the sample volume for Doppler flow analysis near the interatrial septum. RA = right atrium.

b) Time interval histogram (TIH) of the Doppler-shifted frequencies. The frequency shift shown does not indicate presence of any considerable blood flow. The upper part shows an M-mode recording of the fetal heart.

foramen ovale in the sector image, Doppler flow analysis revealed the lack of blood flow across the foramen ovale (Figure 2a and b). The right ventricle was large (Figure 2a) and the pulmonary artery seemed to be dilated. The left ventricular cavity was shown to be small with normal anatomy of the mitral valve apparatus, the aortic root was small with normal opening movements of the aortic valves.

Ultrasound findings of the fetus, the echocardiographic configuration and the 2D DE flow analysis were considered to be typical for a premature obstruction of the foramen ovale and the initiation of birth came into question. An intrauterine puncture of the right pleural cavity was performed and 120 ml of effusion aspirated to facilitate respiration after birth.

The child was delivered by Cesarean section. Birth weight was 3.530 g. Marked edema of the upper half of the body was found. Intubation was performed immediately and artificial respiration started. An echocardiographic examination at this time showed a large right atrium, a large right

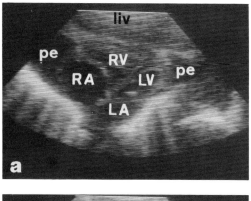

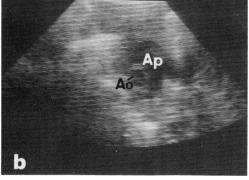

Figure 3. a) Postnatal subcostal four-chamber view. Large right atrium (RA) and right ventricle (RV), relatively small left atrium (LA) and left ventricle (LV). Residual pleural effusion (pe).

b) Postnatal short-axis view of the great arteries. Small aorta (Ao) and large pulmonary artery (Ap) with its bifurcation.

ventricle and residual pleural effusions; the pulmonary artery was dilated (Figure 3a and b). The left heart cavities and the aorta were found to be relatively small. Doppler flow analysis revealed a considerable degree of tricuspid regurgitation (Figure 4).

Therapy with diuretics led to excretion of large amounts of fluid, the edema disappeared, body weight dropped down to 2.600 g after seven days.

Weaning from the respirator was complicated by recurrent pleural effusions and delayed closure of a large persistent ductus arteriosus and was achieved 3 weeks after birth.

Several weeks later both right and left cardiac chambers, as well as the great arteries, had gained normal size (Figure 5). At the site of the foramen ovale, an area of increased echo intensity could be seen.

At cardiac catheterization, a 5F balloon catheter could be passed from the right to the left atrium through the orifice of the foramen ovale. Inflating the

428

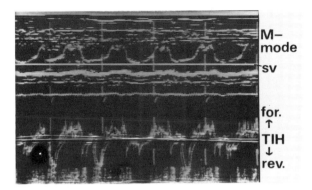

Figure 4. Doppler flow analysis. The position of the sample volume behind the tricuspid valve in the right atrium is marked by the straight line (sv). Considerable tricuspid regurgitation is indicated by the reverse systolic flow (rev.) into the right atrium.

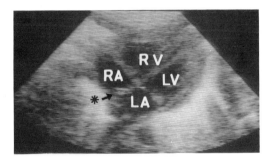

Figure 5. Subcostal four-chamber view several weeks after birth. Normal dimensions of all four cardiac chambers. Asterisk marks increased echoes in the region of the foramen ovale.

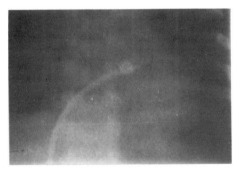

Figure 6. Cineangiogram in the frontal plane showing the 5F catheter in the left atrium. The maximal size of balloon that could be passed through the foramen ovale corresponded to a diameter of 3–4 mm.

balloon stepwise with increasing volumes of contrast medium, a maximal patency of the foramen ovale of 3–4 mm in diameter was found (Figure 6).

3. DISCUSSION

Fetal hydrops may be related to myocardial insufficiency. This has been well documented in cases of Rh-incompatibility and feto-fetal transfusion syndrome of multiples (twins). However, there have been many cases without known cause. Among these we observed two cases with hydrothorax and preferential distribution of edema in the upper regions of the body. In both cases prenatal obstruction of the foramen ovale was demonstrated. In the first case respiratory problems led to death soon after birth; autopsy revealed premature obstruction of the foramen ovale. In the second case presented here this condition was diagnosed prenatally using 2D DE and special precautions could therefore be taken over the delivery. To facilitate expansion of the lungs after birth, an echographically-guided, intrauterine pleural puncture was performed immediately before delivery by Cesarean section. The diagnosis was confirmed by postnatal 2D DE investigation and by heart catheterization and angiocardiography. The child is alive and doing well now.

The typical distribution of fetal hydrops and hydrothorax may be caused by myocardial insufficiency of the right heart. In prenatal obstruction of the foramen ovale, the right ventricle has to cope with by far the largest amount of the combined cardiac output. The higher perfusion rate of the inferior cava blood [1] may prevent accumulation of edema in the lower parts of the body.

4. CONCLUSIONS

We conclude that, in cases of fetal hydrops in late pregnancy, prenatal echocardiographic examinations should be performed to avoid the chance of missing the diagnosis of premature obstruction of the foramen ovale as a treatable cause of this life-threatening condition.

REFERENCES

1. Rudolph A: Congenital diseases of the heart. Year Book Medical Publishers Inc, Chicago 1974.

III. TECHNOLOGICAL ASPECTS OF ECHOCARDIOLOGY

48. M-MODE SCANNING WITH AUTOMATIC GAIN CONTROL

C. T. Lancée and J. A. Blom

INTRODUCTION

After the inspired work of the pioneers during the fifties, M-mode echo-cardiographic analysis has become a routine diagnostic procedure, developing from A-scan to stripchart recording. In our center alone, the annual number of outpatient M-mode examinations is now over 3000. The high patient load soon raised the question of whether or not the scanning procedure could be simplified by decreasing the time-consuming man-machine interaction. We therefore decided to start developing an automatic time-gain-curve (TGC) generator, since most of the interaction between the operator and the M-mode instrument is related to the manual setting of this curve.

There have been several reports in the literature on automatic TGC generation [1, 2, 3]. McDicken [1] describes a system whereby the instantaneous amplitude of the echo signal is used in a feed-back circuit. The basic disadvantage of such an approach is that the wide dynamic range of these signals makes it impossible for the device to discriminate between significant echoes and unwanted signal components (due to noise, reverberation, sidelobes, etc.).

Furthermore, because of the short duration of each echo, the feedback circuitry must be fast, which limits the use of sophisticated signal processing. The performance of such a device will therefore always be moderate.

Powis [2] and Roelandt [3] describe the design and clinical performance of a system in which non-linear processing of the instantaneous signal amplitude is used to compress the initially large dynamic range into a much smaller one.

Because of the natural difference in absolute signal level between the early and the late parts of a scan, due to attenuation, this type of device will never provide consistent performance over the whole scan range. In practice, the performance in the first part of the scan (near the transducer) is sacrificed in favour of better performance at greater depth. Clinical performance of the instrument is moderate, the price is, however, extremely low.

434

One may conclude from the above mentioned reports that an advanced automated system with improved performance should meet the following requirements:
1. Operation should be truly automatic, i.e. controls should be kept to a minimum.
2. Performance should be constant over the whole depth of scanning.
3. Structural echoes should be enhanced with respect to spurious signal components.

From these observations it can be further concluded that:
4. Fixed dynamic range compression will be of limited value.
5. Using the instantaneous value of the signal itself as its own reference for feed-back will be inadequate.

These considerations led us to believe that the most promising approach for the design of a fully automatic TGC would be to use the information within one scan as a whole. Since the repetition frequency of most scanners is of the order of 1kHz, the repetition rate may be considered as being at least an order of magnitude higher than the motion of cardiac structures and hence the information in any scan will be a fairly close predictor of the following scan. It therefore seemed appropriate to use the echo information available in each scan to derive the gain-curve for the next. In this way it became possible to generate a gain for a particular echo by considering it in the context of the signal levels occurring both earlier and later in the same scan. The algorithm to conclude whether or not a particular event in the echo signal is significant could now be made rather sophisticated.

PRINCIPLE OF THE SYSTEM

Figure 1 shows a block diagram of the system. The signals from the transducer are demodulated and digitized in a logarithmic, analog to digital (A-D) convertor and fed into memory 1. The signal amplitude is quantized in 16 steps of 5dB each, yielding a 4-bit binary amplitude code. The potential dynamic range of the system is 80 dB. Sample interval time is 1 μsec, while the scan time is approximately 256 μsec, requiring a memory size of 256 4-bit words. Time between scans is 1000 μsec, which leaves 744 μsec data processing time. After memory 1 is filled, the complete scan information is now available for the processor, which calculates an optimal gain-curve. The gain data is read into memory 2 as 256 8-bit words. At the start of the next scan the contents of memory 2 are read out into a digital to analog (D-A) convertor, which translates the word sequence into an analogue voltage. This voltage then is applied to a voltage-controlled gain amplifier, common to

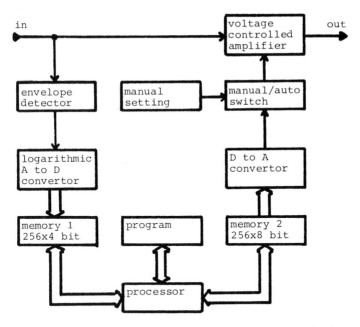

Figure 1. Schematic diagram of the automatic gain control circuit.

most types of M-mode instruments.

In order to evaluate the performance of the prototype instrument, a switch was incorporated in the control voltage path which allowed immediate selection of automatic or manual operation. In this way, the optimal manual setting of the gain curve by an experienced operator was used as a reference for testing the performance of the automatic circuit.

Figure 2 shows a grey scale representation of the digitized logarithmic echo signal from a scan through the aorta. Full black is the maximum level, corresponding to 0 dB, white is the minimum level, corresponding to −60 dB, while the range is here 12 steps of 5dB each. The extreme left section of the photograph shows the full range. In the next section the levels below −40 dB have been suppressed, resulting in a display of the levels between 0 and −40 dB. The next section shows levels between 0 and −35 dB and in each following section the range displayed has been decreased by 5 dB. The extreme right section shows only the levels between 0 and −15 dB. This illustration demonstrates that "noise" in the right ventricular cavity has a much higher level than "noise" in the left atrium and is even of the same order of magnitude as the posterior aortic wall signals.

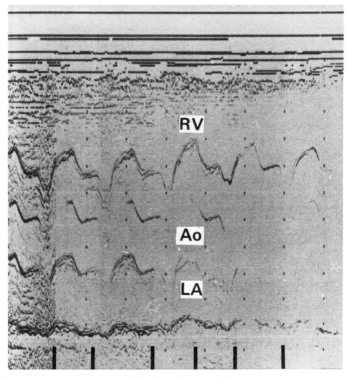

Figure 2. Grey scale representation of the logarithmic A-D convertor output at various range levels. From left to right: 0 to −60 dB, 0 to −40 dB, 0 to −35 dB, 0 to −30 dB, 0 to −25 dB, 0 to −20 dB and 0 to −15 dB.
Anatomical landmarks are indicated in all figures by: Ao = aorta, LA = left atrium, LV = left ventricle and RV = right ventricle.

DISCUSSION OF THE PROCESSING ALGORITHMS

Since the whole information from a previous scan is available, it would be possible to use many approaches to obtain an optimally fitted gain curve. Previous work by McDicken [1] and Broere [4] resulted in the following observations:

1. High quality, grey scale, M-mode tracings result when the strongest echoes of structures are slightly overamplified.
2. The best possible gain curve estimation will be obtained if signal averaging with long time-constants is used (of the order of 50 μsec).
3. Spurious echoes are more disturbing at the beginning of a scan than at the end.
4. Recording of spurious echoes and background noise will be difficult to avoid when these signals occur in large areas without structural echoes.

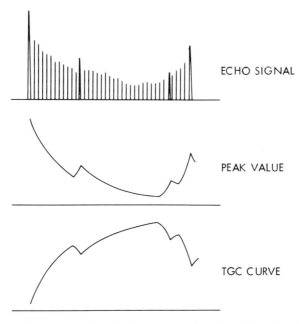

Figure 3. Gain curve estimation based on peak values of the echo signal.

We first tried using a peak-detection scheme in which the strongest echoes defined the final gain curve. The principle is outlined in Figure 3. At the top, a schematic representation of the logarithmic echo signal is seen. The processor searches the complete data set of such points for all maximum values and calculates an envelope curve from an exponential fit of the rise and decay of each maximum.

The resulting envelope waveform is shown in the middle part of the figure. In order to obtain the gain control signal, the peak value curve was then inverted, as depicted in the lower panel of the figure. In this way a constant level of all maximum echoes was ensured.

Two important shortcomings of this procedure can be seen from the figure. The extremely high signal amplitude due to the transmission pulse yields a very low gain at the beginning of a scan. Also, as can be seen in the middle section of the scan, during a relatively long period with an absence of strong echoes the gain curve will tend to adjust itself to the background noise level.

A typical clinical result is shown in Figure 4. During a scan from the aorta to the mitral valve the system was switched from automatic to manual operation. Notice that in the upper part of the automatic scan almost no details are available, whereas in the lower part performance is adequate, except for some noise in the aorta and left atrium. For comparison with existing instruments, a tracing of the same patient made with the Echomatic

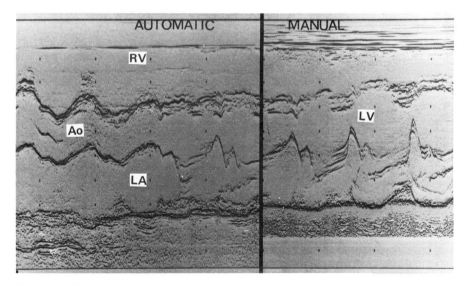

Figure 4. Left side: typical clinical result obtained using the peak detection procedure. Right side: the same scan obtained using manual gain control.

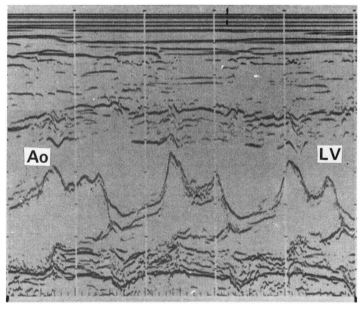

Figure 5. Tracing of the same patient as in Figure 4 obtained with a production model Echomatic from Metrix Teknika.

from Metrix Teknika is given in Figure 5. This instrument also performed worse in the upper part of the tracing than in the lower part, due to somewhat unsophisticated signal processing.

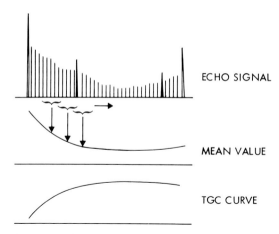

ECHO SIGNAL

MEAN VALUE

TGC CURVE

Figure 6. Gain curve estimation based on mean values within the echo signal.

Our unsatisfactory experiences with the peak-detection approach led us to a different processing scheme, which is illustrated in Figure 6. The basic principle is to construct a signal envelope based on the average signal amplitude within a certain time window. This may be achieved by summing all samples in a time interval and dividing the result by the number of samples. The averaged signal value is then stored as a point of the mean signal envelope at the time corresponding to the mid-point of the time interval. The time window is then shifted over one sample period and the same procedure is repeated, as indicated by arrows in the figure. The result of a complete sequence will be a running mean value versus time. The corresponding gain curve is again obtained by inversion. The general effect of this type of processing will be a combination of overamplified, isolated, strong echoes and underamplified background noise.

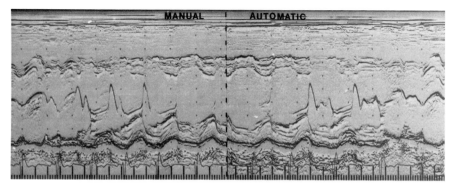

Figure 7. Typical clinical result of the mean value procedure compared with manual gain setting, both obtained using a modified Echomatic.

Extensive clinical trials on fifty, randomly selected, patients (both adults and children) showed a tendency to overestimate the required gain in the beginning of a tracing which gradually changed to a tendency to underestimation by the end of the tracing. This could easily be corrected for by means of an offset increasing with time. After this modification, the instrument performance was considered to be comparable to that of manually operated instruments. A typical tracing of an Echomatic equipped with this type of signal processing is given in Figure 7. A sweep from the aorta to the cardiac apex is shown, first in the manual mode, then (as a reverse sweep) in the automatic mode.

DISCUSSION

After lengthy clinical trials, the automatic mode of the instrument has proven itself to be almost as good as manual operation by expert technicians. Several consistent findings are to be noted. First of all, an automated device will never be able to discriminate between "noise" and significant, but weak, echoes in the same subtle manner as a trained operator. Therefore, the automatically obtained echograms will always be slightly "noisy". A mixed mode was provided in the prototype to allow for slight local corrections in the gain curve. In practice, however, this was not used frequently. Secondly, because of the dynamic nature of the gain curve, the outline of the septal walls is sometimes even better displayed than on manually obtained tracings. These echoes show a tendency to fluctuate in intensity over the cardiac cycle and hence a continuously adapting curve may be of advantage here as compared to a stationary one.

Furthermore the automatic gain curve proved to be extremely convenient when a sweep is performed from the aorta to the cardiac apex. In manual operation, continuous adjustment of the gain settings is required during this procedure in order to obtain optimal results. The reason is, that the cardiac structures along the scanning path change significantly, both in position and in ultrasonic reflection properties, over the whole procedure. In the automatic mode, however, the gain curve, being updated 1000 times per second, adjusts itself to the changes in the anatomy along the scanning path. This enables the operator to concentrate on the transducer manipulation alone.

Finally, the authors believe strongly that any automated scanner should also be equipped with manual operation. The operator can then check whether echoes which are not displayed are really non-existent and whether weakly displayed echoes are really spurious rather than due to, for instance, intracardiac tumors, vegetations and the like.

CONCLUSION

The results of this work have shown that an automated M-mode scanner capable of providing clinical results has been achieved. The interaction between operator and instrument has been significantly reduced without the loss of diagnostic value of the tracings. Operator skill, however, remains a crucial factor, since automation alone will by no means circumvent the necessity for accurate manipulation of the transducer in order to get optimal tracings of the cardiac structures of interest.

ACKNOWLEDGEMENT

The authors wish to thank J. Davidse and A. Willemse from the Delft University of Technology for their co-operation in this study.

Furthermore we are grateful to W. Vletter and J. McGhie at the laboratory of clinical echocardiography of the Thoraxcenter for their critical evaluation of this study. Clinical support has also been given by J.J.M. van Heyst at the Ignatius Ziekenhuis Breda, where part of the evaluation study was carried out.

Finally we wish to thank Organon Teknika for material support.

REFERENCES

1. McDicken WN, DH Evans, DAR Robertson: Automatic sensitivity control in diagnostic ultrasonics. Ultrasonics 12:173–176, 1974.
2. Powis RL: TGC – A function of operator or echo? Clinical Ultrasound Purchaser's Catalogue, McGraphics, Denver, Colorado, 1978.
3. Roelandt J, L Lima, HA Hajar, et al.: Clinical experience with an automatic echocardiograph. J Cardiovasc Pulm Technol 12:27, 1979.
4. Broere C: Het automatisch regelen in diagnostische ultrageluidsapparatuur. Thesis, Delft University of Technology, 1978.

49. PULSED-DOPPLER WITH REAL-TIME FOURIER TRANSFORM

R. FEHR

1. INTRODUCTION

Pulsed-Doppler echocardiography makes it possible to obtain information about blood flow velocities inside or near the heart. This information is encoded in a complex spectrum of Doppler signals. This spectrum can be analyzed by a zero-crossing detector which gives an estimate of the mean Doppler frequency. More information can be obtained from the Time Interval Histogram (TIH), which displays the statistics of the time intervals between zero-crossings of the Doppler signal [1]. The TIH only gives a rather rough estimate of the Doppler spectrum, as was shown in [2]. The complete Doppler information can be obtained by spectral analysis of the Doppler signal. The required spectrum analyzers are, however, rather bulky, expensive, and do not work in real-time.

A pulsed single-channel Doppler instrument is described here, which analyzes the Doppler signal by digitally computing the Fourier Transform in real-time. This computation is performed by a special-purpose, low-cost processor.

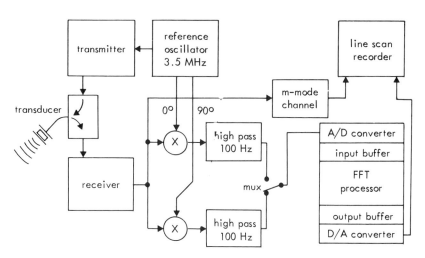

Figure 1. Block diagram of instrument.

Rijsterborgh H, ed: Echocardiology, p 443-447. All rights reserved.
Copyright © 1981 Martinus Nijhoff Publishers, The Hague/Boston/London.

2. DESCRIPTION OF THE INSTRUMENT

A block diagram of the instrument is shown in Figure 1. An ultrasound frequency of 3.5 MHz is used and the pulse repetition frequency (PRF) is variable between 4 and 10 kHz. Two synchronous demodulators convert the echo signal into two quadrature low frequency channels. After gating and fixed echo rejection by 100 Hz highpass filters, both channels are digitized with 10 bits resolution. Sets of 128 complex data points are processed by the Fast Fourier Transform (FFT) algorithm in 18 ms. The Doppler spectrum is displayed together with the M-mode signal on a line scan recorder.

3. REAL-TIME OPERATION

In a gated Doppler system, one sample of the Doppler signal is available after each transmit pulse. The maximum detectable Doppler shift is given by the sampling theorem and is PRF/2.

For a frequency resolution of plus and minus 64 points, 128 data points have to be acquired for one FFT. At a PRF of 7 kHz this takes 18 ms. Operation is understood to be real-time, if the FFT processing is faster than data acquisition. The information is then processed as fast as it is obtained.

4. THE FFT PROCESSOR

The FFT processor is built on three printed circuit boards (Figure 2). The arithmetic unit takes up one board. Two additional boards are required for the analog to digital conversion and the output buffer. A block diagram of the processor is given in Figure 3. The signal is processed in three steps. During the first step, a set of 128 samples is digitized and stored in the input buffer. During the second step this set is transferred to the data memory and

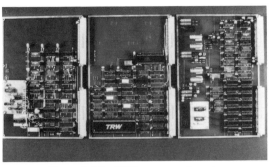

Figure 2. The FFT processor boards.

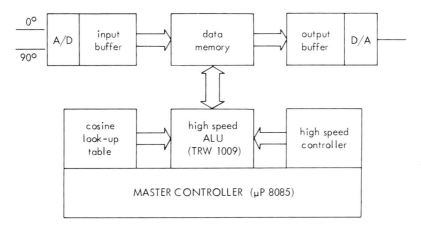

Figure 3. Block diagram of FFT processor.
ALU = arithmetic logic unit, A/D = analog to digital converter, D/A = digital to analog converter.

the spectrum is computed. During the third step the result is available in the output buffer. These three units work in pipeline. During the second step of the processing, the A/D conversion unit is already acquiring data for the next computation.

The arithmetic unit shows a dual processor structure. An 8085 microprocessor controls the program flow of the FFT algorithm. It provides all necessary control information for a 12-bit high-speed arithmetic processor. This processor is built with low-power Schottky transistor logic, around an integrated multiplier/accumulator from TRW *. It is capable of performing the so-called "butterfly" operation (two complex additions and one complex multiplication) in $9 \mu s$. After having computed the FFT, the processor also computes the absolute value of the complex spectrum by an iterative method.

Since we use complex input data and computation, forward and backward flow is separated and can be displayed as positive and negative Doppler frequencies.

5. RESULTS

In Figure 4, the left hand side of the full record shows the time motion records. The upper trace is used to display a conventional M-mode echocardiogram; an indication of the Doppler gate position is included. The lower trace shows the behaviour of the spectrum with time (here, frequency of the

* TRW-products, El Segundo, California.

446

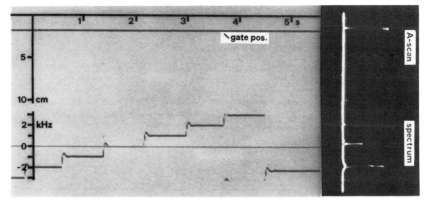

Figure 4. Record with test signal.

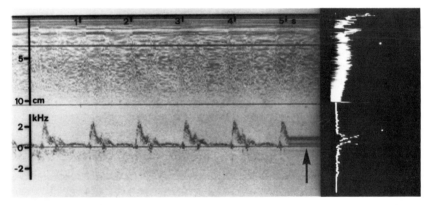

Figure 5. Measurement in the aortic arch. The recorded Doppler spectrum has been frozen on the right hand side of the lowermost trace (see arrow).

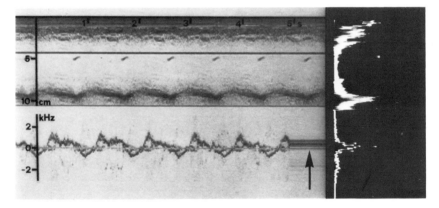

Figure 6. Measurement in the heart (apex view). The recorded Doppler spectrum has been frozen on the right hand side of the lowermost trace (see arrow).

test signal was changed in 1 kHz steps). The spectrum may be stored on manual request or via an ECG trigger. On the right hand side of the record are the signals as shown on an A-scan monitor. Although it is planned to combine this instrument with a two-dimensional (2D) scctor-scanner, initial clinical trials were performed using it as a stand-alone unit with a standard M-mode transducer. The signal processing worked well in cardiological applications but positioning of the sample volume turned out to be difficult.

The signal processing performance is shown in Figures 5 and 6. Figure 5 shows a measurement in the aortic arch. Figure 6 is a recording made in the heart of an adult (apex view).

6. FURTHER DEVELOPMENTS

During testing it was learned that the amplitude of the Doppler signal must be controlled carefully, because signals exceeding the linear range of the processor produce artefacts. A higher frequency resolution might be useful but this would lower the number of spectra per second. Combination with a 2D scanner is probably required in order to control the position of the sample volume. This instrument demonstrates that a real-time FFT processor for Doppler signals can be built at moderate cost. Therefore this feature will probably soon be available in commercial instruments.

ACKNOWLEDGEMENT

We would like to acknowledge the invaluable help of Dr. Schmidt-Redemann during preliminary clinical trials.

REFERENCES

1. Daigle RE, DW Baker: A readout for pulsed Doppler velocity meters. ISA Transactions 16:41–44, 1977.
2. Burckhardt CB: Comparison between spectrum and time interval histogram of ultrasound Doppler signals. Ultrasound Med Biol 7:79–82, 1981.

50. THREE-DIMENSIONAL IMAGING AND VOLUME DETERMINATION USING A SERIES OF TWO-DIMENSIONAL ULTRASONIC SCANS

WILLIAM E. MORITZ, DOUGLAS K. MEDEMA, DANIEL MCCABE, and ALAN S. PEARLMAN

INTRODUCTION

A two-dimensional (2D) ultrasonic scan provides a tomographic view of a structure of interest. A series of such 2D scans could be used to develop a three-dimensional (3D) representation of the entire structure [1]. Critical elements in such an approach are (a) knowledge of the position and orientation of individual scans with respect to a spatial reference system, and (b) a method of identifying the structure borders in a given scan [2].

A new technique for 3D reconstruction has been developed. The spatial position and orientation of multiple, non-parallel 2D real-time ultrasonic scans are determined. As imaged in individual scans, the outline of a structure of interest is digitized, and the data from multiple scans is assembled into a 3D representation whose volume can be computed automatically. The system has been tested using a series of balloons, kidneys, and hearts.

PROCEDURE

The system consists of the following major elements: 1) a real-time, commercial 2D ultrasonic scanner (ATL Mk III); 2) a locating system which determines the position and orientation of a scan plane relative to a reference coordinate system; 3) a method for digitizing the x, y, z coordinates of points on the outline of a structure in a given 2D image; 4) a system for displaying the reconstructed image; and 5) an algorithm that computes the volume of the imaged structure. Figure 1 shows the data acquisition elements of the system (1 – 3 above), while the reconstruction display and volume algorithms (item 4 and 5) are implemented on the PDP 11/34 computer.

The basic operating principle of the locator system is shown in Figure 2. Three small spark gaps are mounted in a plexiglass disk that is attached to the 2D scan head. The spark gaps provide point sound sources. Sound waves emitted by the spark gaps are detected by three point microphones which are mounted on an " L " shaped arm. The system microprocessor (a 4MHz 8080) fires each spark in sequence and measures for each shock wave the respective

Rijsterborgh H, ed: Echocardiology, p 449-454. All rights reserved.
Copyright © 1981 Martinus Nijhoff Publishers, The Hague/Boston/London.

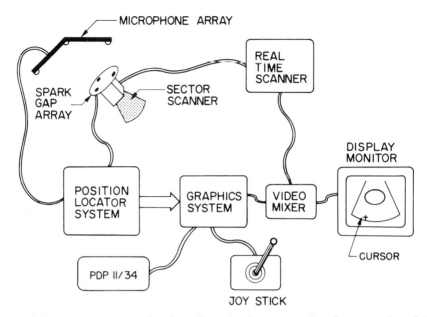

Figure 1. System components for three-dimensional reconstruction from a series of 2D ultrasonic scans.

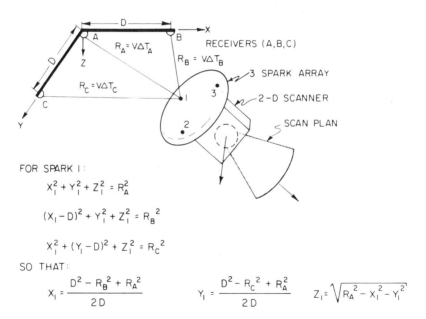

FOR SPARK I :

$$X_I^2 + Y_I^2 + Z_I^2 = R_A^2$$

$$(X_I - D)^2 + Y_I^2 + Z_I^2 = R_B^2$$

$$X_I^2 + (Y_I - D)^2 + Z_I^2 = R_C^2$$

SO THAT :

$$X_I = \frac{D^2 - R_B^2 + R_A^2}{2D} \qquad Y_I = \frac{D^2 - R_C^2 + R_A^2}{2D} \qquad Z_I = \sqrt{R_A^2 - X_I^2 - Y_I^2}$$

Figure 2. Locator principle showing calculations required to determine x, y, z coordinates of each spark. V = speed of sound in air, ΔT_i = transit time.

transit times (ΔT) to each of the three microphones. Ambient air temperature (t) is measured by a thermistor and used to calculate the instantaneous speed of sound (V = $331.5 + 0.605 \cdot t$ m/sec).

The resulting 9 ΔT's and V are used to compute the x, y, z coordinates of sparks 1, 2 and 3 using 32-bit floating-point arithmetic (24 bit mantissa, 8 bit exponent) as shown in Figure 2. These coordinates define the position and orientation of the plane formed by the 3 sparks. Vector manipulation and knowledge of the scan-head geometry permit subsequent determination of the location of the scan plane origin (in this case, the center of the mechanical rotor) and of 2 vectors – one in the scan plane and one normal to it. These parameters define the position and orientation of the scan plane in space. The locator can determine position to within ± 1 mm and orientation to within $\pm 1°$ over a working volume of about 1 m^3 located below the microphone array [3].

Establishment of a "patient coordinate system" (PCS) at the beginning of a study permits serial patient studies. The locator system transforms all position and orientation information from the microphone coordinate system into the PCS. In this way, the spatial coordinates of a scan plane imaged during an initial study can be used to guide repositioning and reorientation of the scan head at the time of a second study.

The scanner video image is mixed with a graphics/alphanumeric system that includes an internal cursor whose position is controlled by means of a joystick. Prior to each study, the scale factor for the ultrasound display is determined by positioning the scan head in a test tank containing wire targets separated by known distances. The system microprocessor uses the scan plane position and orientation information, along with the screen coordinates, to calculate the x, y, z position of the cursor as it is moved within the image. Individual points are stored on the display and in locator memory.

A series of studies have been performed in order to validate the system. Targets included fluid-filled balloons (51–302cc), fixed, excised kidneys (45–220cc) and fixed, excised hearts (30–144cc). Heart specimens were prepared by removing the atria at the atrioventricular groove and excising the mitral leaflets; papillary muscles were left intact. Each target was submerged and imaged in a water tank. To study each target, a series of individual scans were obtained; the cursor was manipulated by the operator in order to digitize the structure of interest, thereby defining a series of x, y, z coordinates describing the structure outline in that scan frame. The collection of points obtained in this way from a single scan was then transferred to the PDP 11/34 computer and incorporated into a display showing the acquired scans. Subsequent scans could thus be selected so that all regions of the structure were imaged (normally 10–20 scans per target).

At the completion of a study, the collection of data points (512 max) were stored on disk in the 11/34. One program permits the operator to reconstruct

452

a 3D image of the structure and to specify viewing angle and distance for display purposes. A second program processes the data to compute the volume of the structure enclosed by the digitized points. This algorithm first determines the long axis of the structure and then generates 12 equally spaced polar planes that pass through the long axis. Intersections between these planes and the data points are used to compute the volume enclosed by each pair of polar planes. Total volume is then determined by summing the 12 section volumes.

RESULTS

A total of 229 studies were performed by three observers using 8 balloons, 6 kidneys, and 6 hearts. Each object was studied between 5 and 15 times. Three-dimensional reconstructions were made for each study and visually compared with the actual target. Figure 3 presents one such reconstruction in 4 separate views (clockwise, starting in lower left corner): 1 each down the z, y, and x axes, and 1 view from a position at 45° to each axis.

To validate the accuracy of the reconstructions, the volume of each imaged target was computed and compared to the actual target volume. Figure 4 shows the results of a volume calculation for one of the excised heart models.

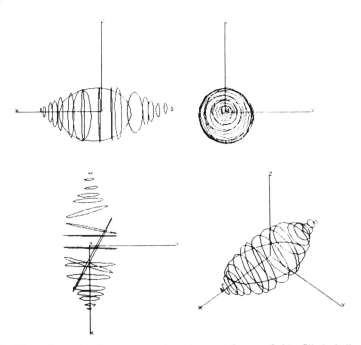

Figure 3. Three-dimensional reconstruction images for a fluid filled balloon (volume = 103 cc).

453

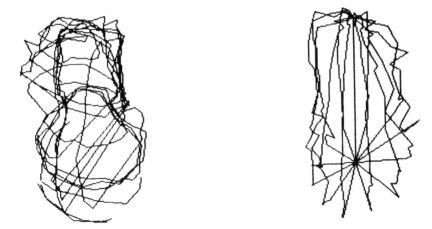

Figure 4. Volume calculation for excised left ventricle. The acquired data set is on the left (note incomplete scans) while the computed volume image is on the right (rotated 180° about the vertical axis). Calculated volume = 30.401 ml (actual volume = 31.7 ml).

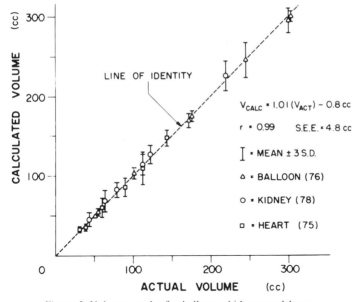

Figure 5. Volume results for balloons, kidneys and hearts.

The collection of acquired scans appears on the left, while the 12 computed polar sections are shown on the right. Note that the algorithm permits the use of incomplete structure outlines.

The combined results for all 229 studies are shown in Figure 5. Calculated volumes are compared to actual volumes, as determined by either fluid displacement (balloons and kidneys) or filling from a graduated cylinder (hearts). For each target, the mean of 5–15 determinations is shown, along with ±3 standard deviations. Using linear regression analysis, the data falls quite close to the line of identity, with a very high correlation coefficient and a small standard error of the estimate.

CONCLUSIONS

The results presented above indicate that our method allows us to acquire and use a series of non-parallel 2D scans to develop a 3D reconstruction of a structure of interest. The reconstruction method permits us to determine the volume of a series of static targets, some smooth and some irregular in shape, with a high degree of accuracy. We believe this technique holds great promise for ultimate application to quantitative analysis of ventricular geometry and wall motion, using multiple 2D scans of the heart imaged *in vivo*.

REFERENCES

1. Eaton LW, WL Maughan, AA Shoukas, JL Weiss: Accurate volume determination in the isolated ejecting canine left ventricle by two-dimensional echocardiography. Circulation 60:320, 1979.
2. Geiser EA, et al.: A framework for three-dimensional time-varying reconstruction of the human left ventricle: sources of error and estimation of their magnitude. Comp and Biomed Res 13:225, 1980.
3. Moritz WE, PL Shreve: A system for locating points, lines and planes in space. IEEE Trans Instr and Meas IM26 1:5, 1977.

51. PRESENT STATUS OF TISSUE IDENTIFICATION

P.N.T. WELLS

1. INTRODUCTION

Ultrasonic tissue characterisation in cardiology is aimed at the actual identification of the histology of the components of the heart. This distinguishes it from echocardiography, which is concerned with the study and measurement of cardiac dimensions and structure motion patterns.

Using conventional pulse-echo methods, the histology can sometimes be deduced from clues which are evident from echocardiographic observations. For example:

a) Blood declares itself by being relatively anechoic and transparent to ultrasound;

b) Valve calification can be recognised by echoes of unusually high amplitude;

c) Hypertrophic cardiomyopathy is evident from the observation of abnormally thick ventricular walls;

d) Left atrial myxoma is apparent from the movement of the mass through the mitral valve orifice.

Although further applications along these lines can be expected to emerge as echocardiographic techniques develop, substantial progress in tissue characterisation is likely to depend on more specific methods. In essence, there are three tissue properties – speed, attenuation and scattering – which are candidates for ultrasonic measurement, and these properties and their dependence on frequency may prove to be of value in tissue characterisation. Although apparently the first experiment to test the possibility of detecting myocardial infarction on the basis of echo amplitude was reported in 1957 [1] it is only within the last five or six years that the idea has been taken up again and that research has begun in earnest.

2. ULTRASONIC TISSUE CHARACTERISATION

A crude index of tissue type is provided by a scale based on ultrasonic attenuation [2]. Thus tissues with higher attenuation tend to have lower water content and higher structural protein content (and, incidentally, higher

Rijsterborgh H, ed: Echocardiology, p 455-460. All rights reserved.
Copyright © 1981 Martinus Nijhoff Publishers, The Hague/Boston/London.

propagation speed). In this scheme, materials such as blood and adipose tissue have low attenuation; liver, muscle and "heart" have medium attenuation; tendon and bone have high attenuation.

This broad approach clearly cannot be expected to provide useful differential diagnoses in cardiology. More detailed studies of cardiac tissue characteristics, however, are discussed in Sections 2.1 and 2.2.

2.1. Data on speed and attenuation

During the last six years, three major reviews of the available data on ultrasonic propagation in biological tissues have been published [3, 4, 5]. Examination of these reviews reveals how little is known about the ultrasonic properties of the materials of the heart.

One exception is blood. For example, in fresh heparinised whole human blood, the speed of 5 MHz ultrasound at 36 °C is 1584.6 ± 2.0 m/sec in blood from males, and 1582.4 ± 2.3 m/sec in blood from females [6]. The speed is substantially independent of frequency. The attenuation in blood is also well known; typical data showing frequency dependence are given in Figure 1.

Figure 1 also presents typical loss/frequency data for solid cardiac tissues. The dog ventricle [7] has a lower attenuation than the cat "heart" [8] but this may be more a reflexion of different measurement methods than of different tissue properties. The cat heart absorption [8] contrasts with the

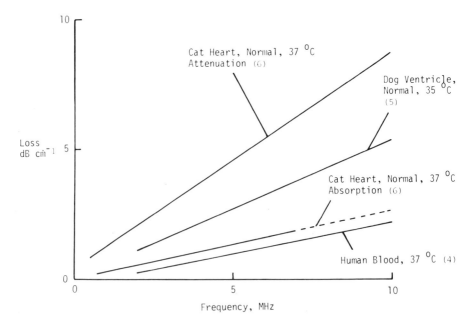

Figure 1. Typical loss/frequency data for blood and solid cardiac tissues.

attenuation; the absorption corresponds to the loss due to direct conversion into heat, whereas the attenuation value also includes losses due to scattering and, possibly, to other mechanisms.

Comparison between the speeds in different cardiac tissues is more difficult, as the data are so sparse. The speed in beef myocardium, measured perpendicular to the fibres at 5 MHz and 22 °C, is 1559 ± 7 m/sec [9]. In blood, the most closely matched conditions for comparison are for man, measured at 4 MHz and 22 °C, the speed being 1530–1540 m/sec [10].

This survey of the world literature does not provide a very encouraging picture of the prospects for ultrasonic cardiac tissue identification on the basis of speed or attenuation measurements. Nevertheless, the results from at least two research groups – at the Mayo Clinic [11] and Washington University [12] – do give grounds for some optimism. Using computed tomography, speed-of-sound images do seem to correlate with myocardial pathology [11], although the practical reservations about the applicability of this approach, mentioned in Section 3, should not be forgotten. Secondly, it has been clearly established [12] that the frequency dependence of the attenuation coefficient is different in normal and infarcted myocardium. This is illustrated in Figure 2, which aims to summarise part of an extensive study in which care was taken to avoid the pitfalls, such as phase cancellation effects in the receiving transducer, which compromise so many of the published data. Other experiments [13] have shown that, although collagen is responsible for not more than 15% of the attenuation observed in normal myocardium,

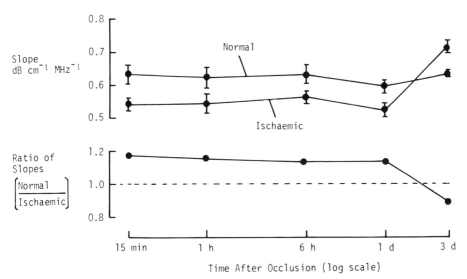

Figure 2. Frequency dependence of attenuation coefficient in normal and in ischaemic dog myocardium, over the frequency range 1–10 MHz, measured at 20 °C [10].

collagen is the principal determinant of the elevated attenuation in regions of myocardial infarction.

2.2. Data on scattering

It has been shown [14] that the backscattering coefficient for myocardium is an increasing function of frequency in the range 3-10 MHz. Quantitatively, at 10 MHz the backscattering coefficient is approximately 0.02 per cm per unit solid angle, and backscattering accounts for about 30% of the observed attenuation. This is quite consistent with the data in Figure 1, which indicate that about 50% of the total attenuation is due to scattering in cat heart at this frequency.

It has further been shown [15], by the results of experiments with dogs with artificially occluded left anterior descending coronary arteries, that, at 2.25 MHz, infarcted myocardium has a backscattering coefficient 1.4–2.6 times that of normal muscle. The best correlation is obtained in infarcts of a day's duration or less, at the time when the electrocardiographic pattern and blood enzyme changes associated with myocardial infarction are often not stabilised. It is tempting to speculate that the raised backscattering coefficient is related to an increase in collagen content, which has already been noted in connexion with attenuation in myocardium [13].

A more empirical – but, from a clinical viewpoint, possibly a more immediately applicable – approach to the study of backscattering in myocardial infarction is based on the use of a real-time electronically-steered array-scanner. The early results [16] were somewhat disappointing, the authors concluding that "... application of methods which have differentiated between normal and ischemic ... myocardium in vitro to in vivo data ... is not likely to be successful due to the triple whammy of limited bandwidth, overlying tissue and cardiac motion ... The substantial changes in ... spectra (suggest) that they reflect the state of contraction of cardiac muscle as well as changes in geometry." Subsequently, however, the same group of investigators [17] have shown that the histogram of echo amplitude distribution is shifted and broadened in damaged myocardium in vivo, as had previously been demonstrated in vitro [15].

3. MEASUREMENT METHODS

In order to determine the propagation speed of ultrasound in tissue, it is necessary to measure the time required for ultrasound to travel along a known path length. In conventional echocardiographic measurements, distances are calculated from measurements of time by assuming the speed to be the same (typically 1540 m/sec) in blood and all soft tissues. In view of the other errors involved in the measurement of distance and of the range of values usually found in similar clinical situations, this assumption of constant speed is quite acceptable.

The identification of different tissues on the basis of their different propagation speeds requires much greater accuracy. First of all, the actual type of tissue is generally evident from its anatomical location, and so differences between speeds in blood and in myocardium, for example, are only of academic interest. The detection of differences in speed in normal and in infarcted myocardium, however, would clearly be of clinical significance. In principle, this might be done by computed tomography. One of the most important limitations of ultrasound transmission computed tomography, which virtually rules it out as a candidate for in vivo tissue characterisation, is that there should be adequate transmission paths in every direction through the object. The presence of bone and lung mean that this requirement cannot be satisfied.

It has been suggested that it might be possible to reconstruct ultrasonic tomographic images of backscatter and attenuation using reflected signals [18]. In principle, this would reduce the required external access aperture to 180°, and this could be approached by scanning the heart from the oesophagus as well as from the anterior chest wall. Computer simulation of reflexion reconstruction has demonstrated the validity of the method for isotropic reflectors, but the degree of anisotrophy which almost certainly exists in real tissues at low megahertz frequencies would probably ruin the results in practice. There is thus no reason for optimism here.

4. CONCLUSIONS

The most promising prospect for clinically useful in vivo cardiac tissue characterisation seems to hinge around the possibility of quantitating differences in backscattered echo signals from normal and diseased tissues. Besides conventional statistical analyses [17], autocorrelation is an approach which deserves further study [19].

REFERENCES

1. Wild JJ, HD Crawford, JM Reid: Visualization of the excised human heart by means of reflected ultrasound or echography. Am Heart J 54:903, 1957.
2. Johnson RL, SA Goss, V Maynard, JK Brady, LA Frizzell, WD O'Brien Jr, F Dunn: Elements of tissue characterization. Part I. Ultrasonic propagation properties. Ultrasonic Tissue Characterization II (Linzer M, ed.), p 19. NBS Spec Publ 525. US Government Printing Office, Washington, 1979.

3. Goss SA, RL Johnston, F Dunn: Comprehensive compilation of empirical ultrasonic properties of mammalian tissues. J Acoust Soc Am 64:423, 1978.

4. Chivers RC, RJ Parry: Ultrasonic velocity and attenuation in mammalian tissues. J Acoust Soc Am 63:940, 1978.

5. Wells PNT: Absorption and dispersion of ultrasound in biological tissue. Ultrasound Med Biol 1:369, 1975.

6. Kikuchi Y, D Okuyama, C Kasai, Y Yoshida: Measurements on the sound velocity and absorption of human blood in 1–10 MHz frequency range. Rec Elect Commun Eng Convers Tohoku Univ 4:152, 1972.

7. O'Donnell M, JW Mimbs, BE Sobel, J Miller: Ultrasonic attenuation of myocardial tissue: dependence on time after excision and on temperature. J Acoust Soc Am 62:1054, 1977.

8. Goss SA, LA Frizell, F Dunn: Ultrasonic absorption and attenuation in mammalian tissues. Ultrasound Med Biol 5:181, 1979.

9. Shung KK, JM Reid: Ultrasonic scattering from tissues. IEEE Ultrasonics Symp Proc 77CH1264–1SU: 230, 1977.

10. Oksala A, A Lehtinen: Experimental researches on vitreous haemorrhages and on the echogram emitted by them. Acta Ophthal 37:17, 1959.

11. Johnson SA, JF Greenleaf, WF Samayoa, FA Duck, JD Sjostrand: Reconstruction of three-dimensional velocity fields and other parameters by acoustic ray tracing. IEEE Ultrasonics Symp Proc 75CHP994–4SU:46, 1975.

12. O'Donnell M, JW Mimbs, BE Sobel, J Miller: Ultrasonic attenuation in normal and ischaemic myocardium. Ultrasonic Tissue Characterization II (Linzer M, ed.), p 63. NBS Spec Publ 525. US Government Printing Office, Washington, 1979.

13. O'Donnell M, JW Mimbs, JG Miller: The relationship between collagen and ultrasonic attenuation in myocardial tissue. J Acoust Soc Am 65:512, 1979.

14. Reid JM, KK Shung: Quantitative measurements of scattering of ultrasound by heart and liver. Ultrasonic Tissue Characterization II (Linzer M, ed.), p 153. NBS Spec Publ 525, US Government Printing Office, Washington, 1979.

15. Gramiak R, RC Waag, EA Schenk, PPK Lee, K Thomson, P Macintosh: Ultrasonic detection of myocardial infarction by amplitude analysis. Radiology 130:713, 1979.

16. Joynt L, D Boyle, H Rakowski, R Popp, W Beaver: Identification of tissue parameters by digital processing of real-time ultrasonic clinical cardiac data. Ultrasonic Tissue Characterization II (Linzer M, ed.), p 267. NBS Spec Publ 525. US Government Printing Office, Washington, 1979.

17. Joynt L, A Macovski, D Boyle: Techniques for in vivo tissue characterization. Abstr 3rd int Symp Ultrasonic Imaging and Tissue Characterization, p 59. National Bureau of Standards, Gaithersburg.

18. Duck FA, CR Hill: Mapping true ultrasonic backscatter and attenuation distribution in tissue – a digital reconstruction approach. Ultrasonic Tissue Characterization II (Linzer M, ed.), p 247. NBS Spec Publ 525. US Government Printing Office, Washington, 1979.

19. Gore JC, S Leeman, C Metreweli, NJ Plessner, K Willson: Dynamic autocorrelation analysis of A-scans in vivo. Ultrasonic Tissue Characterization II (Linzer M, ed.), p 275. NBS Spec Publ 525. US Government Printing Office, Washington, 1979.

52. PRECISION MICROBUBBLES FOR RIGHT SIDE INTRACARDIAC PRESSURE AND FLOW MEASUREMENTS

E. GLENN TICKNER

1. INTRODUCTION

A noninvasive "cath-lab" has long been a dream in the medical community. Two parameters often measured by employing catheters are cardiac pressures and flow. Now the potential for both measurements to be performed noninvasively or minimally invasively exists with the use of precision gas microbubble agents, developed by Ultra Med Inc.*, Sunnyvale California. Microbubbles injected into a convenient vein, such as the median cubital, flow into the heart. These bubbles, in conjunction with specialized ultrasonic equipment, can be used to measure both these cardiac parameters. The purpose of this text is to discuss these methods which have been made possible by the establishment of microbubble technology. Microbubbles are defined as gas bubbles generally smaller than 100 microns in diameter. In some cases, these microbubbles are encapsulated in rigid substances.

2. PRESSURE MEASUREMENTS

2.1. Background

Bubbles exhibit in their purest form a simple, one-degree-of-freedom, damped oscillatory behavior [1, 2, 3]. Their dynamic characteristics are comparable to a simple spring/mass system. The spring constant is represented by the compression of the bubble gas, and the mass is equivalent to some effective mass of the liquid surrounding the bubble. Damping is caused by thermal and viscous effects of the gas and the surrounding liquid.

The free ringing frequency f_r of a bubble which oscillates as a sphere is given by

$$f_r = (3\gamma p/\rho)^{\frac{1}{2}}/\pi d, \tag{1}$$

where p is the absolute pressure of gas in the bubble, γ is the specific heat ratio of the gas, ρ is the density of the liquid, and d is the bubble diameter.

---

* Formerly Rasor Associates, Inc.

Rijsterborgh H, ed: Echocardiology, p 461-472. All rights reserved.
Copyright © 1981 Martinus Nijhoff Publishers, The Hague/Boston/London.

462

Spherical oscillations or volume oscillations create compression waves which readily propagate through body tissue. The oscillatory frequency for a given gas bubble depends solely on the bubble diameter and its absolute pressure. Hence, if the physical properties and diameter are known, then the free ringing oscillation uniquely indicates the absolute local blood pressure.

In order to better appreciate the significance of Eq. (1), let us assume that a bubble of carbon dioxide is near a pressure of one atmosphere. The ringing frequency in kHz when d is in microns is approximately given by

$$f_r = 6500/d. \tag{2}$$

Hence, a 100 micron bubble oscillates at an ultrasonic frequency of 65 kHz. Any bubble smaller than 325 microns will ring ultrasonically, i.e. $f_r > 20$ kHz. Conversely, bubbles larger than 325 microns ring sonically. For this reason, we have taken 325 microns as the break point between microbubbles and bubbles. Sounds of babbling brooks, sizzling ocean surf, or champagne bubbles are examples of sonic oscillations of bubbles. We intend to use microbubbles and the relationship of Eq. (1) to measure cardiac pressures.

Since the bubble diameter $d = \sqrt[3]{6V/\pi}$ depends upon its volume V, the pressure and volume are related by the compressibility equation ($pV^n =$ constant), Eq. (1) yields

$$p = p_o(f/f_0)^c, \tag{3}$$

where the zero subscripts refer to the reference condition (e.g. atmospheric pressure) and c is a gas constant which depends solely upon the polytropic coefficient at the excitation frequency. The constant c is determined experimentally. Differentiating Eq. (3) gives

$$\Delta p/p_0 = c\Delta f_r/f_0. \tag{4}$$

It can be seen, therefore, that local changes in blood pressure Δp can be directly determined by measurement of the change in ringing frequency Δf_r of bubbles in the blood stream. Two important requirements are that the bubbles must ring within the heart chambers and that the bubbles must be extremely precise in order to obtain accurate measurements.

2.2. Method

Gas microbubbles are encapsulated under pressure in a fused saccharide sphere. The strength of the saccharide shell contains the pressurized microbubbles. Carbon dioxide has been selected as the bubble gas because it is nontoxic, has low damping and is rapidly absorbed by the blood. The blood gradually dissolves the saccharide shell in the blood stream. At some critical point the shell becomes thin and is unable to tolerate the built-up stresses caused by the pressurized bubble and suddenly fails. The freed microbubble rapidly expands and rings ultrasonically at its new pressure, the blood pressure. A compression wave is propagated to the chest wall where it is detected by a hand-held transducer. The ringing frequency of each bubble is a direct measure of its pressure at that point in time. Pressure histories are determined by timing the signals relative to the electrocardiogram.

The method that is envisioned in the future is quite simple. The physician would place the transducer on the chest of the patient at the appropriate location. The pressurized saccharide encapsulated microbubbles suspended in a viscous slurry would be delivered into a large vein. The particles would than be carried into the heart by the flush and the venous return. This process would spread out their arrival in the heart over a few heart beats. Cardiac dynamics would thoroughly mix the slurry with the blood exposing all the particles which would then begin dissolving. Shortly thereafter, and for the next few heart beats, free ringing signals would be detected by the hand-held transducer placed on the patients chest. The ultrasonic signals would be decoded electronically and converted into pressure with the use of Eq. (4). Note that the detection system would only be a receiver system. Hence, conceptually, it would be simpler than conventional echographic equipment which involves both transmitter and receiver.

2.3. Experimental results

Before carrying the technology past the research stage into the development stage, three key questions should be answered.

First, can bubbles be made to ring in compressional oscillation? If so, is there a unique, and preferably linear, relationship between this ringing frequency and ambient pressure? If the answers to these first two questions

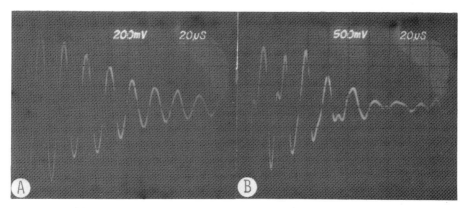

Figure 1. Oscillograph tracing showing free ringing bubble signal. *a)* Ideal damped sine wave signal; *b)* Damped signal with secondary oscillations.

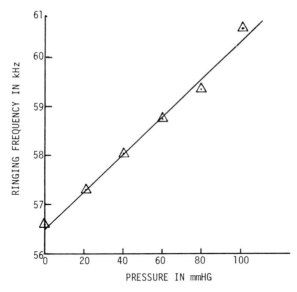

Figure 2. Variation of free ringing bubble frequency with pressure.

are positive, then the third question becomes, is the accuracy of the technique adequate for clinical use?

The first question can be answered by examination of Figure 1a and b. The two oscillographic tracings were taken of two different free ringing bubble signals. Pressurized particles were placed under the surface in a container of water which was being stirred. An ultrasonic transducer was placed on the surface to record any signal that would be created. Figure 1a shows the case of a classic damped sine wave of a 148 micron microbubble. Figure 1b also shows a free ringing bubble signal, but one which is not perfect. This imperfect signal is believed to be caused by the bubble rupture mechanism, which introduces shape oscillations that distort the compressional dynamics. This effect is thought to be the primary source of error. Because this effect exists, numerous data samples are required to obtain statistically significant results. Each particle is extremely small, being approximately 10^{-6} cc in volume, so additional particles are not believed to be a problem for delivery or toxicity. Naturally, toxicity tests must be performed to confirm this.

The same liquid chamber was employed to answer the second question. This time the liquid vessel was placed within a pressure chamber. The pressure within the chamber was varied from 0 to 100 mmHg at 20 mmHg multiples. Data were recorded on magnetic tape and reduced for frequency content at a later time. The results of this test are presented in Figure 2. A linear regression curve was employed to fit the data. This yielded an error in the pressure measurement of ± 16 mmHg. The correlation coefficient for these data was computed to be 0.995. Clearly, the results derived in Eq. (4)

were achieved. If the zero reference frequency is determined, then Eq. (4) can be used to calculate the absolute cardiac pressures. This zero reading is made by placing some of the free ringing material into a beaker of water exposed to the atmosphere and determining the average f_0. The mean frequency is associated with the sum of small beaker pressure and the measured barometric pressure p_0.

The third question still remains to be answered and will be answered as testing progresses. Clearly, there are two routes to take to obtain more accurate pressure measurements. First improve the accuracy of the particles so that they ring more precisely. Second, sample more signals before computing the pressure. For example, injecting four times as many particles would decrease the error by a factor of 2 and would only introduce approximately 0.03 cc of additional material.

3. FLOW MEASUREMENTS

3.1. Background

Cardiac output is often measured using some form of dye dilution technique which involves threading one or two catheters into the heart of a patient. The echocardiographer can see within the heart using various noninvasive devices but cannot utilize existing dyes to measure cardiac flow. It would be highly desirable to echo a "dye" within the heart and thereby eliminate the requirement for catheters. Bubbles have been shown to be superior ultrasonic reflectors [4, 5] and therefore should act as an excellent ultrasonic dye.

In 1978, Bommer, DeMaria et al. [6] suggested a method whereby cardiac output measurements could be made from dilution type curves created from photo-densitometric sampling of the image brightness created by microbubble reflections using two-dimensional echo systems. Their data indicates considerable promise for the approach.

Another potential method also exists and is presently being developed in our laboratory. This approach is based upon the attenuation of an ultrasonic signal passing through a bubbly medium. When sound waves are propagated through a medium containing microbubbles, scattering and absorption remove energy from the incident beam giving rise to an exponentially decreasing sound energy with distance (attenuation). Attenuation is generally expressed in terms of an attenuation coefficient α. Previous investigators [7, 8] have shown that suspensions of sand and clay particles and lycopodium spores increase the attenuation coefficient linearly with volume concentration or particle concentration. Oceanographers [9, 10, 11] have observed the comparable effect with microbubbles. In the past few years, Medwin [12] has used this effect and has developed instrumentation to

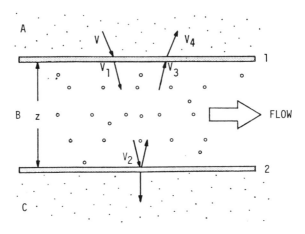

Figure 3. Schematic drawing showing reflection of plane waves.

measure bubble size distributions within the ocean. The bubbles' contribution (α_1) to the attenuation coefficient is then given as

$$\alpha_1 = k\varphi, \tag{5}$$

where k is a bubble constant which is a function of bubble gas, diameter, and ultrasonic excitation frequency and φ is the bubble concentration by volume.

The total attenuation coefficient is

$$\alpha = \alpha_0 + \alpha_1, \tag{6}$$

where α_0 is the attenuation coefficient for blood. It will be shown that this simple relationship can be used to measure bubble concentration.

In order to demonstrate this point, consider a plane wave V passing through medium A as shown in Figure 3. It will encounter two interfaces, walls, identified as 1 and 2, before continuing into medium C.

Medium B, lying between the two interfaces, is blood which may or may not contain the microbubbles. The amount of energy which is propagated through the interfaces depends upon the acoustic impedance of the media [13] and upon the attenuation of the signal by the bubbly medium B. The ratio of the signal strength between 1 and 2 is given by

$$V_2/V_1 = e^{-\alpha z}, \tag{7}$$

where z is the thickness of the medium.

It can be shown that the ratio of the backwall signal V_r for the case with bubbles to the case without bubbles is

$$V_r = e^{-2z(\alpha - \alpha_0)} \tag{8}$$

It also can be shown that, if the ratio of V_r remains near unity when bubbles pass by, Eq. (8) is further linearized and becomes

$$V_r = 1 - 2zk\varphi. \tag{9}$$

The bubble volumetric concentration φ is determined from Eq. (9) because k is known and z and V_r are measured during the test. Also, because precision microbubbles are used, the bubble volume v is known so the bubble concentration C, which is the number of bubbles per unit volume, is simply computed by $C = \varphi/v$.

For steady infusion, cardiac output CO [14] is computed by

$$CO = I/C_{max}, \tag{10}$$

where I is the known bubble infusion rate (bubbles/ second) and C_{max} is the equilibrium (plateau) value of the bubble concentration curve.

For bolus injections, the cardiac output equation takes the form

$$CO = \frac{N}{\int_0^\infty C(t)\,dt} \tag{11}$$

where N is the total number of injected bubbles. It is thus postulated that attenuation of an ultrasonic radio-frequency (rf) signal can be measured in vivo and used to determine bubble concentration and, with the aid of dye dilution technology, cardiac output.

3.2. Method

The basic approach lends itself to either the bolus injection or steady infusion method for measuring cardiac output. Consider here the steady infusion technique. Following the preparation of the bubble-containing syringe or dye-tube and insertion of an intravenous catheter into the median cubital vein of the patient, the ultrasonographer examines a backwall cardiac surface with a cardiac echo unit and, when satisfied with the signal and its stability, starts an infusion pump to deliver microbubbles at a constant and known rate into the vein. When bubbles arrive in the heart, the backwall signal becomes attenuated. This reflected signal decreases with time until equilibrium has been reached and then stabilizes at a constant value. The associated electronics converts the signal into a measurement of mean flow.

3.3. Microbubbles

Microbubbles of gases such as nitrogen and carbon dioxide ranging from 10 microns to 300 microns in diameter have been produced in various encapsulation materials. The encapsulation materials used most often are saccharides and gelatins. The saccharide agents consist of solid spherical precision particles, containing precision bubbles, and are packaged in a sealed container until ready for use. The agent is then mixed with a delivery vehicle on site. Gelatin encapsulated microbubble agents are packed and centered along the axis of a syringe or dye tube and refrigerated until ready for use. A gelatin matrix surrounds these bubbles during storage. All excess gelatin dissolves from the bubbles when injected into the blood stream, leaving only a thin layer of gelatin around each microbubble. The gelatin microbubbles can be made to be very precise, with a standard deviation of ± 0.7 microns. Exact precision of the saccharide encapsulated microbubbles has not been determined yet but is believed to be approximately equal to that of the gelatin agents.

Because the microbubble itself is the echo source, and not the shell, either encapsulation material is acceptable for cardiac output measurements. From a practical standpoint, the gelatin appears to be easier to deliver at slow steady infusion rates and appears to be somewhat more difficult to deliver for bolus injections.

3.4. Experimental results

The prospect of noninvasive cardiac output measurements depends upon the demonstration that (1) a unique and preferably linear relationship exists between bubble concentration and the dimensionless backwall signal level; (2) homogeneous distributions of bubbles exist within the heart; (3) all injected bubbles flow into the heart and do not recirculate; and (4) a stable and suitable echo source can be found within the heart. If these four conditions are achieved, then a device can be designed which would take a modified form of the rf signal from an ultrasonic unit and automatically convert the signal into a measurement of cardiac output.

Previous work [11] strongly suggested that high intensity, long duration ultrasonic pulses are attenuated linearly by bubble concentrations. However, present units have relatively low level signals which are of short duration. Additionally, our own research [15] indicates that a minimum pulse duration of more than ten equal amplitude cycles is required to excite bubbles into steady-state oscillation. Hence, it remained to be shown that bubbles respond to present day ultrasound pulses in a predictable manner. To do this, we used a SKI Ekoline 20A as our ultrasound source. The rf receiver signal was taken from the unit after amplification and before other processing. Tapping this signal did not alter the normal response of the unit. Our cardiopulmonary model was employed for the study. The model was to human scale and had a 2.5 cm diameter "pulmonary artery". Seventy-six micron diameter gelatin-

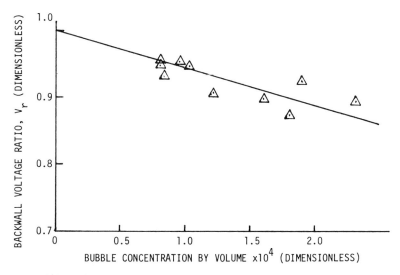

Figure 4. Variation of backwall signal as a function of bubble concentration using gelatin encapsulated microbubbles of 76 micron diameter.

encapsulated microbubbles were infused at a steady rate by a syringe pump into a vein in the model, and the pulmonary artery was insonated from above. The backwall portion of the rf signal was separated from the total signal and its steady-state peak value recorded for five different infusion rates. Figure 4 presents the dimensionless backwall voltage as a function of bubble concentration. A least-squares linear fit with an intercept at unity was made to these data. The correlation coefficient for these data was found to be 0.92. This particular form of a linear fit was chosen because it matched Eq. (8). Our preliminary results look quite promising and suggest that Eq. (8) is valid and can be used to obtain bubble concentration.

Experimental verification of the homogeneous distribution of bubbles was achieved by examination of many M-mode records of the pulmonary artery. One such record is shown in Figure 5. The reader will note a uniform opacification of the lumen by the microbubbles.

An integration effect occurs as sound waves pass through a bubble field. This is characteristic of the microbubble attenuation approach. Hence, even if small areas of inhomogeneity exist, they are averaged by the sound wave. It appears that the requirement of homogeneity can be relaxed somewhat for our particular approach, although our preliminary data do not indicate that it is necessary.

An electronic circuit was developed which would take the reflected backwall signal and convert it into a direct current voltage so that time variations could be recorded. One such recording was taken on the cardio-pulmonary model in pulsatile flow (Figure 6). The time of injection was also noted. One can observe a steady decrease in signal level as more bubbles

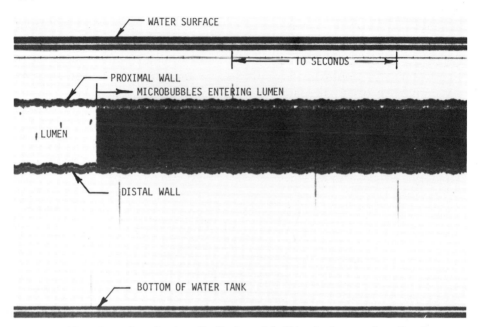

Figure 5. M-mode tracing showing distribution of bubbles in lumen of cardiopulmonary model.

enter the pulmonary artery until equilibrium is reached and a plateau is observed. Note that the lungs of the model capture the gelatin microbubbles as do real lungs so recirculation does not occur. The slight oscillations in the curve are caused by the pulsatile nature of the flow. Note that the baseline does return to its initial no-bubble level following the test.

The fact that a plateau is observed indicates that the bubble infusion rate is constant and that the bubbles are passing below the transducer at a constant rate, i.e. bubbles are not being trapped somewhere within the system. This was easily verified experimentally because much of the model was fabricated from clear plastic.

Testing has shown that there is a specific range of bubble densities which can be used. High concentrations ($\varphi > 10^{-3}$) virtually eliminate the backwall signal as observed by Meltzer et al. [4] and preclude determination of bubble concentration. Somewhat lower concentrations cause the effects to be nonlinear. Further, small bubble concentrations ($\varphi < 10^{-5}$) do not cause significant

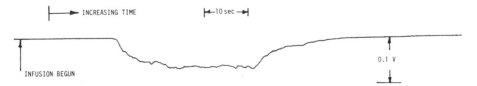

Figure 6. Demodulated backwall signal variation with time for constant infusion rate.

changes in backwall signals, resulting in measurement errors. Laboratory tests are currently underway to optimize delivery rates, bubble gas, size, density and other basic parameters. Currently, we find bubble concentrations by volume of approximately 10^{-4} serve this purpose. Fewer than 435 microbubbles of 76 micron diameter in one cubic centimeter blood volume are then sufficient for measurement. This can be accomplished by selecting the bubble delivery rate relative to the anticipated mean flow.

Peripherally injected microbubbles are trapped by the lungs. The lungs filter microbubbles larger than 8 microns and bubbles smaller than this dissolve in the blood stream before they can traverse the pulmonary circulation [16, 17]. Hence, microbubbles do not recirculate to cause what is sometimes referred to as recirculation error.

3.5. Conclusions

Bubbles are known to be very echogenic and hence act as superior ultrasonic contrast agents. They also exhibit the potential for noninvasive right heart side pressure and flow measurements. Theoretical considerations and preliminary experimental results indicate their potential. Encapsulation materials and bubble gases appear nontoxic. Detailed animal and toxicity studies are planned to insure the efficacy and safety of the materials. Microbubbles now appear to be a key part of a noninvasive "cath-lab." It may even be possible to make one peripheral injection of our pressurized microbubble dispersion and obtain right heart ultrasonic contrast, pressures and flows simultaneously.

ACKNOWLEDGEMENTS

Much of this work would not have been possible without the technical assistance, encouragement and candid comments from various people. The author is grateful to Drs. N. Rasor and H. Rugge for their guidance and foresight throughout this effort, and to D. Griffin, T. Nyren, J. Rasor, and T. Sahines for making many technical contributions. Additionally, the author expresses his thanks to Drs. W. Bommer, A. DeMaria, H. Feigenbaum, G. Goetowski, E. Kinney, R. Meltzer, R. Popp and N. Silverman for their encouragement and medical inputs at various times during the development. Part of this effort was supported by a contract from the National, Heart, Lung, and Blood Institute, Division of Lung Diseases.

472

REFERENCES

1. Devin C: Survey of thermal, radiation and viscous damping of pulsating air bubbles in water. J Acoust Soc Am 31:1654, 1959.
2. Plesset M, A Prosperetti: Bubble dynamics and cavitation. Am Rev Fluid Mech 9:145, 1977.
3. Minnaert M: On musical air-bubbles and sounds of running water. Phil Mag, 16:235, 1933.
4. Meltzer R, G Tickner, T Sahines, R Popp: The sources of ultrasound contrast effect. J Clin Ultrasound 8:121, 1980.
5. Lubbers J, J Van den Berg: An ultrasonic detector for microgasemboli in a bloodflow line. Ultrasound in Med. and Biol. 2, 301, 1976.
6. Bommer W, A DeMaria, et al.: Indicator-dilution curves obtained by photometric analysis of two-dimensional echo-contrast studies. (Abstract) Am J Cardiol 41:370, 1978.
7. Urick RJ: The absorption of sound in suspension of irregular particles. J Acoust Soc Am 20:283, 1948.
8. Stakutis V, R Morse, M Dill, R Beyer: Attenuation of ultrasound in aqueous suspensions. J Acoust Soc Am 27:539, 1955.
9. Urick RJ: Principles of Underwater Sound, p 203 McGraw Hill Book Co., New York, 1967.
10. Gavrilov L: On the size distribution of gas bubbles in water. Sov Phys-Acoust 15:22, 1969.
11. Medwin H: Counting bubbles acoustically: a review. Ultrasonics 15:7, 1977.
12. Medwin H: In-situ acoustic measurement of microbubbles at sea. J Geophys Res 82:971, 1977.
13. Wells P: Physical principles of ultrasonic diagnosis, pp 9–14. Academic Press, New York, 1969.
14. Hamilton W: Measurement of the cardiac output. Handbook Physiology Sec. 2 Circulation 1:551 (Hamilton W, ed.). Amer Physiol Soc, Washington, D.C., 1962.
15. Tickner G, N Rasor: Noninvasive assessment of pulmonary hypertension using the bubble ultrasonic resonance pressure (BURP) method. Annual Report #HR-62917-1A, NHLBI, 1977.
16. Butler B, B Hills: The lungs as a filter for microbubbles. J Appl Physiol 47:537, 1979.
17. Meltzer R, G Tickner, R Popp: Why do the lungs clear ultrasonic contrast. Ultrasound Med Biol 6:263, 1980.

INDEX